MORE DOCTORING

Richard Moskowitz M. D.

Selected Writings, Volume 2, 1977-2014

ISBN: 1502426684
ISBN 13: 9781502426680

Library of Congress Control Number: 2014916862
CreateSpace Independent Publishing Platform
North Charleston, South Carolina

Table of Contents

IV. Reviews.

V. Obituaries.

Preface.

As a companion volume to *Plain Doctoring,* the present collection consists mostly of shorter, occasional pieces: articles, case reports, political statements, obituaries, letters, interviews, and book and seminar reviews. Whereas *Plain Doctoring* featured mainly basic theoretical statements and position papers, these are freer, more informal, and more intimately reflective of the development of my thinking and the actual flow of my career.

In both volumes, the main criterion that I have used for making my selections is that I still like how they sound in my mind's ear as I re-read them slowly to myself, which is pretty much the standard I adopted when I wrote and edited them originally. I've cleaned some of them up a bit, by changing a few words or phrases, or even adding or subtracting a sentence or two here and there; but the meaning has not been altered in any way.

I always write with a broad literate audience in mind, but for now at least the present volume will probably appeal mainly to health care professionals, patients, and laypeople who are already acquainted with, interested in, or curious about homeopathy, a way of thinking about the nature of health and illness that looks and feels radically different from the model that our present medical system still prefers to operate with.

Forty-seven years of medical practice have taught me that these differences can in fact be reconciled far more easily than might at first appear. Reading these texts will help make it clear that homeopathic medicine is best thought of as complementary rather than alternative to the system we already have in place, as simply adding to and fine-tuning the vast body of useful knowledge that we have been amassing with such diligence over the past three centuries or so.

A good example is modern surgery, the epitome of technical mastery in medicine, which could not reliably succeed without the ability to control pain, bleeding, and infection by purely mechanical means, or the precise and systematic identification of the structure and function of the parts of the human body, both truly magnificent achievements. Without consummate skill and effective moment-to-moment control at every point, our surgical patients would regularly die or suffer crippling impairment on the operating table. Neither I nor any other homeopath I know of has the slightest wish to turn back the clock on that, or on a whole lot else that the medical profession still does superbly well.

Homeopathic medicine simply adds a further dimension, a subtler level of causal influence, as I'd prefer to call it, based on a curious empirical finding that has never been satisfactorily explained, that every medicinal agent which can elicit a distinctive symptom-picture in healthy people can also initiate a genuine healing response in sick people who exhibit the same symptomatology, as if they had become highly sensitized to it by virtue of that correspondence. This awesome and unexpected resonance in turn makes sense if and only if the illness that we see and the patient must live through already represents the organism's endeavor to heal itself, to overcome whatever it is trying to overcome, so that the homeopathic phenomenon challenges the life sciences to reimagine living organisms as integrated energy systems evolving through time, just as we intuitively know them to be, rather than simply specimens of this or that disease entity.

The writings here assembled make no claim that homeopathic medicines can heal everybody, much less replace pharmaceutical drugs or surgery where they are needed. But the mere fact that I have used them successfully enough to sustain me in a general practice of medicine for forty years without needing to write prescriptions, and that thousands of colleagues all over the world have been doing the same for over two hundred years, is already sufficient to answer the tired, old default argument that homeopathy can't *possibly* work. From there it's but a short step to take a closer look at its fascinating implications for medicine, all of which follow from the ancient wisdom that self-healing is a fundamental property of all living things, indeed synonymous with life itself, and therefore that all healing, whether aided by drugs or surgery or herbs or nothing at all, must ultimately happen or not happen on that level, so that the proper role of medical and health professionals becomes simply to assist a process that is already under way, rather than to surpass, defeat, or interfere with it. Whatever name we choose to call it, this almost embarrassingly self-evident truth is what all of my writings are really about.

I. Articles.

"What Is Homeopathy?"

"Homeopathic Reasoning"

"Vague, Long-Term Diagnosis: the *Nocebo* Effect"

"Two Childbirth Remedies"

"Vaccinations"

"Illness as Metaphor"

*What Is Homeopathy?**

Homeopathy is a method of treating the sick that was developed by Samuel Hahnemann, M. D. (1755-1843), an eminent German physician and Professor of Pharmacology, and is now practiced all over the world, mainly by physicians and licensed health professionals. Protected by Federal law and supervised by the FDA, homeopathic remedies are economical, deemed safe and effective for first-aid and domestic use, and with a few exceptions are available over the counter without prescription.

The Law of Similars.

In a series of experiments from 1792 onwards, Hahnemann proved 1) that medicines regularly produce in healthy people the same array of symptoms that they cure in the sick; and 2) that the medicine producing symptomatology most similar to that of the illness as a whole is the one most likely to initiate a genuinely curative response, one which can complete itself spontaneously without further assistance.

Hahnemann understood these experiments to mean that the manifest symptoms of illness already represent the attempt of the organism to heal itself, to overcome whatever it is trying to overcome; that the similar remedy acts by reinforcing that attempt in some way; and that true cure involves a concerted response of the whole organism, inasmuch as the remedy acts only if it is correctly chosen, if its essential similarity to the illness as a whole somehow renders the patient abnormally sensitive to it. Otherwise, the minuteness of the dose makes it likely that little or nothing will happen -- an important safety feature.

The Classical Method.

As practiced today, classical homeopathy includes the following elements:

* "What Is Homeopathy?" ***Emanuel Swedenborg: A Continuing Vision,*** Robin Larsen, et al., eds., Swedenborg Foundation, New York, 1988, pp. 475-476.

1) Each remedy is given in small doses to healthy volunteers, and the full range of physical, mental, and emotional responses to it are carefully recorded.

2) Each patient is likewise interviewed at length, and all the signs and symptoms of the illness to be treated are similarly noted in detail.

3) The patient is given only the one remedy whose total symptom-picture most closely resembles his or her own.

4) The remedy is given until a curative reaction occurs, and then stopped for as long as the reaction lasts.

5) The patient is instructed to avoid coffee, camphor, herbs, allopathic drugs where possible, and dental work, and to limit the use of tea, menthol, camphor, and other aromatic substances, as well as tobacco, alcohol, and other stimulants, as much as possible.

6) The remedies, which are mostly of natural origin (herbs, minerals, animal poisons, etc.), are specially diluted and refined, to minimize the risk of toxicity and enhance the depth and completeness of their action.

The Interview.

The homeopathic interview is necessarily detailed and intimate, because it looks beyond the abstract "disease entity" to the illness as a unique set of responses of the individual patient. Special attention is paid to the most unusual, striking, or idiosyncratic features of the case, which are often ignored during the usual diagnostic workup, even by the patients themselves.

Pros and Cons.

Homeopathic remedies are safe and economical, simple to use, and act very gently as a rule, with few side effects. When it occurs, the cure is prompt, thorough, and long-lasting, and does not require often-repeated doses of medication. By utilizing the innate healing power of the organism, it also encourages patients to assume more responsibility for their own health. On the other hand, it is an exacting art, requiring years of study and practice, such that even a qualified and experienced practitioner may need to try several remedies before an effective one is found, while in still other cases there is no benefit at all. Moreover, we do not really understand how the dilute remedies act, so that we cannot always predict exactly how or in what order a given patient will respond to them. In addition, the remedies are somewhat delicate and can be inactivated or antidoted rather easily.

When to Consider Homeopathy.

Although any patient may or may not respond to it, the following are some situations in which homeopathic treatment is most likely to be successful, or should at least be considered before resorting to more drastic methods, or after they have failed:

1) functional complaints with no tissue damage (headache, insomnia, IBS, dysmenorrhea, constipation, anxiety, PMS, CFS, ADD, etc.);

2) conditions for which no specific treatment is available, such as viral illnesses, or to promote wound healing after major trauma or surgery, or for crippling diseases, like MS, emphysema, etc., where great benefit can be obtained and very little harm done;

3) conditions for which elective surgery is indicated, such as fibroids, gall-stones, BPH, hemorrhoids, varicose veins, and the like, provided that immediate operation is not required and the surgery can always be performed later if necessary;

4) conditions for which allopathic drugs would have to be taken for years, like allergies, asthma, eczema, lupus, colitis, hypertension, epilepsy, etc.; and

5) conditions in which the standard medications have not worked, or the patient refuses to take them, including even incurable or terminal cases, where significant relief of symptoms may still be possible.

Homeopathy tends to be much less suitable, although still often worth a try, in severe chronic cases with established dependence on allopathic drugs, especially corticosteroids, antipsychotics, and anticonvulsants, where it could be dangerous or harmful to withdraw them. Nor, it must be said, is it a substitute for trained and experienced professional help.

*Homeopathic Reasoning**

Homeopathic medicine is a difficult and exacting art, requiring years of intensive study and practice; and even today, after almost two hundred years, we still do not know how our medicines act, or how our patients arc cured. It therefore seems entirely reasonable to suppose, as many of our patients do, that they simply cure themselves, and even that they might have done so without our medicines at all. So instead of trying to convince you of its validity, I shall present homeopathy to you simply as a way of thinking intelligently about the world of health and disease that you already know, an attitude and a philosophy that can serve you well whether you ultimately decide to practice it or not.

Although I shall not try to prove it today, I must also tell you that, far from being mere placebos, the homeopathic medicines appear to act with uncanny effectiveness in ways that seem to have as yet no adequate explanation according to the laws of physics and chemistry as we know them, and therefore have something new to tell us about the nature of the healing process in general, regardless of the method we use or the circumstances surrounding it. Far from it being an embarrassment, then, our ignorance of these matters merely proves that mainstream science hasn't yet caught up with the homeopathic phenomenon, or even acknowledged its existence. Nor am I in the least ashamed to ask for your help, or indeed for the help of the entire scientific world, in unraveling the thread of this most intriguing and important mystery. So today I aspire to no higher reward than that your curiosity be aroused and set in motion, just as mine has been.

The Concept of the *Materia Medica.*

Homeopathy is fundamentally a method of treating the sick, rather than a set of hypotheses about the nature of health and disease; it originated simply as a new way of ascertaining the healing powers of medicinal substances. In the allopathic tradition, we are taught to reason from the symptomatology of the patient to the diagnostic category, the pathological

* "Homeopathic Reasoning," ***Homeotherapy*** 6:135, September 1980.

process that they represent, and to give drugs to counteract or oppose that process by producing a contrary state in the body. Thus a patient with headaches, blurred vision, and irritability is found to have high blood pressure; the term diastolic hypertension enables us to comprehend all of these symptoms under a single, unifying concept; and we then give an antihypertensive drug, such as chlorothiazide, reserpine, or propanolol, to lower the blood pressure, and thereby also to suppress or control the other symptoms insofar as possible. The concept of the pathological process enables us to deduce which symptoms are pathognomonic or typical of the disease, and which are merely idiosyncratic for that patient; above all, it indicates the decisive point in his functioning against which we must exert maximum leverage, to reverse the direction of the disease as a whole.

Once the diagnosis is made, the homeopathic physician proceeds in exactly the opposite fashion, to recognize and identify those symptoms which are *atypical* of the disease, and thus distinctive of or peculiar to this patient as an individual, a unique energy system, and to select the medicine which can reproduce the most exactly similar picture when given to healthy people. Thus on further questioning the same hypertensive patient is revealed to be a successful, aggressive, businessman, who is unable to relax or to sleep restfully at night, who doses himself with large quantities of alcohol, coffee, and tobacco, often eats out at restaurants, and prefers a diet rich in animal fat, and in rich gravies, sauces, and seasonings, because of which he is prone to indigestion, heartburn, and constipation. His medicine might well be small doses of *Nux vomica,* a poisonous plant rich in the alkaloid strychnine, which in physiologic or subtoxic doses regularly provokes a general nervous hyperstimulation of this type.

The tissue pathology of this patient, the hypertensive changes in his blood vessels, remains a useful abstraction for helping us to classify the symptoms and risk of further diseases that he shares with many others; but it tells us almost nothing about his actual lived experience, and must therefore be regarded as simply a final common pathway, a morphological end result of a functional illness, a self-destructive life style in this case, which has presented itself only recently for diagnosis and treatment.

That is why we say, treat the patient, not the disease: it is only this patient who stands before you, asking for your help, who can or cannot be cured; and whatever about him is or is not curable is something equally peculiar to him, and cannot simply be inferred from the presence of this or that diagnostic category, of which he can be merely a specimen. For the homeopath, then, the unifying concept is not the disease entity, but the unique totality of lived symptoms and responses which is this patient, here and now, or to put it differently, the medicine which can most nearly reproduce that picture, and therefore help cure it as well. The usefulness of a medicine in treatment is therefore a special case of its power to produce symptoms, to alter health in either direction: to cause or cure, to act as medicine or poison, depending on the dosage, the circumstances, and the sensitivity of the patient. So we might say that homeopathy in its first approximation is the study of *medicines,* rather than diseases.

In allopathic medicine, given the importance of disease processes, the investigation of medicinal substances is necessarily indirect and difficult to interpret, because we must first reproduce an experimental model of the disease being studied in some laboratory animal; then the drug must be administered in high enough doses to have a significant effect in the majority of cases, regardless of the individual sensitivity of the subject; and, finally, the drug must be given a trial in human patients with the disease, once again in sufficiently high dose to override the symptoms in nearly all cases, regardless of the recipients and their circumstances, and the therapeutic benefit must be carefully weighed against the risk of toxicity due to overdose, side effects, or long-term dependence on the drug.

In contrast, homeopathy teaches us that the therapeutic power of a drug can never be tested adequately in a diseased organism, because its physiological responses are by definition altered in various ways, such as morbid cravings, intolerances, and the like, so that the only reliable test of the medicinal powers of a substance is to determine the full range of symptoms that it can provoke or elicit in an organism healthy enough to respond to it maximally and without limitation. Similarly, it follows as the night the day that a medicine for human beings must have the power to affect and act upon every sphere of human life, including those mental, emotional, and spiritual characteristics that are peculiar to our species and therefore cannot be adequately tested on other life forms.

The homeopathic method of investigating a medicinal substance is roughly as follows: to administer it in subtoxic doses to a number of healthy volunteers of various ages, sexes, and constitutions; to record accurately and in detail the full range of their responses to it, including the idiosyncratic reactions of each subject; and finally, to synthesize out of these fragments a composite picture of that substance, consisting of physical symptoms, mental symptoms, emotional symptoms, and their arrangement into a unique whole that is characteristic of that substance, and can be used to distinguish it clearly from the picture of every other substance, especially from those most closely resembling it.

These 'provings,' as we call them, are purely experimental, owing nothing to any hypothesis or speculation about this or that disease entity; and they enable us to investigate systematically the medicinal properties of any substance whatsoever, and to evaluate the claims made for it, either in the folklore, or allopathically on the basis of animal experiments and pathological models, as above. As such, they are interesting and valuable for their own sake, whether or not the medicine is to be used homeopathically, or indeed in treatment of any kind.

I will begin with the example of penicillin, because it is already one of the great medicines of human history, despite having been studied and used by the medical profession for only about forty years. In allopathic medicine, we use penicillin solely on the basis of one property, its ability to destroy a certain type of bacterial cell walls: our understanding of pathogenic bacteria as a cause of infectious diseases has led to the discovery of penicillin and other antibiotics to destroy our bacterial enemies, and inadvertently, a considerable number of friendly species as well. Everything else that penicillin can bring about, e.g., skin allergies, anaphylaxis, fever, Herxheimer reactions, and so forth, are relegated to the fine print as 'side effects,' i.e., undesirable, non-therapeutic actions, idiosyncrasies on the part of the patient.

But for the homeopath, these idiosyncratic reactions are precisely the ones that we must study, because highly sensitive patients are those most highly responsive to the drug, and therefore the best able to exhibit its true, detailed, and most distinctive symptom-picture. So I repeat: if penicillin is to be a drug for human beings, it must have the power to alter the health of human beings, and not merely of bacteria, a truism which explains why in provings there are no side effects.

To the medical profession I therefore propose a great collaborative project, namely, to investigate this medicine as a whole, by recording the full range of symptoms that it can produce, and thus learn to recognize on purely clinical grounds the patient who will respond to it curatively, before the culture reports come back, and before our crude antibacterial dose nearly kills him. We could then cure him with a tiny fraction of the usual dose, and with minimal risk of re-infection or the development of resistant strains, because we would then be treating the patient, rather than merely decimating his bacteria.

The apparent paradox that viral illnesses also not infrequently respond to penicillin, and the uncontested fact that even highly susceptible bacterial populations quickly develop resistance to it, show that we really do not know very much about the fundamental powers of this drug, and that in most cases we must be content with a palliative or temporary action, inasmuch as the host factors are unaffected and the risk of re-infection remains unchanged.

To produce a reliable proving will require a huge co-operative effort over a period of many years; but its obvious interest and importance to regulars and homeopaths alike are more than sufficient to warrant our undertaking this project together as a step toward further communication between us in the future.

From these considerations it follows that homeopathic and allopathic medicine likewise have radically different conceptions of the purposes and values of medicinal treatment. In the allopathic method, the medicine is designed to intervene selectively at key points in the disease process, and to counteract the pathogenetically important symptoms, often but not always those most distressing to the patient, with minimal effect upon the remainder of the organism. The search is always for drugs with a more and more limited range and specificity of action: the ideal drug would be one with only a single action upon a single physiological mechanism, and no effect elsewhere.

Crude drugs of botanical origin tend to be less and less suitable for this purpose, because each of them contains a variety of alkaloids and other medicinal constituents, with diverse effects on the human body. The opium poppy, for example, contains not only morphine, the great analgesic, sedative, and narcotic, and codeine, another potent analgesic and cough suppressant, but also papaverine, a smooth-muscle relaxant, and several other alkaloids for which no medicinal use has yet been found.

The drug industry thus approaches botanical drugs in a definite and predictable sequence. First, it extracts, isolates, and characterizes the individual alkaloids in pure form, testing each of them separately, and reproducing them synthetically if possible. At a later stage, it develops new semi-synthetic or wholly synthetic derivatives, with greater specificity of action, fewer side effects, greater ease of administration, and so forth. Thus we now have a wide variety of opiate drugs to choose from, such as diacetyl morphine, or heroin, which produces a state of euphoria that is very useful in treating terminally ill patients, but presently outlawed because of its addictive potential; meperidine, or Demerol, a totally synthetic opiate with an analgesic potency almost equal to that of morphine, but much less tendency to produce vomiting, constipation, and other side effects, and much greater effectiveness orally; and oxycodone, or Percodan, a potent oral analgesic which is structurally related to codeine but has no action on the cough center.

In contrast, homeopathy prefers to concentrate on the parent drug, the opium poppy itself, because the total picture of its effects tends to be far more striking than the effects of its constituents, either alone or in combination. As you all know, the pathogenesis of *Opium,* as drawn from provings, overdoses, toxicology, and cured cases, features analgesia and insensitivity to pain, progressing to stupor, loss of consciousness, and, in toxic overdose, coma and death from respiratory paralysis. In homeopathy, *Opium* is often used in situations where the patient is already stuporous or comatose and insensitive to pain, such as coma, massive CVA, and so forth.

But another interesting feature of the drug, as indeed of all drugs when they are investigated thoroughly, is its contradictoriness, its tendency to produce diametrically opposite symptoms, sometimes even in the same patient. Thus, most provers of *Opium* are insensitive to pain, but a significant number are hyper-sensitive; many complain of being unable to feel or express any emotion, but quite a few are tormented by anxiety or terror; the majority are constipated, but some have diarrhea; and there is often a paralysis of the bladder, or an inability to retain the urine, i.e., either spasm or paralysis of the vesical sphincter; the muscles tend to be weak and flaccid, but there may also be twitching or convulsions, even in the same patient. I will present a short case to illustrate these dualisms.

Postoperative bladder paralysis. A 32-year-old mother of two whom I first saw in her home for severe abdominal pain of 3 days' duration, she being at the time 'too sick to move.' Three weeks earlier, in September 1977, she had given birth normally to her second child in the Taos Hospital, and was discharged in good health. As I entered her home, the patient lay in the next room with the door shut, but I was instantly overcome by the foul odor of a massive septic infection. With a fever of 102° and pulse of 120 per minute, her abdomen was diffusely tender, with guarding and rebound, and her consciousness obtunded and far away, as if in a dream. I took her to the hospital with a diagnosis of peritonitis, and a total hysterectomy was performed without delay. Postoperatively she did quite well for the first three days, but then the ICU nurse called to say that the patient was oliguric, with an output of only 200 cc. in the past 12 hours. At that time she was still receiving Demerol 100 mg. IM every 4 hours for pain; yet she appeared quite alert and even apprehensive, perhaps only then fully realizing how close to death she had been. I gave her *Opium* 200, 1 dose, dry on the tongue; and within 2 hours she passed 600 cc. of urine. Her output remained normal thereafter, and she made an uneventful recovery.

A homeopathic medicine can be any substance that produces symptoms in or otherwise alters the health of a significant number of the people exposed to it. Whether it causes symptoms or cures them depends on the dosage and the sensitivity of the patient, which tends to be highest when the patient already has the symptoms that the drug is known to produce.

Because the whole of the medicine must be matched with the total symptom-picture of the patient, homeopaths use only one medicine at a time, and only in a very minute dose, because the remedy that can most closely reproduce the illness owes its effectiveness to the patient's abnormally heightened sensitivity to it. Thus the homeopath seeks that medicine to which that patient will be the most sensitive at that particular time, and gives the smallest possible dose of it that will still be a dose. If the medicine is well chosen, it will substitute its own artificial 'drug' disease for the natural illness of the patient, which then gradually wears off; if it is incorrectly chosen, the minuteness of the dose all but guarantees that little or nothing will happen. The proper selection of the remedy accordingly requires a considerable measure of art, which is what makes it so difficult, so time-consuming, and so exciting to practice.

In addition to a number of allopathic drugs, the homeopathic *materia medica* includes herbs, spices, foods, hormones, chemicals, cosmetics, allergens, minerals, bacteria, viruses, disease products, and even a few substances like table salt, chalk, club moss, etc., that are comparatively inert physiologically and produce symptoms only when diluted and prepared homeopathically. All of these substances are capable of producing characteristic symptoms in healthy people, and even pathological changes if taken in overdose. In allopathic medicine, the therapeutic dose is simply an average, one that will produce a palliative effect in most people, albeit totally ineffective for some patients and highly toxic for others, namely, those who are hypersensitive to and therefore potentially curable by it if given in homeopathic dose.

Similarly, any medicinal substance can produce symptoms if taken regularly over a prolonged period of time, not infrequently the same ones for which it was originally taken. Thus, many people appreciate the laxative effect of their morning coffee, and even use it regularly for that purpose; but that is how a good medicine easily becomes a bad habit, when they can no longer move their bowels without it. A nursing mother may give her colicky baby chamomile tea with such good results that she continues to give it preventively, only to discover that the colic soon returns with equal or greater force, and persists until the habit is broken. Similarly, pregnant women are taught to take their iron pills religiously to prevent anemia, but by the second or third trimester quite a few will actually *become* anemic on this regimen, and remain so until the iron is stopped. One could go on and on.

Tobacco began its medicinal career as a tiny shrub with leaves so poisonous that the American Indian tribes who prized it most highly were obliged to dilute it with kinnikinnik and other herbs to keep from vomiting. By the time the council was concluded and the ceremonial pipe reduced to ashes, all further desire for tobacco would have been extinguished for many days. Today the plant is grown commercially as a hybrid with colossal leaves, each one producing dozens of cigarettes of very low medicinal content and often containing insecticide residues and other chemical additives to make them burn continuously without having to be re-ignited. Many habitual smokers no longer actually enjoy the herb, or even remember why they started smoking it; yet there is no end to the craving, in part because they are still seeking the medicinal experience which is no longer there, while the appearance of pathological symptoms makes it almost impossible to break the habit without swearing off this superb medicine of the earth once and for all.

Whether smoked as marijuana, hashish, bhang, or ganja, preparations of *Cannabis* have been esteemed as mild intoxicants for thousands of years in many different parts of the world; in years gone by, it also enjoyed a considerable medicinal reputation as a tranquilizer, and in the Nineteenth Century was used as a near-specific for gonorrhea. The provings of *Cannabis* have amply confirmed both uses, and even hinted at others previously unrecognized. As a powerful irritant of the urethra and the entire genitourinary tract of both sexes, it has been shown both to stimulate and inhibit its functions; and its well-known mental symptoms have also been widely reproduced and clarified: the euphoria and increased fluency of ideas; the anxiety, silliness, and loss of recent memory; the marked slowing of the sense of duration or the passage of time, and the perceived elongation of space or distance, often associated with feelings of hurry, of being late or pressed for time, and of being removed or alienated from familiar experiences close at hand.

But the provings of *Cannabis* have also brought out a number of less familiar but potentially important actions on the cardiovascular system, such as lowering or raising the pulse and blood pressure, and provoking instability of the peripheral circulation (cold hands and feet, dizziness, syncope, etc.). The drug industry is already at work extracting the various alkaloids from the plant, and developing semisynthetic derivatives with more specific actions on the intraocular pressure, for example, and for use against diseases in its usual way. Nor should it occasion any surprise that even this relatively nontoxic herb, when taken in excess or repeatedly over long periods of time, can produce unpleasant or troublesome symptoms and eventually pathological changes in the tissues as well.

Homeopathy recognizes this basic duality as inherent in all medicines, as simply their power to cause or to cure, to stimulate or inhibit, to enhance life or to poison it. To use a substance medicinally, in other words, implies treating it with respect, as a special or occasional experience, followed by periods of recovery and still longer intervals during which no medicine is taken, freeing the patient to integrate the experience without risk of habituation, addiction, or chronic dependence of any kind.

The Concept of the "Vital Force."

It has often been said that modern allopathic medicine is purely empirical, in the sense that it has no general philosophy of health and disease, and indeed no desire for any. But I would prefer to say that its fundamental principles are methodological, rather than having to do with content, and that they consist of the basic experimental methods of physiology, biochemistry, microbiology, and the like, which specify how we can acquire valid scientific knowledge of living beings, and what other types of inquiry are to be avoided. This view was beautifully expressed by Claude Bernard, the great French physiologist, in words written 150 years ago that still ring true today:

> What we call the immediate cause of a phenomenon is nothing but the physical and material condition in which it exists or appears. The object of the experimental method, and the limit of every scientific research, is therefore the same for living as for inanimate bodies: it consists in finding the relations which connect any phenomenon with its immediate cause, or, putting it differently, in defining the conditions necessary to the appearance of the phenomenon. Indeed, when the experimenter succeeds in learning the necessary conditions of a phenomenon, he is in some sense its master: he can predict its course and appearance; he can promote or prevent it at will. We shall therefore define physiology thus: the science whose object it is to study the phenomena of living beings, and to determine the material conditions in which they appear.
>
> As a corollary to the above, we must add that neither physiologists nor physicians must imagine it their task to seek the cause of life, or the essence of disease. That would be entirely wasting one's time in pursuing a phantom. The words 'life,' 'death', 'health,' and 'disease' have no objective reality. Newton said of gravitation, *"Bodies fall with an accelerated motion whose law we know: that is a fact, that is reality. But the first cause that makes these bodies fall is unknown. To picture the phenomenon to our minds, we may say that they fall as if there were a force of attraction toward the center of the earth. But the force of attraction does not exist, we do not see it; it is merely a word used to abbreviate speech."* When a physiologist invokes 'the vital force,' he likewise does not see it; he merely pronounces a word. Only the vital phenomenon exists, with its material conditions; that is the one thing that he can study and know.[1]

The allopathic method is thus essentially analytical:

first, we reduce the symptoms to their lowest common denominator, the disease process(es) that can most fully comprehend them;

then we isolate the mechanism or mechanisms that are most important in the pathogenesis of the disease and the production of its symptoms;

and finally, we select the medicine(s) that can most directly influence or control that part of the process, while having the least possible effect on the remainder of the patient's life.

The homeopathic method, on the other hand, is synthetic, or "holistic:" it views the illness as a complex totality of symptoms or responses that are uniquely expressive of the individuality of the patient, and it matches this *Gestalt* or image directly to the medicine with the most similar pathogenesis, i. e., the power to reproduce that picture in healthy people as broadly and minutely as possible. In other words, the allopathic method gives part of the medicine to part of the patient, all the rest of its actions being discounted as 'side effects,' while homeopathy gives the whole of the medicine to the whole of the patient, such that its effectiveness depends upon the ability of the patient to respond it as a whole and by virtue of that correspondence.

As we saw, in selecting a pharmaceutical drug, the most important symptoms are those pathognomonic or typical of the disease process, and therefore common to most patients bearing that diagnosis, whereas in selecting a homeopathic remedy, the most valuable symptoms are those most uniquely characteristic of the patient, which set him apart from others with the same diagnosis, and those which refer to the patient as a whole, rather than merely to a part of the body. Some examples of these are mental states, such as fears, delusions, moods, and so forth; special times of the day, weather conditions, positions, and movements when the symptoms are consistently better or worse; marked cravings or intolerances for particular articles of food or drink; and any other symptoms that are the reverse of what would be expected from someone with the same diagnosis, and sufficiently odd or striking as to accentuate the uniqueness of the patient.

Similarly, in allopathic medicine the fundamental concept is the disease process, as we saw, whereas in homeopathy, it is the unformulable integrity of the individual patient and the medicine which most closely corresponds to it. Another way of saying this is that allopathic medicine treats each disease process a separate entity with an etiology and pathogenesis of its own that commandeers the physiology of the patient, as if it could be isolated, controlled, or even removed surgically, more or less independently of the health and well-being of the patient as a whole.

Homeopathy, on the other hand, regards the illness that we can see, the illness that the patient must live through, as the concerted response of the organism to its own particular stress-producing factors, whatever they are, so that suppressing any of these symptoms must necessarily weaken that response and detract proportionately from the recuperative powers of the patient. Attempting to separate the diseased parts of the organism from the healthy parts thus merely adds to the disunity which the disease already represents, while strengthening the healthy parts at the expense of the diseased parts simply perpetuates the conflict which created the disease in the first place.

Finally, wherever possible, modern "scientific" medicine tries to assign etiological factors, such as pathogenic bacteria, viruses, cigarette smoking, 'stress,' and the like, to each disease process, to identify its necessary cause(s), just as Claude Bernard once taught. In these same connections, homeopathy acknowledges the complementary truth, that what is stressful or pathogenic for one person may not be for another, and that it is often very difficult to tell why the patient suddenly becomes sensitized to stress factors that had previously been tolerated without any difficulty, or why those stresses happen to cause symptoms or pathological changes in one part of the body rather than another.

So always we are brought back to the irreducible and essentially unformulable integrity of living beings, which respond in characteristic and yet often unpredictable ways, to stimuli that are also uniquely their own. We cannot 'see' this unity directly, and must infer it through its effects; it remains a philosophical assumption rather than a scientific hypothesis as yet capable of proof or disproof. So we may readily accept a positivistic formulation to the effect that living beings behave as if they were animated by a peculiar force or energy that flows through and emanates from them without interruption, until the death of the body. Nor is it unlikely that what homeopaths like to call the 'vital force,' once properly understood, will take its place as yet another important dimension of living organisms, in addition to cells, biochemistry, 'mind,' and the like, rather than the whole of it, which will doubtless continue to elude our grasp.

Nevertheless, the experience of health and disease must remain forever opaque and unintelligible to us as physicians without some concept of the life energy as a whole, whatever we may choose to call it. Homeopathy calls it the 'vital force,' emphasizing its holistic aspect; Walter Cannon termed it 'homeostasis,' emphasizing its biochemical aspect. Undoubtedly in the future we shall invent more names for still other ways of approaching it. What makes the concept of a vital force so appealing, so useful, and indeed so indispensable to us is that it lies wholly outside the classical paradox of mind and body, because it encompasses the integrity of living beings in a purely energetic dimension that is more primitive and undifferentiated than either the anatomization of a body in space or the evolution of consciousness as a sequence of experiences in time. Only the unity of the vital force or something like it enables us to locate all the phenomena of life wholly within the operation of a single, continuous energy field, and to derive both 'mind' and 'body' from it as valid, independent perspectives.

Our need for the vital force is also the reason why the human body can no longer remain the dominant concept in healing, any more than we can afford to limit our life sciences to the study of the material conditions of phenomena, as Claude Bernard had insisted. For even if we know and can satisfy the necessary conditions of phenomena, these may still be insufficient to guarantee that they will actually occur; and, conversely, even if those conditions are lacking, the healthy organism is capable by definition of creating them.

That is why we need a concept of human life that includes love and the striving for transcendence no less than the anatomical and biochemical organization of the body. The vital force is merely our schematization of that need, however inadequate it may some day prove to be. Hahnemann originally coined the term 'vital force' to refer to the totality of the responses of the organism, because the homeopathic phenomenon, the mysterious correspondence between the symptoms of the medicine and the needs of the patient, implies the existence of a force capable of responding at this level of subtlety and complexity. Hahnemann discovered that the organism regularly responds to suppressive medication by relief of symptoms, followed by their reappearance as soon as the drug is stopped, while the curative response to homeopathic medicines, when it occurs, often consists of an initial aggravation, followed by amelioration and recovery.

The healing process was studied even more thoroughly by Constantine Hering, M.D., who discovered that a curative response, as distinguished from a temporary or palliative one, regularly follows certain patterns, which may be summarized as follows:

1) the symptoms proceed *from above downwards,* from the head end of the body to the feet or tail, or caudal end;

2) the symptoms proceed from *inside outwards,* from the center or innermost parts outward toward the periphery;

3) the symptoms proceed *from more vital to less vital organs;* and

4) the symptoms disappear *in the reverse order of their appearance in the life history of the patient,* the recent symptoms disappearing first, followed by the reappearance and disappearance of older symptoms in the reverse order of their original chronology.

I would add that similar patterns can be observed in cases cured with herbs, acupuncture, pharmaceutical drugs, surgery, placebo, and even in patients who recover spontaneously without any treatment at all. So another piece of evidence in favor of a vital force would seem to be the existence and validity of these 'laws' governing the healing process in general, irrespective of the mode of treatment employed, which you can observe and verify for yourselves in your daily practice.

In any case, it strikes me as a major indictment of our present medical system that, notwithstanding all our disease entities and potent drugs for suppressing them, we can no longer accommodate or find much use for the ancient concept of 'healing,' or simply 'making whole' [again], so that instead we have learned to settle for 'disease control', remission, good five-year survival rates, and so forth. Intuitively we all know that healing is always possible, and is in fact going on everywhere, all the time, both because and in spite of our efforts, and whatever treatment modality we use. The problem is that medical science no longer has any room for it, so that healing is reduced to a 'miracle,' a quasi-religious occurrence that lies outside the realm of identifiable causes or rational explanations. Whether you believe in it or not, homeopathy deserves much credit for honoring the phenomenon of healing, which is built right into the concept of the vital force.

I would like to tell you a story from my own medical history to illustrate another aspect of the vital force, which is its unpredictability. In 1974, shortly after being introduced to homeopathy, I suffered a concussion and could easily have been killed in a head-on collision, from which I awoke with several rib fractures and a large scalp laceration, and in which the driver of the other car was unhurt, but his aged mother in the back seat was fatally injured. Lying flat on a Gurney in the emergency room, the chest pain was unbearable; but a single dose of *Arnica* 200 relieved it within a few seconds, to the point that I was able to take my shirt off without assistance and then be driven home, an incredible feat under the circumstances. It never came back.

On the third night after the accident, however, while trying to sleep, I suddenly experienced another kind of chest pain, if anything even more intense than the first one, and quite unlike anything I'd ever felt before, gripping my chest like a vise, and letting go again within a minute or two. Although it didn't happen very often or last very long after that, it unnerved me because it was so sudden, violent, and unpredictable, coming on with equal probability whether I was moving, just beginning to move, or lying perfectly still, and *Arnica* had no effect on it at all; so I gladly accepted the help of a Demerol injection for the night. The following day, I called Nakazono, my acupuncture Sensei, who put an arrowroot poultice on my chest and needled a few points; within an hour or two, the pain had completely disappeared, and I completed my recovery without further trouble.

Early in spring, about six months later, while visiting the Indian ruins at Bandelier, my friend and I impulsively decided to spend the night in one of the caves, although we had no bedding, and it was illegal to build a fire within the monument area. After several cold, sleepless hours, we capitulated and went home; and as I woke the next morning, the right side of my neck seized up with a terrific pain, which I instantly recognized as the viselike grip I described a few sentences back, only now transferred to another place. This time it abated without treatment, and disappeared the following day; I cite it merely as an instance of how we fashion our sicknesses out of materials ready-to-hand, and how we are capable of detaching, transferring, and recombining our old symptoms into new patterns for new purposes of which we are as ignorant as of the old.

The final application of the vital force that I want to discuss with you is the use of the high attenuations, or what we homeopaths sometimes call the 'infinitesimal dose.' Most of you probably know that Hahnemann was a pharmacologist of note, as well as a physician, and indeed the author of a standard text on the preparation of the familiar remedies of his time. Perhaps you do not know that it was the local pharmacists who especially persecuted him and drove him from town to town in the early years of his career, mainly for preparing and dispensing his own medicines. I say this because I want you to keep always in your minds that classical homeopathy was invented by a pharmacist and is imbued throughout with the meticulous exactitude of the apothecary. Almost as soon as Hahnemann used medicines according to the homeopathic law, he began to experiment with serial dilutions to reduce the dose, because his initial aggravations were sometimes quite alarming; and he soon discovered, just as you'd expect, that the more he diluted them, the more these aggravations were reduced in intensity, but so was the benefit. Eventually, and it seems more or less by accident, he discovered that by triturating the solid remedy in a mortar with each dilution, or by pounding or 'succussing' it in a vial if in a liquid state, the therapeutic power was actually deepened and enhanced in a subtle and beautiful way.

If, for instance, you give a nursing infant chamomile tea for colic, he will often calm down and go to sleep; but the following day, once the drug is metabolized, you must start all over again. It is only when you give the higher attenuations of the remedy, and if the totality of the symptoms correspond, that the remedy will act *curatively.* To Hahnemann it seemed as though the healing power embedded within the physical structure of the plant, once freed by the process of succussion or 'dynamization,' could penetrate more deeply into the vital force of the patient, and need no longer be metabolized or excreted as would the plant drug from which it came. After 200 years of chemical science, we can reasonably hypothesize that the higher attenuations of the remedy exist in the form of energy, and that the pattern or blueprint of it still resonates qualitatively with the proved symptomatology of the plant, even after being freed from the electrochemical bonding forces of its molecular structure.

As you can well imagine, this kind of talk cost Hahnemann a good many followers from the beginning, and does so still. But the idea still fascinates and makes a certain amount of intuitive sense. You take the crude substance, say chamomile, and prepare the mother tincture with alcohol; then the dilutions, 1:10 (decimal) or 1:100 (centesimal), succussing each time. After the 30th centesimal dilution, already well beyond the limit of Avogadro's number, according to the atomic theory of matter there should be no more molecules or measurable amounts of the substance remaining; yet this is the level of dilution at which we really begin to see results clinically. I often use a 200th centesimal dilution (i. e., 1:100 diluted 200 times), and sometimes a 1M (1:100 diluted 1000 times), 10M (10,000 times), or a 50M (50,000 times), all of which are literally 'infinitesimal', or out of the ballpark of chemistry entirely. At this level, the remedy can work quite dramatically, within a few seconds or minutes in an acute case, and, if properly chosen, can go on working for a long, long time.

Assuming for the moment that you don't simply have me committed for psychiatric observation, and you can believe, at least hypothetically, that such remedies can and do in fact work, I would like to think about what the phenomenon of the high dilutions tells us about the nature of the vital force upon which they act. We can say, first of all, that it cannot be a chemical action primarily, although in the lower potencies there will be a chemical action as well, and these actions will usually be at least qualitatively similar. Secondly, we know that the medicine works if and only if it is properly chosen, which also seems to mean that the patient is highly sensitive to it. Thirdly, we know from experiments with bacteria, germinating plants, fruit flies, cell-free enzyme systems, and the like, that if the target population is exposed to ascending dilutions of a homeopathic remedy to which it responds, the responses frequently show a band-like effect, with certain dilutions stimulating growth or activity, others inhibiting growth or activity, and still others having little or no effect.[2]

In many cases, this pattern also tends to be repeatable up the scale, at levels and intervals of dilution characteristic of both the substance and the subject population. These graphs suggest a sinusoidal or wave-like pattern, like the overtones of a certain musical note, some of which will send shivers down the spine of a music lover, others perhaps leaving the same person unmoved or even 'turned off, and all perhaps equally uninteresting to somebody who doesn't respond to the music at all. Clinically, most homeopaths have had the experience that a certain potency or dilution is exactly right for a given patient at a given time, while other neighboring potencies may have a slight effect, an adverse effect, e.g., a severe aggravation with little or no improvement, or no effect at all.

So it seems reasonable to suppose that the dilute remedy exists in the form of an energy pattern, that it has the power to resonate with or reinforce or interfere with the existing energy field of the patient, and that, if the change is productive or at least energy-efficient, the patient will take it up and continue to function along these lines; very rarely, these changes will be destructive. The remedy is merely the key that fits in the door, or does not fit: if it succeeds in opening the door, such that the patient can walk through it more easily than before, the life energy, having been thus set in motion, will complete the rest of the healing work without further assistance.

It seems highly probable that these subtle forces will prove to be related to the quantum electromagnetic energies of the atom, and in particular to the action potentials at the cell membrane. Most recently, Kirlian photography offers a practical technique for measuring the 'aura' as an electromagnetic emanation from the body surface, and how it changes in health and disease, and during various forms of treatment.[3] The idea is essentially similar to the etheric or 'subtle' body of yogic philosophy, and the *chi* of acupuncture, both of which map the organism as an energy continuum, the latter consisting of longitudinal or meridional energy currents and a point-for-point correspondence between the surface of the body and various internal organs. We are still very far from a clear scientific understanding of the life energy, which is why we still badly need the philosophical concept of the vital force, at least for the time being.

Purely from a clinical point of view, I can attest to the fact that patients undergoing homoeopathic treatment tend to describe their experience in qualitatively similar ways. Often the first noticeable change is an emotional feeling, a sense of well-being, euphoria, or happiness, or an experience of heightened energy or vitality, or both. Perhaps a few days later, they may experience a brief intensification or aggravation of their physical symptoms, often but not always their chief complaint; but if you question them closely, you will see that, while the sensation may be more vivid or intense, they seem more distant from it, or in some other way it actually bothers them less than before. So it is not yet the symptom itself, but rather their *relationship* to it, that has changed: they notice it, bear witness to it, and record it, but it no longer has the power to overwhelm them or carry them away with it. It is as if they sat somewhere in the center of their symptoms, quite unmoved and undisturbed by them, and indeed sometimes quite elated, as if having penetrated to the core of their illness and found it not quite so threatening after all. From that point on, you have the sense that they have mastered it, and recovery is usually quite rapid after that.

So now, in conclusion, I would like to come back to where we began, to the placebo effect, which is still, after all, the principal treatment modality with which homeopathy has generally been credited. Might it not be the highest compliment that could be paid to a remedy that patients would barely notice that it was acting, would truly and correctly believe that they healed themselves without it, and would continue not to need it in the future? As the Chinese sage once said,

> A leader is best when people barely know he exists,
> Not so good when they obey and acclaim him,
> Worst when they despise him.
> Of a good leader, when his work is done and his aim fulfilled,
> The people will say, "We did this ourselves."[4]

NOTES.

1. Claude Bernard, *An introduction to the Study of Experimental Medicine,* translated by Henry Copley Greene, Dover, New York, 1957, pp. 65-67, *passim.*
2 Cf. *Transactions,* XXXI Congress, International League of Homoeopathic Physicians, Athens, 1976, *passim.*
3. Krippner, S., and Rubin, D.. eds., *The Kirlian Aura,* Anchor. N.Y., 1974.
4. Lao-Tse, *The Way of Life,* translated by Witter Bynner, pp. 34-35.

*Vague, Long-Term Diagnosis: The Nocebo Effect**

I read with great interest the study of mild hypertension reported in the October 14 issue of the *New England Journal of Medicine.*[1] Once the diagnosis is made, the study concludes, even mild high blood pressure should be treated aggressively, because the long-term mortality is significantly reduced by doing so. Unfortunately, the study does not show the long-term effect on morbidity, mortality, and quality of life of simply *making the diagnosis,* which I have good reason to suspect is very considerable. For we all know, as do our patients, that the diagnosis of even mild hypertension amounts to an official prophecy that serious or fatal cardiovascular diseases are much more likely to follow unless something more or less drastic is done to prevent them.

The formidable and essentially incurable anxiety generated by such a prophecy immediately suggests two alternative interpretations of the same data, both of which would have to be refuted by the authors of the present study before their conclusions would merit general acceptance. The first is that mild hypertension is a normal physiologic variant, utterly without prognostic significance, and that it is only our extreme fear of serious or fatal cardiovascular diseases that does indeed make such complications much more likely once the diagnosis is made.

The second is that hypertension *does* confer a somewhat higher probability of developing these complications in the future, but that that probability is *significantly increased* by the diagnosis, thereby adding the substantial burden of intractable lifelong anxiety to the underlying illness that the patient already has to bear. Even if both of these hypotheses could be proven untrue, at the moment either one of them is just as plausible as the one proposed by the authors to justify their major intervention into the lives of these many millions of people.

---

* "Vague, Long-Term Diagnosis: the *Nocebo* Effect," ***Journal of the American Institute of Homeopathy*** 76:26, March 1983.

Indeed, there are compelling reasons for believing that one of these alternative hypotheses is in fact the correct one. Chief among them is the formidable and well-documented effect of chronic anxiety on all types of cardiovascular disease.[2] What greater anxiety can a patient suffer than to be told that he is quite likely to develop a serious or fatal disease unless he agrees to take powerful and toxic drugs for the rest of his life, and quite possibly even then?

Unfortunately, it is almost impossible to design another study to test these two hypotheses without introducing ethical and methodological dilemmas every bit as troubling as the hypotheses themselves. Such a study would require a third group of patients who were diagnosed but not told that their blood pressures were abnormal and perhaps even a fourth group who were not diagnosed or even examined. What doctor among us is courageous or foolhardy enough not to diagnose even mild hypertension, or not to tell his patients that they had it? What patient would be willing not to know if he had it, or be less anxious for not knowing? Even if such people could be found, informed consent would require us to notify the patients that some of them would not be diagnosed or told, which would vitiate the whole point of the study, to eliminate the anxiety caused by making the diagnosis.

In other words, the diagnosis of hypertension is anxiety-provoking *by its very existence,* because it causes every person to wonder if he has it, even if he never goes to a doctor. This type of anxiety can never be eliminated by any study, because our whole system of clinical and experimental research ultimately rests upon the independent validity of the pathological diagnosis itself in providing accurate information about the "objective reality" of the disease, including its natural history, abnormal physiology, and prognosis, quite apart from the subjective or lived experience of the patient. Indeed, this assumption is itself untestable within the system that we have developed for discovering medical truth. It often functions in much the same way as a religious commandment: obey it without question; ignore or transgress it at your peril.

Yet there is mounting evidence on all sides that pathological evidence is often a very poor guide to what our patients' lives will be like, let alone whether they will recover, worsen, or die. A good case in point is the article by Susan Love, et al., in the same October 14 issue of the *New England Journal.*[3] The authors reviewed several studies on so-called "fibrocystic disease" of the breast, and could find no convincing evidence that this condition was anything other than a normal variant, for which they proposed the more descriptive and less threatening names of "lumpy breast" or "physiologic nodularity."

What they *did* find, however, was that the incidence of histologically "proven" cases of breast cancer correlated very significantly with a prior breast biopsy, regardless of how the pathologist read it. The clear implication was that making this "precancerous" diagnosis created a different attitude in doctors and patients alike, and in both pathologists and surgeons as well, such that, for whatever reason, the result was more biopsies and mammograms, more positive diagnoses of breast cancer, more mastectomies, more chemotherapy, and ultimately more deaths, thus not only in a sense *justifying* the original diagnosis, but also in fact fulfilling its prophecy.

In the end, the reader is left with the further possibility, again in effect untestable, that the histological diagnosis itself, the procedure with seemingly the highest degree of accuracy, may be giving exceedingly poor prognostic information when measured against what nobody dares to measure, namely, what would have happened if the examination was not done, the lump not detected, or the patient told simply that we do not understand the cancer process, and sent home without treatment. It is precisely *because* we don't understand it, and can't realistically know how a given patient would have done without all our intervention, that making the diagnosis might not serve a useful purpose until the patient herself becomes capable of making it.

So what I am really asking is, when and under what circumstances is a pathological diagnosis useful? Clearly, it seems useful and indeed often life-saving in the management of acute diseases, infections, heart attacks, etc., where it helps both the doctor and patient to know what they are up against, and what they have to do next.

But, I submit, it is far less useful and often clearly injurious when the illness is permanent and incurable, or the patient has to be kept on a certain regimen of drugs throughout life, most especially when the patient is not ill, presents with few or no symptoms, and is told that he or she has "hypertension" or "fibrocystic disease of the breast," purely on the basis of a laboratory specimen that has nothing to do with how he or she feels or functions. In such a case, we can expect that the anxiety provoked by making the diagnosis will predispose both doctor and patient to discover the very diseases that they are trying to prevent. Under these circumstances, when a woman has spent most of her adult life anticipating that she will one day develop breast cancer, she may actually experience profound symptomatic relief on all levels when that expectation is finally validated.

I therefore propose the term "nocebo effect" to refer to the pathogenetic effect of making such diagnoses, by inflicting pain and suffering on our patients. It comes from the Latin *nocebo,* literally "I shall harm, or injure," the exact opposite of the "placebo effect" (the Latin *placebo,* meaning "I shall please"). The latter denotes the healing or curative power of giving our patients blank pills and persuading them that they are real; it works because they want our help and trust us, however unwisely. We now know that the placebo effect is about as good a model currently available to us of the healing process in general, whether we choose to co-operate with it or not.[4]

The "nocebo" effect, on the other hand, indicates the damaging and sometimes catastrophic effect of telling a patient what they "really" have, of redefining his reality in such a way that he must forever after live in its shadow, substituting *its* law, or rather *ours,* for his own. I doubt that we can devise a simpler or wiser rule for our profession than the one announced by our illustrious progenitor 2500 years ago:

> Declare the past, diagnose the present, and foretell the future; but, as to diseases, let us try to help, or at least to *do no harm.*[5]

NOTES.

1. Hypertension Detection and Follow-up Program Co-operative Group, "The Effect of Treatment on Mortality in Mild Hypertension," ***New England Journal of Medicine*** 307:976, 14 Oct. 1982.
2. Cf., for example, Selye, H., ***The Stress of Life.***
3. Love, S., et al., "Fibrocystic Disease of the Breast—A Nondisease?" ***New England Journal of Medicine*** 307:1010, 14 Oct. 1982.
4. Cf. Cousins, N.. "The Mysterious Placebo," in ***The Anatomy of an illness as Perceived by the Patient,*** chapter 2.
5. Hippocrates, ***Epidemics,*** Part I, Section 2, Chapter. xi.

*Two Childbirth Remedies**

While many remedies are useful in the treatment of painful uterine contractions, only two have been shown to produce contractions at regular intervals simulating labor. Both were introduced into homeopathy from Native American medicine, and both are still used primarily for complaints of or in relation to the female reproductive cycles of pregnancy, childbirth, and menstruation. Because their symptom pictures closely resemble two major subtypes of dysfunctional labor, they are also useful standards against which other possible remedies can be measured, and can reasonably be tried when other more specific indications are lacking.

Caulophyllum.

Tincture of the root, *Caulophyllum thalictroides,* N. O. *Berberidaceæ,* blue cohosh, squaw root.

1. Uterine dysfunction.

The muscle fibers of the mammalian uterus have the unique ability to relax isometrically at their contracted length, such that each contraction further reduces the volume of the organ. In labor, rhythmic contractions of this type, centered in the fundus or upper segment, accomplish the splendid athletic feats of effacing the lower segment, dilating the cervix, and pushing the baby into, through, and out of the vagina. After labor, similar contractions expel the placenta and any remaining clots and placental fragments, compress the decidual vessels, and thus minimize further blood loss.

The symptomatology of *Caulophyllum* is dominated by abnormal uterine contractions of a familiar and easily recognizable type. While often extremely painful and distressing to the patient, they are centered primarily in the *lower* segment, and tend to be sharp and spasmodic in character, brief in duration, and very unstable, often flitting about or extending into the bladder, groins, and thighs. Above all, they fail to

* "Two Childbirth Remedies," ***Homeopathic Medicines for Pregnancy and Childbirth,*** North Atlantic, Berkeley, 1992.

dilate the cervix, which remains thick and spasmodically closed, and in emptying the uterus, which reverts after each contraction to its former length, like any other muscle.

Such contractions are commonly seen in prolonged or difficult labors that get "stuck" in the dilatation phase, when the vaginal exam reveals so little objective progress that the attendant is apt to feel embarrassed at having to break the news, and may indeed have been misled by the intense pain and accompanying exhaustion and insufficiently attentive to the flabby tone of the upper segment to suspect that the labor was not progressing satisfactorily.

Case 1. After a splendidly healthy first pregnancy, a woman of 24 settled into a slow, desultory labor that never progressed beyond the latent phase. Within minutes after a dose of *Caulophyllum* 200, she went into good, active labor and gave birth speedily, without further impediment.

2. Muscular weakness, trembling, and nervous excitement.

Almost invariably, the contractions of *Caulophyllum* are associated with a sense of marked weakness or muscular exhaustion, sometimes to the point that the patient can hardly move or speak. At the same time, there is usually evidence of trembling, shivering, or some other form of jittery, nervous excitement, such as retching or vomiting. In both respects, its closest analogue is *Gelsemium,* which often succeeds where *Caulophyllum* seems indicated but does not help.

Case 2. A woman of 32 completed her first pregnancy and labor without any trouble until the placenta separated, and an hour went by without the slightest contraction or urge to expel it. After 6 drops of *Caulophyllum* tincture, she began to have painful contractions, her right arm shook, and she fell back into a dreamlike state, but still no placenta. Asking everyone else to leave the room, I spoke to her softly in a soothing voice, until the contractions subsided and the placenta slid out, soft and glistening. Thus ended my experiments with *Caulophyllum* tincture.

3. Neuralgic and arthritic pains.

Caulophyllum has also relieved neuralgic pains in various parts of the body, especially the bladder, vagina, and intestines. Much like the uterine pains, these are short, sharp, spasmodic, and tend to fly about rapidly from place to place. The remedy also has a rheumatic tendency, with pain, swelling, and stiffness in muscles, and particularly in the fingers, toes, and smaller joints.

4. Miscellaneous symptoms.

All symptoms of the remedy tend to appear more frequently and with greater intensity during pregnancy, labor, and menstruation. It can also produce or relieve weakness of the pelvic muscles, and excessive laxness of the suspensory ligaments of the uterus to the point of actual prolapse. At times there may be a profuse, irritating vaginal discharge, especially in the last trimester, as the labor draws near.

> **Case 3.** A woman of 22 had no trouble with her first pregnancy until the 39th week, when she complained of urinary frequency and Braxton-Hicks contractions that awakened her at night and left her with a feeling of residual soreness low in the pelvis. These symptoms were also accompanied by an itchy discharge with irritation of the vulva, and tenderness and swelling of the fingers that made her rings uncomfortable. After a few doses of *Caulophyllum* 30 she swiftly overcame these difficulties, giving birth a week later with no problems of any kind.

Caulophyllum patients are apt to be thirsty, chilly, and sensitive to the cold, with a marked intolerance of coffee. While often delicate and nervous, with rapid changes of mood, they rarely exhibit emotional symptoms as vivid or distinctive as those of *Pulsatilla* or *Ignatia,* for example. The flavor is more what would be expected in someone exhausted and overwrought from a supreme effort upon which she has staked a great deal, and for which she finds herself insufficiently prepared.

5. Therapeutics.

Caulophyllum should always be considered and will often be useful in typical or early cases of uterine dysfunction in which the predominant flavor is one of muscular weakness or exhaustion and nervous excitement, with no more specific indications to suggest other remedies. Most often encountered during labor, including premature or false labor, this pattern may also appear immediately after labor, around expulsion of the placenta, or in the immediate post-partum period, in the form of after-pains and/or bleeding from the hypotonic uterus, as well as during and after miscarriage or abortion, and in difficult menstruation and dysmenorrhea, from the teen years through menopause.

Finally, the remedy corresponds to a whole range of chronic cases in which nervous excitability and general weakness of the female reproductive system loom as major predisposing factors in chronic infertility, repeated miscarriages, and a tendency to premature or dysfunctional labors, or to postpartum complications secondary to uterine atony, especially retained placenta, postpartum bleeding, and subinvolution.

For women with a history of this kind, *Caulophyllum* 6 or 12 given daily for the last 2 to 4 weeks of pregnancy will often facilitate a speedier and more efficient labor. With the same indications, a similar regimen may also be used to prevent miscarriage or premature labor if these conditions have occurred repeatedly in the past, or are imminent or threatening.

Because of its well-documented effectiveness in such situations, some homeopaths have advocated giving *Caulophyllum* routinely in the last month, especially for first pregnancies, when lack of experience with the labor process and the normal excitement of giving birth for the first time could be regarded as additional risk factors. Some reputable studies have shown that such a regimen does indeed shorten the average length of labor and reduce both the intensity of pain and the risk of significant complications.

Personally, I tend to shy away from using remedies routinely without definite indications over long periods of time. More like a proving than a treatment, this strategy can predictably elicit the same symptoms that the remedy is known to relieve. One patient who took *Caulophyllum* 6 daily for the last month gave birth unattended in the hospital corridor and bled heavily enough that the midwife who prescribed it was called on the carpet for possible disciplinary action. Such reactions are rare, to be sure, and even the one just cited could have been avoided or minimized if the staff had been forewarned and attentive to the danger. Yet the fact that women are entitled to participate in such experiments if they wish simply underscores the decisive importance of the unique birth mythology that each pregnant woman must create for herself.

If the typical symptom-picture is present, *Caulophyllum* will also be effective in the treatment of established uterine dysfunction during or after labor, miscarriage, or menstruation. In such cases, the fundus feels relatively flabby even during the contraction, and the usual signs of generalized muscular weakness, exhaustion that seems disproportionate to the effort expended, and trembling with nervous excitement will ordinarily be present; *Caulophyllum* 12 or 30 may then be given up to every 15 to 30 minutes until there is definite improvement. It tends to work best in the early stages; in more advanced cases, other more distinctive symptoms will often point to another remedy, such as *Gelsemium.*

Given the same general features, it has proved useful in the treatment of neuralgias, arthritis, and rheumatism of the fingers and toes, particularly toward the end of pregnancy, or after labor, miscarriage, or abortion. It has also been helpful in selected cases of vulvovaginitis with a profuse, irritating discharge, especially in late pregnancy, and in young girls before the age of puberty.

It is difficult to present vivid individual cases of this remedy, which tends to be most useful in the lower dilutions, such as the 12th, either preventively or in typical or early cases before reaching their full development. Because it has few distinctive mental or emotional features, and even its well-known physical symptoms are rather nondescript and pretty much what would be expected under the circumstances, its action is apt to be unsung and predictable rather than spectacular or memorable. But I would not want to be without it.

Cimicifuga.

Tincture of the root, *Cimicifuga racemosa* or *Actæa racemosa,* N. O. *Ranunculaceæ,* black cohosh, black snake root.

1. Uterine Dysfunction.

Like *Caulophyllum, Cimicifuga* produces abnormal uterine contractions closely resembling those of dysfunctional labor, and all of its other symptoms are likewise intensified during and after pregnancy, labor, and menstruation. The contractions themselves are similarly brief, sharp, and spasmodic, and just as painful as those of *Caulophyllum,* often darting about from side to side or down the hips and thighs, and also tend to be felt predominantly in the lower uterine segment and the cervix, which remains closed and fails to dilate.

The remedy also resembles *Caulophyllum* in featuring neuralgias, rheumatic and arthritic pains, trembling, nervous and emotional agitation, and an overall sense of instability and mutability, of symptoms traveling from place to place, or changing from one to another or back and forth.

2. Dejection, Fear, and Mental Fragmentation.

Yet from its minutest details to their overall flavor and style, the symptom-picture of *Cimicifuga* is fundamentally different and, when fully developed, not easily mistaken for that of any other remedy. This "essence" is perhaps most readily approached through the mental and emotional state, which has two important and interrelated features. By far the more obvious and easier to recognize is a feeling of moroseness, gloom, or dejection, readily apparent on the behavioral level as a persistent negativism, defeatism, or pessimism that sees the worst side of everything, often with a fixed presentiment of failure or misfortune about the pregnancy, the labor, or the parenting to follow. "I can't do it," or "I can't go through with it," would be an accurate verbal rendering, doubtless easily overlooked in the throes of a difficult labor, when such sentiments are rarely absent.

> Case 4. A young woman in her second pregnancy appeared to be sailing through her labor without any problems, except for her often-repeated conviction that she wouldn't be able to finish it. In this fashion she achieved full dilatation and brought the baby's head halfway down the vagina before her labor did in fact come to a complete stop, her prophecy seemingly fulfilled. With a single dose of *Cimicifuga* 30, the birth followed in a few minutes, as if nothing had happened.

Sometimes the dejection seems almost tangible or palpable to the patient: she may say something like "I feel as if I were enveloped by a black cloud," and convey by her gestures or body language that an actual physical presence is meant. Indeed, this kind of somatization or extension of mental states into physical symptoms is a striking feature of the remedy in all its guises. The "black-cloud" sensation in particular has been verified repeatedly in headache, depression, and many other circumstances.

But underlying these depressive phenomena may lurk bizarre, disabling fears that something terrible is going to happen, that she will die or be poisoned by the remedy you are about to give her, or that she will go insane and never be the same again. Sometimes these fears may only be hinted at by speech, gestures, actions, or physical symptoms that are incoherent or freaky enough to alarm the people around her. At bottom the *Cimicifuga* state includes the threat or actuality of a mental breakdown in which the nexus or common thread of experience dissolves away or is fragmented into a jumble of disconnected thoughts and feelings, a truly pitiable state justly to be feared by doctor and patient alike.

Case 5. A woman of 29 became pregnant again soon after a miscarriage. After two episodes of second-trimester bleeding she grew to term in stable condition, but at 42 weeks she was still not in labor. Faced with the prospect of a hospital birth, she could no longer keep secret the memory of her D & C, its pain already intense enough to give rise to the fixed idea that the actual labor would push her over the edge once and for all. When she appeared at my office a few days later, she was already 6 cm. dilated, but wild-eyed and indeed out of control, just as she had feared, with her speech fragmentary and her gestures disconnected and woeful. Although remaining clinically psychotic throughout the labor, she made excellent progress on a few doses of *Cimicifuga* 200, gave birth normally, and made a full recovery afterwards.

In my experience, alarming and sometimes prophetic fears of insanity, arising out of an unbearably painful or terrifying memory of pregnancy, labor, abortion, or menstruation in the past, are a genuine and important keynote of this remedy, repeatedly verified in practice, and often helpful in explaining other symptoms as well. On the other hand, fear of losing one's mind cuts so deep as to be well guarded by most patients, even from themselves, and will seldom be volunteered or elicited readily.

Case 6. A 37-year-old woman was 15 weeks pregnant when she came in for treatment of spotting and anxiety. Ever since her first pregnancy miscarried at six weeks, she had been haunted by the memory that her mother was four months pregnant with her when her older sister died in a car accident, for which she was always made to feel somehow responsible. No matter how often she heard the baby's heartbeat, every ordinary headache or drop of blood was enough to revive her fears of a tragic retribution.

After one dose of *Cimicifuga* 200 the bleeding stopped, and she felt much calmer, although still convinced that "it will all be taken away in the end!" After *Cimicifuga* 10M at 24 weeks, she felt the baby kick for the first time and pronounced her womb "officially safe for motherhood." At 37 weeks she repeated the 200, and at 42 weeks the 10M, finally going into labor and giving birth at home without a hitch.

3. Fragmentation and Alternation of Physical and Mental Symptoms.

A similarly fragmented quality generally characterizes the physical symptoms as well. Equally intense in both remedies, the pains of *Caulophyllum* are more finely-textured and tend to follow or change into one another more easily, rather like *Pulsatilla,* while those of *Cimicifuga* are coarser, involving larger "chunks" of experience that tend to replace one another more abruptly in a jumbled or random fashion. Thus a labor pain might begin well enough, with good focus and intensity, only to vanish before reaching its peak or pass off into a disabling obturator neuralgia or sciatica, or alternate with negative or psychotic behavior. Like *Ignatia, Lilium tigrinum,* and *Platina, Cimicifuga* is one of the main remedies for physical symptoms that alternate back and forth with one another or with mental and emotional states.

4. Nervous Excitation and Choreiform Movements.

In analogous fashion, the nervous system is every bit as hyperexcitable as with *Caulophyllum,* and as prone to trembling, convulsions, and the like; but the involuntary movements of *Cimicifuga* are coarser and jerkier, typically involving the basal ganglia and extrapyramidal system, as in chorea, athetosis, grimacing, and the like. On the physical no less than the mental level, the fragmentation and alternation of large chunks of experience abruptly and at random makes the *Cimicifuga* picture not merely changeable or unstable, but positively freaky to the patient herself and to everyone else around her. Whatever the symptom, the underlying impression is one of disintegration, of experience coming "unglued" in Humpty-Dumpty fashion, which in turn clouds the prospect of full restitution in the future.

5. Pain: Headache, Neuralgia, Rheumatism, Arthritis.

Diverse, intense, and often disabling, the headaches of *Cimicifuga* are often centered in the back of the head, extending down the neck, or in the vertex, "as if the top of the head would fly off." The neuralgias can be equally severe, often darting or lancinating, and described like "needles pricking" or "electric shocks here and there." These too may occur anywhere and change abruptly from one place to another without warning or continuity. Other patients are bothered by numbness or rheumatic-type sensations of bruised soreness, whether diffuse or localized in particular bones, muscles, and joints; many of these symptoms are intensified by movement but also shift to the side or part lain on, making it very difficult for the patient to remain comfortable for any length of time.

6. Miscellaneous Symptoms.

In general, *Cimicifuga* patients tend to be chilly, and many of their symptoms are intensified in cold, damp weather, except for the headaches, which may be better in the cold; and typical nervous phenomena, like nausea, insomnia, palpitations, numbness, and the like, are also commonly present. As with *Caulophyllum,* the uterine complaints may be accompanied by bearing-down sensations, with or without actual prolapse, and in some cases by excessive bleeding as well.

7. Differential Diagnosis.

With its unique combination of uterine dysfunction and physical and mental fragmentation, the fully-developed picture of *Cimicifuga* will rarely be confused with that of any other remedy. Although its uterine and nervous symptoms are broadly similar to those of *Caulophyllum,* their freaky and disjointed arrangement and tendency to alternate with or change abruptly into other symptoms will generally set them apart. While *Bryonia* is equally arthritic, *Pulsatilla* at least as volatile, *Natrum mur.* comparably morose, and *Aconite* even more fearful, the "essence" or flavor of *Cimicifuga* is unmistakable and equally distinct from all of these.

Perhaps its closest analogue is *Ignatia,* which is similarly motivated by dejection and fear, and features a comparable inventory of headaches, neuralgias, and elusive female symptoms that never quite add up or stay put. But whereas *Ignatia* ailments arise from grief and therefore often seem contradictory or impossible, those of *Cimicifuga* are like frightful premonitions of insanity and convey the impression of fragmenting and dissociation. Both stylistically and in its minutest details, there is no other remedy quite like it; yet *Cimicifuga* is relatively unknown, seldom thought of, and in less advanced cases easily missed.

8. Therapeutics.

Cimicifuga should always be considered for uterine dysfunction with nervous agitation, neuralgic or rheumatic pains, and the characteristic sense of physical and mental fragmentation underlying them. Such a pattern can be seen during prolonged or difficult labor, including premature or false labor; after labor, with typical postpartum complications (bleeding, retained placenta, after-pains, subinvolution, etc.); and similarly during or after miscarriage or abortion, menstruation, or menopause.

Case 6. After giving birth to her second child at home, a woman of 28 developed severe, nauseating after-pains which subsided promptly after a few doses of *Cimicifuga* 30. At 6 months of age the child developed fulminating acute leukemia and died after weeks of admittedly hopeless chemotherapy that nobody could bear to withhold from her. In her grief the mother told me that she had always felt undeserving of the pregnancy and often had premonitions that the child would be taken away. Soon she conceived for a third time and had another successful home birth, but almost immediately she developed a nasty, disabling arthritis in her right wrist that persisted for weeks, had few definite keynotes or modalities to prescribe on, and didn't respond to any of the remedies I tried. Although neither of us could find the words to talk about it, my own prayers led me to acknowledge the fear for the new baby that we both shared, on the basis of which I gave her *Cimicifuga* 200 as a last resort, solely on the strength of that inference, and after a few doses her wrist cleared up quickly and easily, as from a minor injury over which too much had been made.

The remedy may also be used preventively where similar complaints have appeared in the past or appear imminent or threatening. In premature labor or threatened miscarriage, for example, *Cimicifuga* 12 or 30 may be given up to 4 times daily and for days or even weeks at a time.

Case 7. At 22 weeks in her first pregnancy, an environmentally-sensitive woman of 37 went into premature labor and continued to suffer from frequent and painful contractions in spite of enforced bed rest and IV terbutaline drips in the hospital. Apart from occasional doses of *Pulsatilla, Caulophyllum, and Gelsemium,* I gave her mostly *Cimicifuga* 30 once a day for many weeks, nothing elegant or fancy; but she was tickled pink to give birth to a healthy boy at 37 weeks, and so was I.

Cimicifuga is also unrivalled in the prevention and treatment of premature labor in women who have borne malformed or defective children in the past. Under these circumstances, *Cimicifuga* 30 or 200 may be repeated weekly as needed at the beginning of the pregnancy and also throughout the period of greatest risk. In acute situations, such as actual miscarriage, difficult labor, or postpartum bleeding, *Cimicifuga* 12 or 30 may be given as needed up to every half- hour, or even oftener, preferably for at least 4 doses before changing it. When indicated, it is also an important remedy for postpartum depression, although by no means the only one, and may be of considerable benefit even in severe cases requiring psychiatric help. An appropriate professional should be consulted immediately.

Finally, *Cimicifuga* may also be given for acute physical complaints such as headaches, neuralgias, and the like, as well as prophylactically after each occurrence; and it must not be overlooked for the treatment of chronic complaints such as headaches, arthritis, neuralgia, depression, infertility, or repeated miscarriage, premature labor, or dysfunctional labor that began with an acute episode but have never resolved.

Case 8. A woman of 38 developed severe pain in her left ankle following the birth of her daughter by C-section five years earlier. Described as sharp and stabbing, "like a pinched nerve," the pain was connected with her learning of the baby's clubfoot, the mere mention of which still evoked strange grimaces and ominous forebodings that she couldn't or wouldn't identify. More symptoms uncannily reminiscent of her mother's stroke appeared when the latter was hospitalized and subsequently committed suicide. Upbeat and optimistic as long as we avoided these unpleasant subjects, she became unnerved and disjointed whenever I returned to them, as if needing an exorcism. After a brief aggravation, her pains quickly yielded to *Cimicifuga* 10M and 30, as did the fears that soon rose up in their place. Recently she called to report that she has been in good health ever since and has rarely needed or taken the remedy for over six years.

*Vaccinations**

The justification for vaccinating healthy children rests on the twin premises of efficacy and safety:

1) that vaccination simulates the true immunity that follows recovery from the corresponding natural disease, and

2) that the procedure is in no way injurious to health.

But recent evidence indicates that both premises are seriously flawed and deserve closer scrutiny.

The proponents of vaccination demonstrate efficacy in two ways. First, they point to dramatic reductions in the incidence of such diseases as poliomyelitis and measles since the introduction of the vaccines. Second, by detecting specific antibodies in the serum of vaccinated children, they can plausibly connect the clinical events to these microscopic vaccine-induced events.

But natural immunity means far more than the presence of specific antibodies in the blood and a lower incidence of the corresponding diseases. Children who recover from the measles will *never* contract it again, no matter how often they are re-exposed. Yet measles continues to break out in highly-vaccinated and serologically "immune" populations, such as college students. Vaccinated children are also more likely to develop atypical cases that can be more serious than the "wild type" and are always more difficult to recognize. Finally, once the original vaccine "wears off," there is good evidence that re-vaccination is ineffective. All of these data suggest that the "immunity" conferred by vaccines may not be genuine.

Second, true or natural immunity also primes the immune system non-specifically, to respond acutely and vigorously to other infections in the future. Recovering from an acute infection like the measles presupposes

* "Vaccinations," ***Encyclopedia of Childbearing: Critical Perspectives,*** Barbara Katz Rothman, ed., Oryx Press, Phoenix, 1993, pp. 414-415.

the collaboration of lymphocytes, macrophages, serum complement, and every other component of the immune mechanism. The illness that we call the measles is in fact the process by which the virus is expelled from the blood. Specific antibodies appear only when this magnificent outpouring is well under way, and persist afterwards as a kind of "memory" for the experience. The technical feat of manufacturing antibodies without the experience of the acute illness to guide them may well prove a reckless thing to have done, since very little is understood about how vaccines really act inside the body, or how, if at all, the body manages to get rid of them.

The prevailing argument as to the safety of the vaccines likewise rests upon the relative infrequency of severe toxic reactions occurring within a few days of their administration. But this narrow standard completely overlooks the obvious possibility of chronic, long-term effects.

There can be little doubt that the ability to mount a vigorous, acute response to infection and to recover from acute illnesses like the measles is the *sine qua non* for the maturation of a healthy immune system. Yet vaccinated children appear to be more vulnerable to *chronic* infections such as otitis media and sinusitis, for example, and to undergo more relapses, require more antibiotics, and show less capacity to recover completely than their unvaccinated counterparts.

These data arouse the suspicion, likewise borne out by clinical experience, that vaccinated children are less able to respond acutely to *any* foreign stimulus, i.e., that vaccines act by promoting chronic instead of acute responses generally. Such a trade-off would be consistent with the fact that vaccine particles are *designed* to survive as parasites inside the cells of the immune system for decades and to commandeer their function. "Latency" phenomena of this type are well-known in microbiology, and have already been linked to auto-immune phenomena and other chronic diseases, including cancer. To resolve these issues will require studies of a radically new type, comparing the overall health status and other particular variables of vaccinated and unvaccinated children for a whole generation.

For the present, given these major uncertainties, it seems medically, ethically, and politically prudent to make the childhood vaccinations optional, and freely available to those who want them, as many European countries have already done. The rationale for compulsory vaccination is simply that the diseases in question pose a clear and urgent threat to the public, and that their health and welfare would be better served in this way than in any other. But is difficult to see how these conditions could apply in the U. S., since most of the diseases we routinely vaccinate against are not usually life-threatening. Furthermore, even if the vaccines did confer true immunity, then the unvaccinated kids would be a threat to nobody but themselves.

On the other hand, the equation is different enough for each disease to warrant looking at the individual vaccines one by one. Seemingly the least popular and the least necessary are the vaccines against diphtheria, a disease now rare in the U. S., and measles, mumps, and rubella, which have long been viewed as routine diseases of childhood. Yet measles is in fact making a serious comeback in the school-age population, which is already well over 90% vaccinated; and the current hype for compulsory re-vaccination seems predestined for failure.

At the other end of the spectrum, tetanus and poliomyelitis are still widely feared, even though the actual risk of contracting them remains very small. Yet these vaccines continue to be requested by most parents, and are generally accepted by the public as relatively harmless.

The pertussis or whooping cough vaccine has become the logical battleground and rallying-point for the most zealous vaccine proponents and opponents alike, because, on the one hand, the disease is still common and troublesome, and on the other hand, the vaccine has been linked with so many serious complications that pediatricians are increasingly questioning its use.

At present, nearly half the states allow parents strongly opposed to vaccinations to waive the requirement for their children. The others exempt only those belonging to a few religious denominations, like Jehovah's Witnesses and Christian Scientists. No state as yet permits parents to choose some vaccines and not others, i.e., to make informed medical decisions for their children. The growing anti-vaccination movement has lately begun asserting that right, while the medical establishment continues to reserve for themselves the prerogatives of technical expertise and the authority to make such decisions for the public good.

*Illness as Metaphor (with Apologies to Susan Sontag)**

The idea for this talk came to me while reading Susan Sontag's essay of the same title, which begins as follows:

> Illness is the night-side of life, a more onerous citizenship. Everyone who is born holds dual citizenship, in the kingdom of the well and the kingdom of the sick. Although we all prefer to use only the good passport, sooner or later each of us is obliged, at least for a spell, to identify ourselves as citizens of that other place.
>
> My subject is not physical illness itself, but the use of illness as a figure or metaphor. My point is that illness is *not* a metaphor, and that the most truthful way of regarding illness, and the healthiest way of being ill, is the one most purified of and most resistant to metaphoric thinking.[1]

Touched by Ms. Sontag's heroic and so far successful battle with breast cancer, yet also challenged by her words, and hopelessly addicted to metaphorical language in my own work as a homeopath, I turned for guidance to the *Oxford English Dictionary,* my final authority in such matters, where I read the following:

metaphor, n.,

> 1) A figure of speech in which a name or descriptive word or phrase is transferred to an object or action different from but analogous to that to which it is literally applicable.
>
> 2) A thing considered as representative of some other, usually abstract thing; a symbol.[2]

---

* "Illness as Metaphor (with Apologies to Susan Sontag)," ***Journal of the American Institute of Homeopathy*** 94:176, Autumn 2001.

In her short essay, Sontag focuses on the metaphorical coloration of cancer and tuberculosis in modern Western culture, exposing seductive myths and dangerous prejudices that writers, artists, and other cultural figures have imputed to them, including such staples of pop psychology as that we create our own cancer in ourselves through predisposing emotional weaknesses. To this extent, it is difficult not to agree with her that illness is best understood and healed as an experience both concrete and literal, like pain, suffering, and disability, equally purified of the temptation to romanticize and glorify them, like tuberculosis in the Nineteenth Century, or to uglify and demonize them, like cancer in the Twentieth.

On the other hand, one of homeopathy's greatest contributions to medicine may well be its lesson that illness is indeed profoundly metaphorical in a different sense, one that can help our patients understand their own experience more fully and discover a more effective healing path for themselves. With its roots in patients' ordinary speech, and using their own figurative language and imagery wherever possible, the homeopathic interview extends far beyond the diagnostic category to discern the unique flavor of illness in its total symptom-picture, to which quasi-metaphorical analogies often furnish the most accurate description and the closest approximation available.

In what follows I will present a variety of cases to illustrate how metaphorical thinking, or thinking by analogy, as we are more apt to call it, goes straight to the heart of the homeopathic endeavor, as indeed, I would argue, to what all doctoring is really about in a great many instances at least.

Subjective Sensations.

I begin with a case where the main theme of both the illness and the curative remedy was provided by the patient's subjective sensations, particularly the vividness and consistency with which she described the pains in various parts of her body.

> Referred by her employer, a former patient, a woman of 38 came in for treatment of stomach ulcers and chest pain. Her illness began three years earlier, after receiving threatening phone calls from a woman who turned out to be her husband's mistress and the mother of his child, as a result of which she eventually divorced him, and miscarried in the process.

Despite cheering herself up by landing good jobs and even buying a house, she was laid off from each position, and in time became clinically depressed and unable to function. Although she improved a little on Prozac, she gained so much weight that she had to stop taking it, whereupon her depression came back full force, and she started taking St. John's Wort and developed an ulcer at about the same time.

Already prone to "nervous stomach" in times of stress, she was usually able to ignore these symptoms; but this time around her epigastric pains were so severe that she felt "as if I'd been kicked in the stomach," and it made no difference whether she ate or tried not to eat, especially in the morning, when they doubled her over and made her nauseous. While these pains had lessened somewhat on Zantac and Prevacid, she still could not eat raw fruit or salads without serious penalty.

In recent weeks she had also developed intense pains in her chest that felt "as if I were held in a vise," and were accompanied by violent palpitations, hyperventilating, sweaty palms, and other anxiety symptoms. An EKG and ultrasound showed nothing out of the ordinary, but she remembered experiencing similar symptoms when performing on stage, or hurrying frantically to prepare for a trip that she was excited about. Based on this and other information, I gave her *Cactus grandiflorus* 200, which is known for gripping, constricting, vise-like pains in the heart and elsewhere, and six weeks later she reported, more than a little incredulously, "It's working!" Within two days, her ulcer pain was gone, she had cut back on her medications, and was eating raw fruits and vegetables again with impunity. Her heart symptoms and chest pain had also completely disappeared, and did not come back, even when she appeared in a play, "a big test!" Finally, she stopped taking St. John's Wort two weeks before her follow-up, and had felt more energetic and slept better since. "The remedy was great, *a miracle!*" she announced.

I did not repeat it, and she continued to feel well for many months. The chest pain never came back, and she stayed off Prozac and St. John's Wort as well. When her stomach pain and ulcer symptoms returned during a stressful period at work, and Zantac had no effect, I repeated the remedy, and it worked even better the second time. She hasn't needed to come in or take it again for more than two years.

In this case, the patient's own imagery, like the metaphors we all have recourse to in describing our experience of pain, provided the key to understanding her illness bio-energetically, as was confirmed by the prompt and long-lasting relief of her condition by the remedy that was chosen on the basis of that correspondence.

The next case was likewise solved by paying attention to the patient's own imagery, which he first used to describe a particular sensation, but later applied to important life situations as well, such that it became in effect a metaphor for his condition as a whole.

> Coming in reluctantly at his wife's insistence, a 57-year-old engineer was bothered especially by muscle cramps in his feet and legs after heavy physical work, and was aware of general tension or tightness in all of his muscles that made him feel "locked up" a lot of the time, especially in cold weather, but even from a draft or a fan. If he neglected to keep his throat warm, for example, and well protected from catching cold, his muscles would tighten up even more, while his feet remained icy cold even in summer. For years, he had also been troubled by sciatica in his left hip and leg that pulled, tugged, and tightened up at bedtime, making exercise uncomfortable, and in relation to which X-rays had shown degenerative changes in the joint.
>
> A mechanical engineer by training, he had been testing various materials for an electronics firm, including toxic chemicals, and felt driven to finish any project that he started, no matter how late he had to work to do so. Born and raised in Nazi Germany, he came to America at the age of eleven, after his father died in the War, his mother was left traumatized, and the politics of his homeland were "all locked up" in the tense atmosphere of the Cold War. Taking pride in his "squeaky-clean" personal habits and almost fanatical devotion to keeping his house and yard in tiptop shape, he seldom allowed himself the luxury of relaxing and enjoying life.
>
> Most of all, he felt stymied by the defiant backtalk and rebellious acting-out of his teen-age daughter, whom he could not influence or even bring himself to talk to most of the time, yet another "locked-up situation," the oft-repeated phrase thus becoming a central metaphor linking up his physical problems to the character of his life as a whole. Six weeks after a single dose of *Causticum* 1M, he was better. Though he couldn't say why, and even wondered if the tiny dose might have been a placebo, his feet felt warm almost immediately after taking it, and still did, while the "bounce" had returned to his leg muscles, and he felt much less sensitive to cold in general, albeit not quite as good in recent days.
>
> After a few weekly doses of *Causticum* 30, he again felt much more relaxed and limber, as well as warmer and more tolerant of the cold. Even his sleep became calmer and less restless, although he'd never thought to mention it as a problem

before. That was a year and a half ago, and his wife recently told me he hasn't needed or taken the remedy again.

Animal Totems, Archetypes, and Relationships with Humans.

In the next case, again involving subjective sensations as reported by the patient, the important clue was the obvious resemblance between the stinging character of her pains and the experience of being stung by bees, further corroborated by the renal involvement for which the remedy *Apis,* made from the honeybee, is well-known.

After a six-year battle with chronic fatigue syndrome, a 41-year-old woman had had very little relief from either conventional or alternative treatments. Ever since an acute illness consisting of fever, back pain, and extreme weakness that sounded like a kidney infection from which she'd never fully recovered, she had had recurrent bouts of fever with exacerbation of her chronic symptoms, chiefly prostration, weakness, and a sharp, stinging pain in the area of her right kidney that "wrapped around" to the front and forced her to sit down. In the past year, numerous red cells were found in several urine samples, and IVP's showed deformities of the left kidney, for which she had taken antibiotics for weeks, until severe numbness and tingling in her face and legs forced her to stop them.

Meanwhile she had also developed nasty, stinging pains in various other sites, including the right leg, which swelled up and hurt for nearly a month after a dog bite; her right ovary, which felt hot and swollen, "like a fireball;" and elsewhere on the right side. While slowly improving over the years, fatigue still laid her low whenever the fevers returned, typically when overheated or before the menstrual period. At such times she also became awkward and clumsy, dropping things and forgetting well-known phone numbers.

Beginning with *Apis* 30, once a week, after two menstrual cycles she felt much more energetic, with milder symptoms in general and low fever confined to the day before the flow. To test the waters, she had even begun working full-time on assignment from a temp agency. In spite of the increased stress, she had not been sick or had kidney or urinary symptoms to speak of. No remedy was given, and 3 months later she reported several "really good" periods followed by relapse, "like a car that really gets going and then stalls out," for each of which she had repeated the remedy with splendid effect. Although one dose of *Apis* 200 worked beautifully for a month, it was followed by fatigue more profound than any since the early days of the treatment, and she had needed the 30 five times in two months, whenever she tried stretching the limits of what she could do.

Within a few days after a dose of *Apis* 1M, she developed fever and lesions of oral and genital herpes, old complaints from long ago, but these quickly subsided, and she felt very well for quite a while after that, better than in years, until her kidney hurt again following major dental work. Again I gave *Apis* 30, and after seven months she felt almost fully recovered, needing the remedy only twice more for herpes and stinging pains after dental work.

Eventually repeating the 1M, she relapsed well over a year later with a slight fever and similar symptoms, for which I gave her a third dose. Despite continuing to spill a few red cells in the urine occasionally, she was assured on a repeat IVP that her kidneys were completely normal. Since finding and keeping a good full-time job in her field, she has not needed to come back or take remedies in the past three years.

In this case, the experience of being stung by the honeybee was the central metaphor that not only best described the illness, but also provided a curative treatment for it, as though the insect were a kind of totem for this patient in her peculiar situation. The next case had to do with another stinging insect, the hornet, which I thought of only after the more familiar *Apis* had failed.

With virtually her entire face disfigured by clusters of itchy, bright-red pustules, a 41-year-old wife and mother was desperate for relief. In the midst of her third such attack in as many years, what began with a few small lesions had rapidly grown and spread into ever larger and more confluent patches that left little normal skin visible. Worst of all, she was tormented day and night by nasty stiletto-like pains that were hot, itchy, and stinging, rather like bee bites, as well as worse from heat and better from ice, and often made her irritable and angry at everyone and everything, especially her husband and children, and unable to concentrate on anything else.

Repeatedly afflicted with impetigo throughout her childhood, at thirteen she came down with severe chicken pox, again followed by persistent *Staphylococcus* infections. In college she developed eczematous lesions that also tended to suppurate, obliging her to resort to antibiotics several times. But her skin didn't flare up really badly until after the death of her father, a talented and attractive man who had been convicted of fraud, done time in jail for arson, and finally left at her mother's insistence when my patient was in her 20's. Since then, these recent and even more flagrant outbreaks of crops of pustules involving large areas of her face had begun when she was pregnant with her second son, who was 3 at the time I first saw her.

Although happily married to a "wonderful" husband whom she adored and often fantasized about in sexually explicit dreams, she disliked and generally refused having intercourse with him. This curious state of affairs she dated back to the age of 24, when she aborted his child and vowed to abstain from further sex outside of a fully-committed relationship; but her aversion and her vow had both continued in force even after they were married and indeed ever since, like an old grudge that for some profound and inscrutable reason she could neither forgive nor set aside.

The remedy I chose was *Apis 200,* which worked quite well for a time, and even helped restore her sexual desire briefly, a respite for which both she and her husband were most grateful. But she could tell that the remedy wore off after dental work a few months later; and with her sister and brother-in-law moving in for the final weeks of a high-risk pregnancy, she was too preoccupied with caring for them and helping them sort out their relationship to travel so far to see me. Indeed she didn't even tell me all of this until coming back over a year later. When her sister finally gave birth and moved out, her skin flared up worse than ever, and taking *Apis* 30X on her own was only minimally helpful.

After *Tarentula cubensis* 200 was no better, I went back to *Apis* 200, which helped once again, but not nearly as much as before; and meanwhile she had developed a huge, painful boil behind her right ear, her eczema drove her to scratch and tear at her legs for brief periods every day, and large crops of new pustules had appeared that stung as intensely as the time she was attacked by a swarm of yellow-jackets in her teens. This new bit of history led me to study *Vespa crabro,* the hornet, and I gave her the 200, 3 doses in 24 hours, followed by one dose weekly for up to two more weeks as needed, with well-nigh miraculous results.

Within 24 hours her entire face was flaming red and hugely swollen, "as if I'd been stung by ten bees," followed by rapid disappearance of the pain, redness, swelling, and other signs of infection. At her next visit, six weeks later, she reported that her skin looked clearer than it had in a very long time, and that her sexual appetite had been whetted as well. Although her treatment is still too fresh to predict the long-term outcome with certainty, I feel confident that she will continue to improve on this remedy for a long time to come.

Occasionally we think of animal remedies when patients embody familiar traits of the common domesticated species that we keep as pets, servants, and friends. In one such case, the girl's overt affinity with dogs tallied perfectly with T. S. Eliot's whimsical definition:

Now dogs pretend they like to fight;
They often bark, more seldom bite;
But yet a dog is, on the whole,
What you would call a simple soul.
The usual Dog about the Town
Is much inclined to play the clown,
And far from showing too much pride,
Is frequently undignified.
He's very easily taken in —
Just chuck him underneath the chin
Or slap his back or shake his paw,
And he will gambol and guffaw.
He's such an easy-going lout,
He'll answer any hail or shout.[3]

Brought in by her grandmother for chronic bronchitis that often lasted all winter, a chubby, red-faced girl of five seemed quite pleasant at first, but sniffled and sulked whenever she felt left out of the history-taking. Raised by her grandmother, both parents had been drug addicts and were murdered when she was a small baby.

Described as "a happy child who got along with everyone," she constantly blew her nose, hawking up thick, green mucus from her throat, and still wet the bed at night. When she smiled, I noticed that most of her upper teeth were rudimentary, brown-stained, and broken off in places. Her eyes turned in, alternating from side to side, and she craved salt, milk, and dairy primarily, and was quite allergic to cats.

One month after a round of *Calcarea sulph.* 200, she was no better, sniffling loudly as she arrived, and wearing a sweatshirt covered with pictures of dogs of every type and description. This time she got dog's milk, *Lac caninum* 1M, and by her third visit she was greatly improved, rarely coughing at all since a bad spell the second night after the remedy, only wetting the bed once every few weeks, and breathing much more easily through her nose. Six months later, we repeated the remedy for the fall season, and that winter was her best so far, with no bronchitis, minimal coughing, and even her residual sinus congestion had subsided to the extent that the grandmother felt no further need of remedies. I haven't seen her for more than three years, but another patient and friend of the family assures me that she is thriving.

In this case, her loud sweatshirt instantly reminded me of her alternating strabismus, because symptoms that alternate sides are characteristic of the remedy made from dog's milk, and that unlikely and serendipitous correspondence clinched the prescription. In another case, details of the patient's character and even her physique uncannily resembled the animal that furnished the curative remedy, an almost spooky coincidence that was practically all I had to go on, since the information then available about the remedy was still fragmentary and incomplete.

> With a history of benign fibroadenomas of the breast and four surgeries to remove them, a 46-year-old artist came in with pain from a fifth one, as well as seeking a way to prevent them in the future. As big as an egg and growing rapidly, it felt heavy and sore, "like a lump of lead," if she moved too fast; but it could no longer be correlated with her menstrual cycle since her hysterectomy some years ago for multiple fibroid tumors of the uterus and ovaries as well.
>
> She had also been bothered with chronic back pain since being thrown from a horse and crushing three lumbar vertebræ in her teens, but her fractures all healed well, and she never stopped riding, having grown up with horses as a child. She still felt mystically attracted to them, and featured them in her paintings as well. After years of smoking pot in her teens and a major lesbian relationship in her twenties, she became a born-again Christian at 25, still believed in angels, and sensed Christ's presence in the world, but favored Buddhist meditation to dispel her fears that she was really a "witch" in view of her propensity for mystical experiences like ESP and soul travel. Nor could she deny the existence of a darker side to her nature, like the intense hatred she still harbored against her ex-husband for never paying her back for her share of the property after he conned her into signing it all over to him.
>
> But perhaps the hardest of all to exorcise was the rage she felt at sexually and physically abusive relationships in her family, which had driven her mother and brother insane, and left her and the other children to be cared for by a series of foster parents when her father moved out. Alone in the woods most of the time as a child, she grew up seeing herself as an Indian brave riding her pony in the wilderness, not a proper little girl winning ribbons in horse shows, as her grandmother intended. Lean and lanky, with a long, graceful neck, two buck teeth jutting out in front, and a strong craving for lumps of pure cane sugar, constitutionally and even in her physique she seemed to embody and conjure up both the image and archetype of the horse as a kind of personal totem.
>
> With nothing else to go on, I chose *Lac equinum* 200, mare's milk, recently proved by Nancy Herrick in California. In six weeks, the cyst had shrunk to the point that neither she nor her gynecologist could feel it. In some respects the interview itself had had a powerful effect, she felt, particularly when she heard herself exaggerating her rage in order to describe it. Since then she had felt

much calmer, substituting fruit for her sugar lumps, and feeling in good health otherwise. I haven't seen her for three years, but she recently phoned to tell me that her cysts and tumors have never come back, and that she has remained in good health and not needed remedies again for any reason.

Quasi-Objective Signs Noted by the Observer.

With the next case I proceed to applications of metaphoric language that are noticed and used mainly by the homeopath, by grouping together a variety of both subjective and other symptoms that require some interpretation. One notable example is the so-called "never well since" phenomenon, in which the present condition is traceable to an acute illness, injury, or traumatic event in the past from which the patient never fully recovered, such that the event becomes a kind of metaphor that defines and gives human shape and meaning to the whole illness, which would otherwise seem a jumble of unrelated complaints.

Disabled with chronic ovarian pain, a woman of 40 traced her problems to a tubal ligation six months earlier, complicated by a pelvic infection requiring IV antibiotics and an extended hospital stay. Ever since that illness, she had been plagued with severe burning pains in her right ovary with each period and repeated attacks of cystitis in between. However restrained and dignified in the telling, she could not conceal her anger and resentment against the doctor who had performed the surgery and seemingly ruined her health. Radiating down her right leg, the pain was relieved somewhat by heat and pressure; but it had recently spread to the left side and was even bothersome at odd times between the periods. After one dose of *Staphysagria* 200, her next period was the worst ever, but the pain lasted only a few hours, and was much more localized. From then on, her periods were only minimally painful, her cystitis cleared up, and she had no further problems.

In this instance, the remedy *Staphysagria,* often indicated for unexplained ailments that originated after a surgical procedure, matched the guiding metaphor of her history almost perfectly. In another case, the contradictory or "impossible" nature of the symptoms, in seeming defiance of well-established anatomical and physiological principles, gave me the metaphorical clue that led to the remedy.

A girl 10 was brought in for a nasty sore throat that had been interfering with her sleep for weeks. Complaining of a lump there in the morning, especially before lunch, she said that the pain was actually better after eating and hurt most when *not* swallowing. This unlikely pattern led me to elicit the further disclosure that her best friend's mother was receiving chemotherapy for breast cancer, of which a close family member had recently died, and that the girl herself had been troubled for a long time with thoughts of illness and death, and woke in a panic if her mother was not there to comfort her. After a round *of Ignatia* 200, she bounced back from this embryonic illness in a few days. When it recurred in a milder form about a year later, she asked for the remedy herself, and this time it acted immediately and did not have to be repeated.

A related case of the same remedy is a typical case of somatization, in which the patient's reluctance about leaving home became not so much a "cause" as a kind of metaphor for the physical ailments that ensued, showing the same kind of contradictoriness as the previous one.

A few weeks before leaving for her junior year, a 20-year-old college student consulted me for frequent colds and acute illnesses that lasted for weeks and kept her from going to class. Very homesick in her freshman year, she had considered transferring but eventually settled in, made friends, and performed well academically.

Taking a more difficult load as a sophomore, she did poorly at first, and felt depressed and inadequate about her career prospects, but with the support of her father and a college counselor, she finished the spring semester in good shape, but promptly fell ill soon thereafter, developing a high fever soon after her best friend took a leave of absence, followed by a flu-like illness that lingered on for weeks and left her feeling weakened and prone to other minor illnesses in its wake. Ironically, she slept very well at school and badly at home, where she rarely got sick at all. Although her periods were fine, she had lost them while traveling in Europe the summer before. In high school she became similarly ill with infectious mono, fever, and both liver and spleen involvement, not long after her father remarried and her new stepmother moved in.

One month, after a dose of *Ignatia* 1M, she wrote to report a typical cold, so I sent her another. Six weeks later she reported, "We may have had success. I haven't had a cold since I last took your medicine." A year and a half later, she wrote again in the midst of another episode to ask for a third dose: "Since taking your medicine, I went from being sick 70 to 80% of the time to not being sick for a year and a half! I hope the medicine you send will help me like that!" It did. I haven't seen her in more than ten years, but her stepmother assures me that both her health and life have continued to blossom in every way.

Finally, in a third case of *Ignatia* with its typical grief in the background, what stood out and provided the metaphor for her illness was simply the feeling-tone of the interview itself, a global energy state characterized by typical acting-out behavior without any particular physical symptoms to back it up, while the patient herself disclaimed any knowledge of why she was there and came solely at the insistence of her mother:

> Insisting on coming in alone yet sitting as far away from me as possible, a sulky, petulant 14-year-old girl had been urged to come by her mother and couldn't say what she wanted help with. "Is this confidential?" she asked, with a glance over her shoulder. Sent to boarding school after her father's death two years earlier, she had no desire to live at home, but was always in trouble while away, showing up late for class, talking back to her teachers, playing hooky with her boyfriend, and even, she whispered conspiratorially, having sex with him in the dorm.
>
> Generally in good health, she had recently been ill with a sore throat that she couldn't shake until going back to her mother's for the holidays. The next summer she felt depressed and had trouble sleeping, having fallen in love with a boy in college who was only "toying" with her while actually sleeping with somebody else. Ever since the age of 4, when her parents divorced, she had had no contact with her father, a neglect which her mother blamed on his alcoholism, so that when he called in later years and left his number for her, she felt reluctant to use it. At his funeral, his second wife told a very different story; but as much as she regretted not giving him another chance, she refused to shed tears over it either: "It's stupid to wish for what could never happen!"
>
> A talented dancer, she had already been accepted to apprentice with a ballet company, but soon left to go away to boarding school and began taking singing lessons instead. After a period of anorexia in middle school, she became vegetarian, ate erratically, and often felt nauseated at the thought of food, but was also capable of "force-feeding" herself at times. Fond of alcohol and getting drunk, she quit smoking after breaking up with her first lover, hated prescription drugs, even Tylenol, and preferring smoking pot as "more natural." Her periods were similarly inconsistent, but caused her no trouble.
>
> At her first follow-up visit, 6 weeks after a single dose of *Ignatia* 10M, she reported that she hadn't noticed anything, but her mother said she had improved a lot, both academically and in her conduct, a fact that all of her teachers confirmed. Contradicting at every turn, and finally asking her mother to leave, she recounted in lurid and salacious detail how she had announced her sexual relationship at her mother's wedding a few weeks before, which convinced me to give her the remedy again on the spot.

Six months later, she told me excitedly of her acceptance into a top school for the performing arts, while her mother added that she seemed "calmer, more settled, and mature," and that the two of them were getting along better, an assessment that for once she did not disagree with. Over the two and a half years since then, she has continued to flourish, needing no remedies at all for over a year, and eventually moving on to *Natrum mur.* for deeper, more chronic issues that she herself was able to articulate clearly and without prompting.

Keynote Symptom or Global Modality.

Another kind of guiding symptom may be provided by a single keynote symptom, such as a grand modality attributable to the bioenergetic system of the patient as a whole, rather than to a single symptom or part of the body in isolation. Although not necessarily encompassing every last symptom, it can serve as a central organizing principle for the whole case, and thus as a readily comprehensible metaphor or symbolic representation of the whole "totality of symptoms." As we have already seen, the relevance and accuracy of the metaphor are elegantly confirmed by the almost magically curative action of the remedy selected on the basis of it.

Recently diagnosed with rheumatoid arthritis, with a history of the disease in her mother and brother as well, a 39-year-old housewife had had stiff, achy, sore finger joints for a few years, but always managed to ignore or work around them until the last month or so, when they began hurting a lot for days at a time, especially the right index finger, which was also swollen at times; and the hips and toes had recently been acting up as well. Fond of running and jogging, she had also noticed her sacrum aching of late, especially at the end of her run and for some hours afterward. Gay and sprightly in my office, she clearly preferred rocking back and forth in her chair and even dancing around the room to sitting still, an old habit she related to her joint symptoms, which felt "like a rusty gate" as she started to move, but improved once she got going. Though not so clear about the effect of weather and climate, she was consistently frozen and hated the cold weather, especially when damp or windy, and loved the sun and warmth of every kind.

What she dreaded most about her illness was its interference with her freedom of movement, which felt vital to her emotionally as well as physically. Her only fear was about violence, especially involving her children, which often figured in her dreams and had become especially acute recently, when her cousin was found murdered. A lover of dairy, especially cheese, she had never had poison ivy, in spite of repeated exposures to the plant.

After a single dose of *Rhus tox.* 1M, which is made from poison ivy and was chosen on the basis of its classic keynote symptom, the general aggravation of her condition from rest or beginning to move, followed by improvement as the movement continued, she didn't come back for more than three years, insisting that she had been fine and needed no remedies or medical attention the whole time. Some months ago she came back for another flare-up with the same symptoms and in the same joints as before, this time with the beginning of the hot weather, and documented with an elevated sedimentation rate and rheumatoid factor in the blood. I gave her another dose of the remedy, and once again she responded to it magnificently, needing no further treatment.

Metaphor Within Metaphor.

In the following case, I arrived at the remedy as another instance of the rubric "ailments from surgery," itself a prototype of the more generic "ailments from suppressed anger," in that the body of the surgical patient is not only violated by the knife, but also deeply anesthetized and thus rendered unable to express pain or feel anger on the operating table.

Gay and lively, a 48-year-old college professor consulted me for recurrent bladder and kidney infections that spanned her long and arduous reproductive career, dating from a C-section for the birth of her son 17 years earlier. Complaining of severe pain in the incision, she kept politely insisting that her obstetrician pay more attention to it, but no diagnosis was made for more than 2 months, until it grew into a flagrant case of PID requiring emergency hospitalization and IV antibiotics. Although her HMO eventually fired the doctor for negligence, she mainly blamed herself for tolerating the pain too well and hesitating to make a scene.

Pregnant again three years later, she had severe right lower quadrant pain and felt intuitively certain that it was a tubal pregnancy; but once again nobody listened to her until it ruptured and the ovary and tube were removed. After several years of trying, she finally conceived again with IVF, but only after repeated laparoscopies had perforated her bladder and initiated a cycle of recurrent UTI's and kidney infections, one of which provoked an anaphylactic reaction to sulfa drugs that almost killed her. Ever since that time, she had been tormented with frequent burning pains, urging soon after urinating, and the maddening feeling as if her bladder were "solid and swollen like a football" a good deal of the time. Other shooting pains extending upward and to the right were reminiscent of her dreaded IVF cycles, for each of which she had been made to wait with a full bladder for two hours a day over a ten-day period.

Temperamentally, her father's repeated abuse of an older brother had taught her to avoid giving him cause to humiliate her, and even as an adult she had never learned how to get angry in a convincing way. Within a few days of a dose of *Staphysagria* 200, she noticed "quick and dramatic improvement" in the bladder sensations that had always made her feel on the verge of an infection. At her second visit two months later, her bladder felt completely healed, after a touch of constipation that reminded her of a rectal prolapse in the wake of an IVF cycle that led to another surgery and was followed by the worst pain in her life. No further remedies were given, and she has remained well since.

Pathology Itself as Metaphor.

As the preceding examples make clear, homeopaths often use one or more subjective sensations or objective signs quasi-metaphorically to stand for the whole array of signs, symptoms, and pathological abnormalities that constitute the portrait of the illness as a whole. These figures of speech are more or less apt in proportion to their degree of similitude, as measured, first, by their usefulness in elucidating the nature of the illness on a deeper level, and, second, by the effectiveness of the remedy chosen on the basis of such hypotheses.

As I began studying and writing up these cases, it slowly dawned on me that even pathological or diagnostic categories can function quasi-metaphorically in almost the same sense, by substituting pathognomonic signs and symptoms of the "disease" as a kind of shorthand to represent and even purportedly "explain" the array of subjective experiences and objective signs that every illness consists of. As the following case illustrates, even the language of pathology itself sometimes furnishes the best available imagery for understanding the patient's total symptom-picture.

A 19-year-old college student consulted me for treatment of recently diagnosed Crohn's Disease of both the small and large bowel, complicated by the development of a rectal fistula draining into the perineum at roughly the same time. After the fistula was repaired, she was given Asacol for the rest of the school year, and Purinethol in the summer; but while still on vacation she developed a perianal abscess and yet another fistula that opened into the vulva, close to the vaginal opening.

Her bowel troubles had begun in High School three years earlier, when diarrhea and intense pain with every bowel movement led to the discovery of a rectal fissure. In her last year, she neared the breaking point during cross-country ski season, when she became terrified of losing control of her bowels during competition; and despite vigorous efforts by her doctor, the fissure continued to reopen, discharging a mixture of blood, fecal material, and clear, straw-colored fluid, and stubbornly refusing to heal.

After some improvement in her freshman year of college, she developed her first abscess and draining fistula near the anus while home on vacation, with a diffuse, throbbing pain that was even more intense than ever. When her doctors couldn't agree on the diagnosis, she felt troubled, confused, and "invaded" by their repeated examinations of the area, which made her blush in the telling. Her hyperacute sense of shame and self-disgust were heightened by the increasing difficulty of hiding her ailment from her roommates, whose habit of sleeping late threatened to expose her irresistible urge to evacuate in the morning and the huge, explosive stools that resulted from it.

Because there were few distinctive symptoms to prescribe on apart from the nature and persistence of her pathology, I looked up "Rectum, fissure" and "Rectum, fistula," and found *Pæonia* listed prominently in both. In Boericke's *Materia Medica,* I read the following about this little-known remedy, which I had never used before: *"The rectal and anal symptoms are most important. Burning in anus after stool.* Fistula ani *with diarrhea. Fissures of the rectum with ulceration of the anus and perineum. Atrocious pains with and after each stool. Painful ulcer, oozing offensive moisture on perineum."*

Based on this information, which seemed to fit the case admirably, I gave her *Pæonia* 30X, the only attenuation I had at the time, 3-5 pellets three times daily until noticeably better, and as needed after that. Two months later she wrote me the following letter from college:

"The pills that you prescribed are helping my Crohn's disease significantly. Since taking them I've experienced significant decrease in abdominal pains, higher tolerance to gas-producing foods, and a smaller number and more regular consistency of the stools. I attribute these positive changes to the pills, which have not only helped me in these specific ways, but have also improved the whole quality of my life. I feel much healthier than I have in the past. Most important, I do not think about my condition as often and feel freer as a result. Thank you."

That was the last I heard from her until recently, ten months later, when she came back over the summer vacation. At that time she told me that she had stopped the remedy soon after sending the letter and began drinking heavily for the first time and cutting back on her medications, with the predictable result that her symptoms and food intolerances gradually returned, although not as bad as they had been, and another fistula appeared. Repeating the remedy worked even better the second time.

Another case illustrates the usefulness of pathological categories in advanced or terminal disease, where cure is out of reach but considerable palliation is still possible:

With a long history of emphysema, gastritis, and a two-pack-a-day cigarette habit, a much-older-looking man of 56 hobbled in on crutches, daring me to "SAVE MY TOE!" in a jaunty, almost flippant tone, although his prospects were certainly no laughing matter. Ten days earlier, after stubbing his right fourth toe, it had become gangrenous; and by the time I saw it, the tip and under side were swollen and completely black, with severe burning and cutting pains emanating from it whenever he lifted the foot to walk or tried to dangle it over the side of a chair.

The remedy I chose was *Vipera redi* 200, 3 doses in 24 hours, and within a week he was able to walk more easily, and the blackened area was smaller and less painful; but it still hurt a good deal at times, especially in cold air and from going too long without eating. Switching to *Carbo animalis* 200, I saw him again two weeks later, by which time the whole toe appeared normal except for a small black spot on the tip that looked ready to slough off, and it hurt him only when covered with a sock or blanket.

On that indication I gave him *Secale cornutum* 200, and after another three weeks the whole toe and foot were painless and of normal color, although it still stung and turned blue when the leg was dangled. Once more *Vipera* 200 acted beautifully, and the toe was saved; but I told him and his wife that the gangrene indicated a serious underlying vascular pathology that could itself be fatal, and urged him to return for constitutional treatment and remain under close medical supervision.

This he neglected to do, inasmuch as the toe was now healed, and he felt well enough to go back to work part-time. In six months he was back, this time short of breath even at rest, but especially from overeating and hot, humid weather. In spite of considerable help from *Carbo vegetabilis* 200, he had to be hospitalized for congestive heart failure, was placed on digitalis, heparin, bronchodilators, diuretics, oxygen, and prednisone, and soon developed osteomyelitis with deep bone pains in his bad leg, but still insisted over the phone that he was quite well and in no real danger. That persuaded me to give him *Arnica* 200, which worked splendidly for a few weeks every time, but I never saw or spoke to him again. Two years later, his wife called to tell me that he had recently died peacefully in his sleep, and that of all the treatments he had had, "only the remedies really helped!"

As all these cases indicate, what metaphor provides is essentially a mythology or working hypothesis that can help both doctor and patient understand and treat the illness. How powerful and even decisive such myths can be is perhaps best appreciated by cases like the following, where the interview itself had such a profound effect as to cast doubt on whether the remedy played a necessary or important rôle, or indeed any rôle at all:

> A girl of ten was brought in for treatment of enuresis, which began when her parents separated for a year at the age of three, and had continued ever since, but only at home in her own bed, never while visiting relatives or sleeping over at a friend's house. In addition, she was prone to bouts of acute cystitis, with stinging pains in her urethra that often woke her at night and made her scream. After her father returned, she became frightened of him and his booming voice, especially after he didn't believe her story that a neighbor boy had sexually molested her. Ever since then she had been hypersensitive to teasing or criticism from her father or older brother, or whenever her friends told secrets or did anything to exclude her, often to the point that she would leave the scene in tears and vent her anger and humiliation to her mother.
>
> Four weeks after a single dose of *Staphysagria* 10M, her mother wrote that the wetting was even worse than before, and that the girl felt quite discouraged at times and impatient for the remedy to work, but had also "talked a lot about our visit and the way you listened, and seem relieved to have been able to share the sexual stuff with you." That was the last I saw or heard of her for two years, at which point her mother brought her back for a different complaint and told me that the bedwetting had stopped a few weeks after sending the letter and never returned.

These cases, then, are my answer to Sontag. While I admire and endorse her attempt to separate our experience of illness from the highly charged cultural myths that have accrued to it, metaphor also provides doctors and patients with the indispensable healing capacity of imparting personal meaning to illness. She is perfectly right that we use it at our peril, that myths and metaphors are dangerous to the extent that we give them power over us, or in other words, that we may use them well or badly. But beyond that, I can only ask her to enlighten us further: if illness is not metaphor, what *is* it?

NOTES.

1. Sontag, S., ***Illness as Metaphor,*** FSG, New York, 1977, p.3.
2. ***The New Oxford Shorter English Dictionary,*** Clarendon Press, 1993, Vol. 1, p. 1756.
3. Eliot, T. S., "The Ad-dressing of Cats," from *Old Possum's Book of Practical Cats,* in ***Complete Poems and Plays: 1909-1950,*** Harcourt, Brace, New York, 1958, p. 170.

II. Cases.

"Plague and Pregnancy"

"Drug Reactions and Biological Individuality"

"Homeopathic Remedies vs. the Placebo Effect"

"Peculiar and Characteristic Symptoms"

"A Wound Heals -- After 25 Years"

"A Sampling of Animal Cases"

"A 42-Year-Old Man with Bronchiectasis, Among Other Things"

*Plague and Pregnancy**

A 28-year-old woman in her 5th month of pregnancy was examined for chills, fever, and a painful right inguinal swelling. After moving to a house on the edge of Santa Fe, she had dusted her dog with flea powder, as advised by the NM Health Department, but not her cat. Five or six days before being seen, she noted several itchy lesions on her legs which she assumed were flea bites; these subsided in a few days. On the evening before admission, she experienced the sudden onset of high fever, shaking chills, and headache. By the following morning, she complained of severe pain in the right groin, which caused her to limp and seek medical attention. Six previous pregnancies had resulted in four abortions and two live births.

On physical exam the patient appeared acutely toxic, with a temperature of 104°, pulse 120 per min., blood pressure 90/60 mm., and respiration 20 per min. Skin lesions, presumably healing flea bites, were noted on the right calf, with no evidence of purpura, ecchymosis, or petechiæ. A dry, irritating cough on deep inspiration was associated with decreased breath sounds and fremitus over the right base posteriorly. A soft flow murmur was heard over the apex; the liver and spleen could not be felt. The fundus was at the umbilicus; no fetal heart tones were heard, but fetal movement was observed. The right inguinal canal was markedly swollen and red, exquisitely tender to palpation, and contained two tense, marble-sized buboes. The sensorium was clear.

The State Health Department was notified, the patient was hospitalized with a presumptive diagnosis of bubonic plague, and an aspirate of the infected nodes was sent with her serum to the State Lab in Albuquerque with a police escort. The white count was 16,500, with 86% neutrophils, 10% bands, and 4% lynphocytes; the hematocrit was 35%, and the platelets were adequate. The urine contained 1-3 red cells and 35-45 white cells per high-power field, with a trace of albumin and no bacteria. The chest X-ray was normal. The diagnosis of plague was confirmed by the State Lab,

* "Plague and Pregnancy," *Journal of the AMA* 237: 1851, 25 April 1977 (with Jonathan Mann, M.D., New Mexico Health Department).

which demonstrated fluorescent-antibody staining of the aspirated fluid, and *Yersinia pestis* was subsequently cultured from her blood as well. Throat cultures were negative.

She was treated with Streptomycin sulfate 500 mg. IM every 8 hours for five days, and her symptoms improved rapidly; by her fourth hospital day she was afebrile. On the third day, her platelet count dropped to 111,000, with an abnormally high titer of fibrin split products; but there was no bleeding or evidence of renal impairment or placental dysfunction. She was discharged on the sixth hospital day with no further medication, and the buboes regressed slowly over the next several weeks with the aid of *Silica 30,* a homeopathic medicine.

The remainder of the pregnancy was uneventful. On January 30, 1976, she gave birth at home to a healthy six-pound boy after a short labor requiring no medication. There were no complications; the placenta delivered spontaneously and was grossly intact. Both mother and baby continued to do well throughout the postpartum period.

Unless treatment is begun early, plague acquired in pregnancy usually leads to miscarriage, which then in turn exerts a most unfavorable influence on the outcome of the disease.

*Drug Reactions and Biological Individuality**

I want to talk about a type of case that is fairly common in homeopathic practice, in which the curative remedy turns out to be a substance to which the patient has already been exposed, and there is reason to believe that the present illness represents in effect a proving of the remedy in a person abnormally sensitive to it. These cases seem striking to me in several respects:

1) because they exemplify in extreme form the very same sort of individual sensitivity upon which the success of our art depends;

2) because they are useful prototypes for studying and treating a wide range of illnesses attributable to environmental and industrial poisons; and

3) because they provide an optimal model of the homeopathic method in general, since both the cause and the cure of the illness are known to us as completely as they can ever be.

I will begin with three cases from my own practice that illustrate the general situation I have in mind.

Case 1. Previously in good health, a 27-year-old man first consulted me in September of 1975 for an itchy, crusty seborrhea of the scalp of about five years' duration. He failed to respond to *Sulphur* and other seemingly well-indicated remedies, and his scalp condition continued unabated until he consulted me again in December of 1976. At that time he was crippled with acute lower-back pain that prevented him from walking or straightening up, although once he did get moving the pain was relieved. He then told me that he had always been highly sensitive to poison ivy, and that once as a child he had been hospitalized for shortness of breath after a neighbor had burned a large stand of the plant not far from his home. I also learned that he had had chronic lower-back trouble intermittently for many years. A single dose *of Rhus tox.* 10M fixed his back, whereupon the scalp lesions also began to improve.

Case 2. In the eighth month of her first pregnancy, a 35-year-old woman felt her lower back give way suddenly while carrying a heavy pail of water to her

* "Drug Reactions and Biological Individuality," ***Homeotherapy*** 3:1, August 1977.

chickens. Unable to straighten up or sit down, she obtained some relief once she forced herself to move. She was otherwise in good health, and her pregnancy had been uneventful throughout, although she did notice a strong desire for milk that seemed quite unusual for her. In recent years she had also had occasional episodes of bursitis and patchy, scaly eruptions on the trunk. She denied ever having been bothered by poison ivy; in fact she remembered quite vividly how she would walk through large fields of it to impress her friends. One dose of *Rhus tox.* 200 gave her prompt and lasting relief, and not long after she gave birth at home without incident.

Case 3. An 11-month-old girl had had a series of unexplained fevers. During the first episode her temperature exceeded 105°, and she was hospitalized, worked up for meningitis, and placed on IV antibiotics by her pediatrician; but nothing definite was ever found. Thereafter at approximately one-month intervals she would run a fever of 104-105° for several days, but these episodes would invariably subside without further treatment, and from one episode to the next she appeared to be perfectly healthy. All that the mother could add was that the episodes reminded her of the fevers that the child had run following each DPT injection, and that the first episode had occurred about one month after the third and final injection. A single dose of *DPT* 10M six months ago has so far put an end to this cycle.

The two *Rhus tox.* cases are noteworthy for exemplifying totally opposite ways of responding to the same substance. Thus, at least retrospectively, the first one could be regarded as a simple proving that began in childhood and was reactivated by each subsequent exposure, whereas in the second we would have to postulate a latent type of hypersensitivity that remained more or less inapparent for several decades and only achieved full expression during the added stress of pregnancy. The third case raises an entirely different problem, having been provoked by a foreign protein injected routinely into our entire pediatric population.

In all three cases there was prior contact with the offending substance; the present illness was consistent with the provings of the substance; and the same substance, when homeopathically prepared, proved curative as a remedy. I should also say that in all three cases the connection had to be elicited by careful questioning and was totally unsuspected by the patient or informant. All of this led me to wonder whether in fact a great many of our commoner illnesses might also have originated from simple idiosyncrasies of this type — whether at least some cases of arthritis or rheumatism in adults, for example, could have arisen from clinical or subclinical *Rhus* dermatitis in childhood, and indeed whether a whole array of illnesses might be attributable to involuntary provings of DPT and other agents by large numbers of unsuspecting subjects both before and after the age of consent.

It is at this point that my subject becomes part of toxicology, or the study of poisons, because, as we already know, the distinction between remedies and poisons is mainly one of dosage and individual sensitivity, and many of our greatest remedies in their crude state are poisons and even diseases of greater or lesser virulence. Certainly it is no secret that the process of industrialization has itself threatened the persistence of life on the planet, at least in part by bringing a number of highly toxic substances into common use. I will therefore present three cases of "poisoning" in this broader sense.

Case 4. A 55-year-old psychologist consulted me for a painful exostosis of the right wrist of several months' duration. He had been in good health all his life until interned in a German prison camp during World War II, whereupon he developed a persistent arthritis and a number of other complaints that have persisted with only minor variations until the present day. All else that I could glean from him was that the camp had been located in Silesia, not far from a large radium mine. The exostosis rapidly disappeared after two doses of *Radium bromatum* 6X, the only potency of it I had at the time, given one week apart.

Case 5. A 35-year-old woman came to see me doubled over in pain and passing bloody urine. Three weeks earlier she had had a severe bout of the "stomach flu," followed by a deep, persistent cough productive of blood-streaked sputum, and continuing nausea and prostration. On the day of her visit she had awakened with extreme frequency, urgency, and burning on urination; the urine was grossly bloody and accompanied by clots. I found out that she had been taking a silk-screening class for the past several months, and that even before her illness she had several times been overcome by turpentine fumes and forced to leave the class. She responded promptly to a single dose of *Terebinthina* 200, the remedy made from turpentine.

Case 6. A 67-year-old author and environmentalist first consulted me in September of 1975 for a severe and occasionally bloody diarrhea of ten years' duration. Previously diagnosed with chronic ulcerative colitis at several university medical centers, he had been treated aggressively with the most advanced allopathic drugs, all to no effect. For the past three years he had also suffered from the most intractable itching; his whole body was covered with ulcerating skin lesions that had been diagnosed as "neurodermatitis" by several specialists, but similarly failed to respond even to massive doses of corticosteroids. He improved temporarily under infrequent doses of *Sulphur* and other seemingly well-indicated remedies; but his symptoms invariably recurred, and his general condition continued to deteriorate. In September 1976 he underwent a total colectomy and ileostomy, but after a brief improvement the itching became as intolerable as ever, and the skin lesions were now frankly hemorrhagic.

Recently his wife happened to mention that the itching was invariably worse from 8 to 10 in the evening, and I noticed that in Kent's *Repertory* only *Kreosotum* has "itching in the evening" in black type. This struck me because I had recently visited his home, and he had made a point of showing me all the woodwork that he had stained himself over ten years ago with his own home-made mixture of creosote and crankcase oil; it was in fact quite beautiful. I regret that his colon could not be given another chance, but a single dose of *Kreosotum* 200 has so far put an end to the itching and bleeding.

Again in all of these cases the same criteria were met: there was prior exposure to the substance; the symptoms of the illness were consistent with the provings of it; and the illness was cured or significantly relieved by a homeopathic dose of the same substance. What is so striking about them is precisely that all three criteria are present in each patient. For had the remedy been given solely on the basis of prior exposure, without typical symptoms of the remedy, we would be justly accused of isopathy and nothing more. Conversely, repertorization alone may also fail to lead to the proper remedy, particularly if the symptoms are common, because they will usually turn up the same small group of well-proven polychrests.

Furthermore, the connection between exposure and illness is often unsuspected by the patient and is either discovered by accident or has to be elicited by the most careful and detailed questioning. Even then, it remains an unproven hypothesis until it can be confirmed by a successful treatment. This suggests that there is and can be no simple or infallible rule or method for recognizing such cases, or for finding the offending substance once a connection is suspected. The best that can be done is to be aware of the possibility and to take the case with it always in mind.

All of these cases suggest that each of us is uniquely sensitive to a variety of natural and synthetic substances, and that these sensitivities, however they may change from time to time, are nevertheless as basic an expression of our innate biological individuality as, say, our genotype or fingerprints or horoscope, or the illnesses that we create, for that matter, each in our own way.

That is precisely why we cannot simply identify the substance or germ as the "cause" of the illness in the narrowly mechanistic sense of allopathic theory and practice. For something to act as a cause for us, we must already be sufficiently attuned to it to receive it and make it our own, by manifesting its characteristic action. Thus the colitis patient's wife lives in the same house with the same creosote but shows no symptoms of it, while the rest of the silk-screening class likewise failed to come down with turpentine poisoning.

Illness then, like any other life process, cannot be simply a chain of cause and effect, because at every point we find ourselves surrounded by these odd correspondences and synchronicities that exist as if miraculously and without further explanation. It also seems to me that these considerations apply equally to Hahnemann's theory of the chronic diseases and thus to the homeopathic process generally. Hahnemann says that each of the three chronic miasms originates in exposure to a corresponding morbid stimulus, namely the itch mite and the "viruses" of syphilis and gonorrhea respectively. Yet the miasm cannot simply be imposed by the stimulus; it represents a living interaction between the stimulus and the already-disordered and thus receptive constitution of the patient.

Therefore the special importance of the various miasmatic agents must be that something quite profound in the nature of human life itself is receptive to them, such that the diseases they instigate are more or less universally distributed and hence more durable and difficult to eradicate. So in these cases we would have to say that the morbid sensitivity itself is modified and handed down from generation to generation, until the original exposure lies deeply buried or forgotten in mythology and has to be inferred from the persistence of the symptoms.

Likewise, in the case of the "polychrest" remedies corresponding to them, most human beings can be presumed to be sensitive to a variety of them, even without prior contact, precisely because of their correspondence with the fundamental diseases of our species. Thus at this point we must go beyond the vantage point of the individual to the sensitivity of families and nations and ultimately to the human species as a whole; and even at this level we must sometimes resort to biographical clues in prescribing, in addition to simple repertorization of symptoms. Here are two cases of this type.

Case 7. A 53-year-old man first saw me in September of 1976 with a 6-year history of severe right-sided trigeminal neuralgia, partially controlled with large doses of Tegretol. He described the pain as pulsating, like a sharp ticking centered in his lower teeth, and worse from the least motion of the jaw, such as talking or chewing. He improved quite dramatically after *Spigelia*, *Bryonia*, and *Colocynthis;* but each time, after impatiently reducing the dose of the Tegretol, he suffered a relapse and had to resume it. In January of 1977 a large number of warts began to appear on his face, causing him considerable discomfort. Since then he has improved steadily on a single dose of *Thuja* 200, with continuing reduction of the Tegretol.

Case 8. A mother and daughter have been my patients since October of 1975, at which time the mother was 29 years old and four months into her second pregnancy. Her chief complaint was severe nocturnal itching and burning, especially of the palms and soles, which responded well and promptly to a single dose of *Sulphur* 1M, but recurred twice more during the pregnancy. On physical examination she appeared thin and nervous, even hyperactive; her history was overshadowed by her mother's suicide and her father's alcoholism and death from a stab wound.

There was no known history of TB in the family, but her father's parents were Native American and their medical history unknown to her. Her appetite was enormous, and she had a strong craving for meat and especially bacon. In her last trimester she developed a thick cough productive of greenish sputum that persisted until the birth. This occurred in January of 1976, about four weeks prematurely. The baby girl weighed 4½ pounds and had to be hospitalized for respiratory distress, but did well on oxygen and supportive treatment.

In April of 1976 the mother developed a severe case of acute bronchitis, with high fever, chills, cough, and stiff joints, which responded beautifully to a few doses of *Bacillinum* 200. In September she returned with sinusitis and a thick, greenish nasal discharge similar to what she had expectorated in the past. She also recalled having had repeated episodes of bronchitis and pneumonia as a child. One dose of *Tuberculinum* 200 cured her, and she has been well since.

In March of 1977 she brought in her daughter, then just over a year old, for recurrent colds and respiratory infections, including an episode of viral pneumonia for which she had been hospitalized. The mother stated that most of her illnesses centered in the chest, and were always associated with much coughing and thick expectoration. She had also apparently inherited her mother's inordinate love of bacon. On physical examination the child was very slight and delicate of build, and of exceptional beauty. A single dose of *Tuberculinum* 200 likewise put an end to her coughing, and she too has remained well since.

The first case is an example of miasmatic sensitivity, in which the indicated remedies acted but failed to cure until the underlying miasm came to the surface and presented itself for treatment. In cases like this, involving a polychrest remedy, sensitivity to it had to be inferred from the empirical connection between *Thuja* and the sycotic "style" rather than from any prior contact. The second case is that of a familial sensitivity to tuberculosis handed down from mother to daughter, where prior contact with the organism is similarly lost in the history and had to be assumed.

I will conclude with a brief postscript regarding the *Cannabis* drugs, because they are being extensively and voluntarily proved by large segments of especially the teen-age and young adult population, and because I have found them to be of great value in treating a limited range of conditions. I will consider the two drugs together, although in the *indica* variety -- "hashish" -- the mental and circulatory effects tend to be more important, whereas with the *sativa* -- "marijuana," "ganja," "reefer," etc. -- the genito-urinary symptoms are apt to predominate. I've learned to ask about cannabis usage routinely in this age group, and very rarely does this one question fail to yield interesting and useful information. I will present two cases that illustrate the scope of *Cannabis* fairly well.

Case 9. A 34-year-old nuclear physicist consulted me in January of 1975 for a variety of neuropsychiatric symptoms that he traced to an episode of prostatitis and urethritis some seven years previously. When I saw him, he was suffering mainly from ataxia, incoördination, and associated tremors, dizziness, and confusion, as well as some residual dysuria, spermatorrhea, and impotence. I treated him with several remedies to no avail, and was about to give up on him, when he confessed with much embarrassment that his original illness had been preceded by a period of continual marijuana smoking, which particularly impressed me because he had since become almost fanatically opposed to the practice. At that time his pulse was 60 per minute, and his blood pressure 130/80 mm. A single dose of *Cannabis indica* 200 cured him, and he has been well since.

Case 10. A 28-year-old woman first consulted me in the early months of her second pregnancy as a precaution, having had rather severe toxemia at the time of her first birth, with blood pressures as high as 170/110 mm. At that first visit her blood pressure was already 150/95 mm., and her pulse 54 per minute; but apart from certain other minor symptoms of pregnancy she appeared to be quite well. She told me that most of her toxemia symptoms had actually originated at a time of heavy marijuana smoking several years earlier, and had persisted even though she had avoided the drug entirely ever since. Four powders of *Cannabis indica* 200 given at weekly intervals have reduced her blood pressure to 120/70 mm., and she continues in good health.

Of the many well-known mental symptoms of *Cannabis* I will mention only one, the slowing of the passage of time, so that minutes seem like hours, and the duration of the present moment is greatly prolonged. This symptom I have repeatedly confirmed in my practice, and I am convinced that it is correlated with slowing of the pulse rate, the metronome of our internal time sense. Of all the physical symptoms of *Cannabis,* slowing of the pulse has been in my experience by far the most reliable.

On the other hand, just as we might expect from the Arndt-Schultz Law, *Cannabis* can also accelerate the pulse. Indeed, the drug has a marked affinity for the heart and blood vessels generally; and it is also capable of either raising or lowering the blood pressure, and of producing concomitant sensations of heat or chilliness, especially in the hands and feet.

Its other major area of specialization is its affinity for the genito-urinary tract and the reproductive and sexual functions. Known for provoking irritation, inflammation, and discharge along the entire length of the tract, *Cannabis* has been quite useful to me in the treatment of urethritis, cystitis, prostatitis, and even pyelonephritis where the other symptoms agree. In addition, it can either stimulate or depress sexual desire, sexual performance, and fertility in either sex; and recent allopathic studies have shown definite reductions of the sperm count, motility, and serum testosterone levels following high or repeated doses of the crude substance. In former times it was used in the treatment of acute gonorrhea, and I have come to regard it as essentially a sycotic remedy.

It has even occurred to me that the popularity of *Cannabis* use in recent years might be as both cause and effect to the worldwide epidemic of gonorrhea and related illnesses through which we are now passing. In any case, my own experience with it shows how difficult it is either to establish or rule out any drug sensitivity on the basis of exposure alone. There is a natural tendency to confuse sensitivity to a drug with habitual usage of or affinity for it. In both of my cases, for example, sensitivity manifested rather as an extreme aversion to or intolerance of the remedy. So in case-taking it is most important to individualize by letting the patient tell his or her own story.

In this paper I have been advocating a biographical rather than purely symptomatic approach, because I am impressed by the large number of cases where the present illness has proved to be essentially a drug disease in the Hahnemannian sense, and simple repertorization of symptoms may not lead to the indicated remedy until a history of prior exposure can be established. The theoretical interest of such cases also lies in the fact that they suggest a Paracelsian model of correspondence between different levels of the physical world that is quite universal in scope.

Thus for any natural or synthetic substance we can imagine and even predict a complete spectrum of human sensitivities in relation to it, such that some people will react strongly or even violently to even minute quantities of it, and that some of these will go on to develop a drug disease that expresses their own pre-existing miasmatic structure. Others will be relatively indifferent to it, or will even desire and use it regularly without any ill effects at all. Still others and perhaps the majority will be more or less moderately affected, depending on the dosage and other modifying factors; these we might call the 'wild type.'

Presumably the same would also be true of herbs, vitamins, and other substances commonly thought of as beneficial, because as we know the very fact of their curative power also implies the existence of hypersensitive individuals who could become ill even from minute doses; indeed these are apt to be the very people for whom those same substances could be effective remedies. In the same way, we must assume that the current debates between proponents and opponents of, say, nuclear energy or any other physicochemical agency reflect real and different biological sensitivities that must be respected and ultimately reconciled, if we are all to live together in peace. So once again our obligation to heal and be healed transcends the purely personal realm and looks to the planet and the cosmos for truer guidance.

*Homeopathic Remedies vs. the Placebo Effect**

The art of homoeopathic medicine today is all but unknown to the general public; and I would venture to say that a large majority of those who *have* heard of it, including most of our patients, believe in their hearts that the tiny granules that taste so sweet are in fact nothing but sugar pills, and that whatever results we may achieve clinically could just as well be attributed to our own personal or shamanic powers, or the patient's belief in them, or some combination of the two.

Nor does such a view necessarily imply any hostility to homeopathy. Quite the contrary, it often reflects a deepening skepticism about *all* forms of treatment, especially the more aggressive modalities of conventional medicine, and even a humanistic preference for the "placebo effect," i. e., the ancient *vis medicatrix naturae,* the unassisted and indeed innate healing effort of the patient, as a model of the healing process itself.[1]

Moreover, it is a view that homoeopathy has never quite refuted, partly because we still do not know how our medicines act or how our patients are cured, and also because our history as a persecuted minority makes us almost not *want* to know, or indeed to do anything to attract further attention to ourselves. Nor is it by any means a simple matter to demonstrate the efficacy of the high dilutions even to someone who is prepared to examine the evidence with an open mind.

Nevertheless, while it may be quite difficult to *prove* that our remedies actually work, there is a very substantial body of evidence that they do; and in order to refute the argument that they are placebos, it is not necessary to prove that they act *curatively,* which is of course a more complicated matter, but only that they act at all, that *something* happens as a result of their action, rather than simply on account of the interaction between the physician and the patient. Conversely, if it could be proved that our remedies were in fact nothing but placebos, let us by all means admit it with good grace, since, quite apart from having deluded ourselves all these years, knowingly giving

---

* "Homeopathic Remedies vs. the Placebo Effect," ***Homeotherapy*** 6:99, July-August, 1980.

placebos or just saying that we don't know would be incalculably simpler and less expensive than the elaborate rigamarole that we actually practice!

As many of you know, there have been a substantial number of experimental studies demonstrating that homeopathic remedies in high dilution can stimulate or inhibit the growth of various bacteria, plants, molds, fruit flies, etc., as well as the enzymatic activity of some *in vitro* or cell-free systems. But inasmuch as these have already been described fairly extensively in the literature, I will focus on actual cases from my own practice.

In fact, there are a considerable number of clinical situations in which we can show quite convincingly, although necessarily short of formal *proof,* that dilute homeopathic remedies do indeed act. In what follows, I will attempt to group these situations into categories and present cases from my own records to illustrate them.

A. *Where a positive outcome is unlikely in the short time actually observed:*

> Case 1. *Respiratory distress of the newborn.* A full-term, 8-pound baby girl was born at home in February, 1976, after a prolonged second stage. Covered with thick meconium, she took one gasp, but didn't breathe after that. Brisk suctioning of the oropharynx yielded a large quantity of the same thick meconium, and endotracheal intubation was unsuccessful; her vocal cords were not visualized. With a heart rate of 60 per min., and color pale, almost white, the child lay limp and motionless. Responding weakly to mouth-to-mouth resuscitation, she didn't breathe on her own when it was stopped. I gave *Arsenicum album* 200, one dose, dry, on the tongue. She awoke almost instantaneously, with her heart pounding vigorously at 140 per minute, took a huge gulp of air, and began breathing normally, with good muscle tone and normal reflexes, the skin glowing pink with the flame of new life. The whole evolution occupied no more than a few seconds, and from then on the child remained perfectly normal in every way, as if nothing had happened. Hospitalized for observation, she was discharged after 24 hours with no further distress, no evidence of aspiration, and no medication being required.

I should add that the child was full-term, well-formed, and would probably have recovered eventually, even if the remedy had not been given; but I know from experience that her situation would have earned her 24-48 hours in the Newborn ICU, with oxygen, some form of assisted ventilation, and possibly other drugs as well. What was so unforgettable about this case was the rapidity of its evolution, from a life-threatening emergency into a completely normal, stable pattern in the space of a few seconds. What convinced me most of all was the look of utter disbelief on my nurse's face, because she had her ear glued to the stethoscope the whole time, and had not seen me give the remedy. Within two seconds after I gave it, she looked up at me in amazement and handed me the stethoscope, demanding to know, *"What happened?"* Experiences like these are inscribed for life in every practitioner's mind.

Case 2. *Breech presentation.* A 23-year-old woman was due on January 8, 1976. At her regular prenatal visits she was in good health, with the baby in a normal vertex presentation.

December 15, 1975. At her routine checkup, she complained of increased pressure and fetal movement in the suprapubic region. Fetal heart tones were heard at 138 per minute in the right upper quadrant, indicating a breech presentation. I gave *Pulsatilla* 6X, two tablets 3 times daily.

December 18. The mother reported violent movements on the night of the 16th and again on the 17th. The presentation was now vertex, with the fetal heart tones heard at 150 per minute in the left lower quadrant. There were no other complaints.

January 5, 1976. After a short labor at home, she gave birth to a baby girl who weighed 7 lb. 6 oz., born vertex, in the Right Occiput Anterior position, with no problems.

This was the first breech presentation I ever saw turned with remedies. In the old literature I'd read a number of accounts recommending their use prior to engagement, or at least before labor; on the other hand, I also knew that a fairly high percentage of breech babies revert spontaneously in the final weeks. It was purely circumstantial evidence that led both me and the patient to believe that the remedy had acted. I used a low dilution because the patient otherwise had no symptoms, and I was looking for what could be described as a physiologic effect.

Case 3. *Breech presentation.* 24-year-old woman, due on February 8, 1980. She had been feeling well throughout the pregnancy; no major complaints.

November 16, 1979. At her routine visit, the fetal heart was heard in the right upper quadrant, indicating a breech presentation.

December 13. There were no complaints, but the baby was still breech. At that point I gave *Pulsatilla* 6X two tablets 3 times a day for 4 days, but there was no change.

January 11, 1980. With the baby still breech, we discussed the possibility of a hospital birth. No other complaints. Again I gave *Pulsatilla,* this time the 30C, three times daily for 4 days; again there was no change.

January 17. A pelvic ultrasound confirmed the single fetus in a breech presentation.

January 21. With the baby still breech, I gave *Pulsatilla* 200, once a day for 4 days.

January 25. The mother reported that after waking from a normal sleep the baby "felt different." Routine examination revealed that the baby had indeed reverted to a normal vertex presentation. There were no other complaints.

February 4. After an average labor, she delivered a 7-pound baby boy at home, vertex, in the Left Occiput Anterior position, with no problems.

Although here again the evidence was purely circumstantial, neither the patient nor I had the slightest doubts about the remedy having turned it, even though from November on the patient had also been doing special exercises for converting the breech, and was receiving regular acupuncture treatments for the same purpose; these measures had been taken continuously over a two-month period. In this case, it was the degree of dilution that appeared to make the difference: both the 6X and the 30C produced markedly increased fetal movements, but no change in position, whereas the 200 had no effect on fetal movement, but the patient awoke from a sound sleep with the abnormal position corrected.

B. *Where drug treatment hasn't worked, or elective surgery was the only option:*

Case 4. *Epilepsy.* A 4-year-old boy from Hobbs, NM had had a long history of febrile convulsions, as well as minor seizures occurring spontaneously in the past 7 months. When his mother was 5 months pregnant with him, the parents separated; they divorced shortly after his birth, which was normal and uneventful, and the mother promptly remarried. At 4 months of age, he developed febrile convulsions, followed by a rash, possibly roseola, and again several times after that, with acute tonsillitis, otitis media, etc., all grand mal and treated successfully with phenobarbital.

Otherwise, he appeared to be in good health and developing normally, until March 1976, when an ordinary URI with low fever developed into a pattern of persistent grand mal seizures, for which he was hospitalized. The EEG was equivocal, the seizures were well-controlled on Dilantin and phenobarbital, and he was discharged on maintenance doses. After a few weeks, he began having many brief episodes of petit mal type, when his body stiffened, his head was thrown back, his back arched, and his mind went blank for a few seconds; in about half of them, he would also fall to the ground. Zarontin was substituted for Dilantin. When he first saw me, he was having 15-20 such episodes daily, his mother having stopped all the meds for 2 weeks at my request.

October 5, 1976. At his first visit, the child was extremely hyperactive, continually interrupting, and with slurred speech. The physical exam was normal, but twice interrupted by hyperactive episodes. I gave *Calcarea phos.* 200, one dose, plus 6X tablets as needed for seizures or any other acute symptoms, up to 4 times a day.

November 25. The mother telephoned to report that he had improved a lot for 2 weeks, but then relapsed, with all his old symptoms returning, especially in the past 3 days. This time I gave *Hyoscyamus* 200, one dose.

December 20. Again the mother phoned to say that his speech, appetite, hyperactivity, and general condition had all improved considerably, although the petit mal episodes were still fairly frequent, averaging 6 per day, with generalized clonic seizures at rare intervals, but no loss of consciousness. I gave *Opium* 200, one dose.

January 18, 1977. The mother phoned to report several more clonic episodes, as above, but continuing improvement in his general condition; his speech she described as "back to normal." Then, one week ago, he had a severe grand mal seizure, followed by a long, deep sleep, and no seizures at all since. Naturally, I waited, giving no remedy.

April 2. The mother wrote to say that he had a good appetite, and was doing well in public school, with no seizures of any kind.

August 26. The mother wrote to request his medical records, because they were moving to Florida. She described him as "perfectly healthy in every respect," with no seizures of any kind since her last letter.

This case was noteworthy because of the suppressive effect of the anticonvulsant drugs, which abolished grand mal activity, allowing the petit mal to squirt out in its place, such that the treatment was obliged to proceed "backward," so to speak, to its original grand mal form, before he could complete the cure.

Case 5. *Renal calculi; obstructive uropathy.* A 31-year-old surveyor consulted me for renal colic and a long history of kidney stones.

January 24, 1976. At his first visit, he told of having passed stones spontaneously in 1972, followed by intermittent flank pain ever since. For the past 5 days, the pain had been especially intense, radiating from the left costo-vertebral angle to and from the bladder, with obstructed urination, as well as passing large amounts of sediment resembling shreds of tissue. An IVP showed 2 large calculi completely obstructing the left uretero-pelvic junction, with hydronephrosis of the left renal pelvis and calyces; his family doctor was recommending immediate surgery. I gave *Berberis vulgaris* 200, one dose, and 6X tablets as needed, up to 4 times daily.

January 26. The pain had lessened considerably and was now almost gone, essentially a dull ache. I gave *Ocimum canum* 200, one dose, followed by *Calcarea renalis* 6X tablets, up to 4 times daily as needed.

February 16. The pain was now mild, residual, and mainly in the bladder, with some stinging and dysuria in the urethral meatus. I gave nothing further.

February 26. He reported feeling much better still, with only occasional twinges of pain; he felt that the obstruction had been removed. Again I gave no further treatment.

March 25. A repeat IVP showed one stone in the lower pole of left kidney, with no hydronephrosis or other evidence of obstruction, and the other in the bottom of the left ureter, near the uretero-vesical junction. No treatment was given.

November 15. After weeks of hard work and drinking excessive amounts of coffee, he called because of a recent episode of intense pain in the left lower quadrant, near the bladder. This time I gave him *Nux vomica* 200, one dose, and 6X tablets, up to 4 times a day as needed.

November 17. He telephoned to report "much improvement:" the pain was almost gone. No further treatment was given.

January 11, 1977. He called, having passed a large stone of conglomerate type, 6x3x5 mm., and now feeling well in every respect. He refused further treatment and follow-up IVP's.

Experienced homeopaths will doubtless excuse the hasty, symptomatic type of prescribing that could have prolonged or even spoiled this case. I cite it merely to show how surgery can often be avoided, even in threatening situations.

Case 6. *Pelvic trauma.* A 27-year-old weaver consulted me for a long history of repeated, well-documented yeast infections intermittently over the past two years, treated repeatedly with Mycostatin, with only temporary relief.

June 23, 1977. At her first visit, she complained of constant burning in the vagina, with pain on intercourse; the labia were flaming red, with a sticky white substance clinging to the folds, but no discharge. I gave *Sulphur* 200, one dose.

July 1. The pain had lessened, and the irritation was gone; but she was still very dry with intercourse: "lovemaking has become an ordeal!" she wept, complaining bitterly. Her symptoms had begun soon after a car accident 2 years ago, in which she was thrown from the car and landed on her buttocks; there was no fracture, but a large hematoma took a long time to heal, in the course of which her present symptoms developed. On the strength of that bit of history, I gave her *Arnica* 200, one dose, and 6X tablets to take as needed, up to 4 times a day.

December 22. The dryness was gone, and she had no other complaints; she felt well in every respect.

This case is memorable to me, first, in showing very clearly the flaw of conventional prescribing, aimed purely at the microbial flora, the tissue changes, etc., and giving no thought to the patient's story. In addition, it illustrates how homeopathic remedies can search back in time, through the life history of the patient, to locate and overcome chronic symptoms traceable in this case to mechanical trauma in the distant past.

C. Where the patient was skeptical, hostile, unconscious, comatose, or otherwise immune to suggestion (infants, pets, etc.):

Case 7. *Recurrent mastitis.* A 30-year-old woman had her first birth at home in February 1975, with a doctor friend in attendance. Traction on the cord extracted a placenta that was torn in several places, with heavy postpartum bleeding and manual removal of retained placental fragments. At 5 weeks postpartum she developed acute mastitis with a high fever, and was treated once with Ampicillin and twice with Keflex; but the illness recurred three more times, within days after finishing each course. Only then, and most reluctantly, did she decide to try remedies.

May 6, 1975. Making a home visit at her request, I found her with a fever of 102° and pulse of 120 per minute, lying in bed quite motionless, as the slightest movement or change of position brought on nausea and a violent headache; even moving the eyes provoked intense retro-orbital pain, as in all prior episodes. Needless to say, I gave her *Bryonia,* one dose of 200, plus 6X tablets 4 times a day as needed; but as I got up to go home, she pleaded with me not to leave, having no experience with and little if any faith in me or my remedies. So I stayed overnight, and the next morning her fever was gone, her breast was no longer swollen or tender, and the headache and orbital pains were greatly diminished. Within 12 hours she had recovered completely, her symptoms never reappeared, and I attended her second birth, which was beautiful and free of complications or sequelæ.

Case 8. *Urethritis.* A 33-year-old mother of two came in complaining of vaginal discharge, itching, and constant urging to urinate.

July 26, 1979. The patient became quite agitated, suspicious, hostile, and scornful when she discovered that I was a homeopath and gave no drugs or antibiotics. Her illness was only 6 hours old: after separating from her husband some weeks ago, she had recently gone back to him, but their passionate lovemaking gave way to violent, angry scenes when he announced that he had been exposed to gonorrhea during his absence. Her main physical symptom was intense burning in the urethra at the close of urination; her cultures proved negative for gonorrhea and VD. I gave her *Staphysagria* 200, one dose, plus 6X tablets as needed, up to 4 times a day.

July 27. I phoned her, and she reported that her symptoms were almost gone.

July 28. Again I had to call her myself to find out, but she no longer had any symptoms at all.

My only reason for reporting these two cases is to show that patients need not believe in remedies for them to be effective. The second patient was as surly, ill-mannered, and uncoöperative a patient as I have ever had. She knew my name only because I had played volleyball with her husband a few times. She didn't know anything about homeopathy, but was so desperate for relief that she reluctantly agreed to try it when I told her I didn't use drugs or write prescriptions.

D. Where patients loved the remedies, had faith in me, and showed clear, well-defined symptom-pictures, but experienced no benefit whatsoever:

This group is exactly the converse of the last; and cases of this type are, alas, far too common to be particularly memorable, or to deserve specific mention here. I cite them merely to show that it is possible for remedies *not* to work sometimes, even for patients who would be especially likely to benefit from the placebo effect if it were the decisive factor.

E. Where patients developed new symptoms typical of the remedy prescribed:

Case 9. *Premenstrual syndrome.* A 43-year-old lady consulted me for a long history of premenstrual complaints.

November 7, 1979. At her first visit, she said she felt well for 3 weeks out of 4, but that, from 7 days before to the start of her period, she was plagued with painful, lumpy breasts, a ravenous appetite, and nervous irritability. Quite haughty in her demeanor, she waxed eloquent about her love of hot drinks, her inability to tolerate dry spring winds and dry weather in general, and the aggravation of all of her symptoms on waking for the day. I gave *Lycopodium* 200, one dose.

January 10, 1980. Her next period had come just 2 days after onset of her premenstrual symptoms, which were quite mild, and this time only her right breast was tender. Indeed she was struck by the coincidence that *all of her symptoms were right-sided,* which was very unusual for her, such as aching and stiffness of the right side of her neck, which was quite new to her, and even a right-sided earache, which she had not had since childhood. Despite these complaints, she had continued to feel quite well, and had remained so ever since.

This type of case is quite common and to my mind represents some of the most direct and convincing evidence we can have that the remedy is what's doing the job, rather than simply the suggestibility or desire of the patient to be healed. The provings of *Lycopodium clavatum*, a species of club-moss, have shown it to be markedly and predominantly a right-sided medicine. It is this almost spooky correspondence between the experimentally-proven symptoms of the remedy and the actual symptoms of the patient that immediately distinguishes homeopathy from all other methods of treatment. When new symptoms appear in the course of a treatment, when they are known to be characteristic of the remedy given, and above all when they are accompanied by a significant improvement in the general condition and particular symptoms of the patient, one can be virtually certain that the remedy is acting.

Many homeopaths teach that the appearance of a typical homeopathic aggravation of the chief complaint, followed by amelioration and a curative response in accordance with Hering's Laws of Cure, are the surest proof that the chosen remedy is acting. But I have also witnessed these phenomena following allopathic drugs, surgery, acupuncture, faith healing, placebos, and even in the course of spontaneous cures without any treatment whatsoever. These are simply curative reactions, and cure is always miraculous in the sense that it can always occur or fail to occur, whichever modality we use.

F. Where remedies actually did harm, by activating a latent destructive process:

Case 10. *Rectal fissure.* A 27-year-old wildlife photographer consulted me because of a 4-month history of rectal pain and bleeding, which his GP had diagnosed as a rectal fissure, and for which he had recommended elective surgery. His past history included migraines, which had not bothered him for the past 2 years; amœbic dysentery; recurrent prostatitis; and chronic ophthalmic infections, with redness, soreness, and crusting, for which he had been using mercuric oxide ointment an average of 3 times a week for the past 5 years.

October 9, 1975. At his first visit, he complained of sharp, stinging rectal pain that was most severe after prolonged sitting. I gave *Nitric. acid.* 200, one dose.

October 21. The pain and bleeding had almost completely subsided within a few days of taking the remedy, and he felt revitalized and full of well-being; but after one week, his original symptoms reappeared and slowly regained their previous intensity. In addition, his eyes had become increasingly sore in the last 24 hours, with occasional brownish "floaters" in the visual field of the left eye. I repeated the *Nitric. acid.* 200, one dose.

October 22. The vision in his left eye had totally "browned out;" he now saw only fuzzy blotches. Diagnosing retrobulbar neuritis, a local eye specialist referred him to the University of New Mexico Medical Center for a full neurological workup.

November 2. The UNM retinal team diagnosed optic neuritis, a common precursor of multiple sclerosis, finding a large scotoma in the left eye, with a gray penumbra surrounding it; he could still see some light on the edges of the field peripherally. There was also considerable fuzziness of vision in the right eye.

November 20. The vision in his right eye was almost back to normal, but now he was almost totally blind in the left, except for a narrow, crescent- shaped arc at the periphery of the field.

I present this case lest you assume, as most of us do, that homeopathic remedies are simply harmless, that is to say, ineffective. To be sure, such cases are extremely rare, and the safety record of homeopathic remedies, when compared with allopathic drugs, is quite extraordinary. I would also agree that the remedy in this case almost certainly elicited a latent tendency that probably would have come to light in time even without it. Nevertheless, I must continue to live with the fact, as must the patient and his family, that he would have been much happier had he never consulted me in the first place; and I can imagine no clearer demonstration of the real power of remedies than such vanishingly rare instances where they appear to catalyze or activate a latent destructive force of which the patient was previously unaware.

For all of these reasons, I have little doubt that those taking the trouble to practice classical homoeopathy, no more nor less than their patients, will soon be convinced that such remedies at the very least do *something,* and in addition are quite capable of working beneficially and even curatively when used properly, although we still don't really understand *how* they do it, an enigma which of course keeps things interesting. At the same time, we may cheerfully agree with our critics who charge that we are merely using placebos, since the "placebo effect" is thought to measure the patient's own spontaneous healing effort, the ancient *vis medicatrix naturæ,* which after all remains the simplest model of the natural healing process, and which operates continuously throughout life, no matter which modality is used, and whether or not the physician is ready and willing to co-operate with it. In the words of Paracelsus,

The art of healing comes from Nature, not from the physician . . .
Every illness has its own remedy within itself . . .
A man could not be born alive and healthy were there not already a Physician hidden in him.[2]

NOTES.

1. Cousins, N., *The Anatomy of an Illness as Perceived by the Patient,* Norton, Chapter 2, 'The Mysterious Placebo", pp. 49-70.
2. Paracelsus, *Selected Writings,* translated by N. Guterman, ed. J. Jacobi, Bollingen, Princeton, pp. 50, 76, *passim.*

*Peculiar and Characteristic Symptoms**

We all tend to remember those cases in which the symptoms that led us to the remedy were especially distinctive and well-defined. Sometimes these are "strange, rare, and peculiar;" but just as often they are simply characteristic of the remedy, making the selection very easy. What they have in common is that elusive something that all of us are looking for in every case: that sudden insight that illuminates it, or the loose end that helps us unravel it, piece by piece.

Case 1. A young girl of 15 consulted me for back pain, which she had had since the start of her periods a few years before. It turned out that her chief symptom was menstrual cramps, which usually occurred before and during the first few days of her flow, at which time the back pain was also at its worst. The most remarkable feature of the case was the cramps themselves, which she described as intense and knifelike, and often so severe as to cause her to faint. She described several incidents at school where she actually lost consciousness and fell down, causing much embarrassment and concern all around.

Under **Generalities** in Kent's ***Repertory*** I found the rubric, "Faintness before menses, from pain," with only two remedies listed: kali s., *lap. a.* The account of *Lapis albus*, or calcium silicofluoride, in Clarke's *Dictionary* contains the following passage: *"The pains come on before the flow and cause swooning. Pain so severe, she would fall unconscious, the swoon lasting half an hour at times."* That seemed to fit the bill pretty closely; so I gave her *Lapis albus* 30X, the only potency I had of it at the time, to be taken as needed for severe pain, up to 3 times daily till better. That was in September 1978. By November, she was much better; and one year later, she reported that the dysmenorrhea and the back pain had completely disappeared, and she felt very well indeed.

Case 2. Shortly after coming to Boston, I was consulted by a lady of 36 who had suffered from recurrent attacks of bronchitis for many years, with a marked susceptibility to catching cold, such that she felt obliged to keep her neck and throat covered, even from the gentlest breeze. Her personality and many of her underlying constitutional symptoms seemed like *Phosphorus,* which is also quite sensitive to the cold; but this woman's response to cold was so extreme, so

* "Peculiar and Characteristic Symptoms," ***Homeopathy Today,*** April 1983.

unusual, and so well-delineated as to lead me in a different direction. When, for example, she went for a walk in the cold air, which she did only when absolutely necessary and under numerous layers of clothing, she could actually feel the inspired air as a piercing jet of coldness far down into her throat and beyond; and some sort of infection or general devastation would almost invariably follow. What was especially striking about this symptom was not merely that it was *unusual,* but that it clarified and even completed all of the others, so that it could almost be allowed to stand for the whole case.

In Kent, under **Throat,** I found the rubric, 'Coldness, sensation of, on inspiration,' and just two remedies listed for it: *'cist.,* sulph.' With *Sulphur* being quintessentially hot or at least on the warm side in most cases, I looked up *Cistus canadensis* in Clarke, and found the following passage: *"It is most suited to scrofulous subjects who are very sensitive to cold air. 'Sensitive to cold air' runs through the pathogenesis, and also feelings of coldness. Inhaling the slightest cold air causes sore throat. Inhaled air feels cool. Cold breath."*

I gave her *Cistus canadensis* 1M, one dose, which produced a marvelous effect: she returned in November, a month later, invigorated, *warm,* much to her amazement, and her respiratory symptoms and associated weakness no longer perceptible to her. Since then, these improvements have held, and her basic *Phosphorus* picture has begun to emerge.

This case taught me not to begin with the big polychrest, if a lesser remedy covers it better. It also fell out that the 'strange, rare, and peculiar' symptom was itself *characteristic* of the remedy, not in the sense that every patient will have it, but because it highlighted and clarified a number of its essential features.

Case 3. A few years ago, a 36-year-old lady came to see me 8 days after giving birth to her second child, because of a sharp pain in the right breast that made it extremely difficult to nurse on that side. There were no cracks, fissures, or lumps, but only a small, hard whitish spot on the nipple itself. She described the pain as a sharp 'pins-and-needles' sensation, mostly inside the nipple, which came on violently as soon as the baby latched on, and lasted as long as he nursed on that side.

Under **Chest** in Kent, I found the rubric 'Pain, stitching, mammæ, while nursing,' which listed only 2 remedies: *'calc., sil.'* I gave her *Silica* 200, one dose, and some 6X tablets to take as needed. The pain subsided almost entirely within a few hours, came back briefly a few days later, and then again 3 weeks later, this time very suddenly, and worse than ever, until in a minute or so the place on the nipple where the spot had been discharged a flat, ribbon-like caseous material, followed by immediate and total relief of the pain, which never came back.

Silica is a major remedy for cracked nipples and other problems of breastfeeding, and the symptoms in this case were common enough to be characteristic of it. Thus what is most distinctive about a case need not be unusual; and conversely, even a strange, rare, and peculiar symptom may rightly be discarded, if it is merely incidental to the crucial disturbances of the case.

Case 4. A baby boy of 18 months was brought in breathing rapidly, with cough and coarse rattling on inspiration. The pulse was 144 and bounding, the temperature 103.8°. He seemed remarkably calm and affectionate in the office, but I heard fine, moist râles all over the right lung, indicating broncho-pneumonia. The only other symptom the mother reported was a peculiar jerking of the legs during sleep. I don't recall what made me think of *Veratrum viride,* other than that I knew that it was sometimes used in pneumonia; the Kentian rubrics 'Jerking, legs, during sleep,' 'Trembling, legs, during sleep,' and 'Twitching, legs, during sleep' all fail to mention it. But Clarke's account contains the following passage: *"In chorea,* Verat. vir. *has had many successes: 'twitching during sleep' was a characteristic of some cases."* That was good enough for me! I gave *Veratrum vir.* 30C, four times a day. Two days later he was much better, and went on to make an excellent and speedy recovery after a few more doses.

Case 5. Another baby, a twin girl of 11 months, was brought in for scaly eczema of 4 months' duration, beginning in the right shoulder, then proceeding down the right side of the body, and up the left. The mother repeatedly called my attention to the fact that the itching was severe only when the body was *uncovered,* which was the opposite of what she had expected. Under **Skin** in Kent, the rubric 'Itching, undressing agg.' is rather sizeable, with the principal remedies as follows: *'cocc., dros., nat. s., olnd.,* **Rumx.**, *staph., tub.'* Of these, *Rumex* seemed the best, chiefly because of the following passage in Clarke: *"This symptom of Paine's has led to many cures of skin cases:'While undressing, and for more time after, considerable itching. Where exposure to air is the exciting cause.'* "This was in January of 1981. I gave her *Rumex* 200, one dose, with prompt and dramatic relief. The symptoms came back briefly a month later, and another dose was enough to chase them away for good.

Case 6. My last case was that of a 38-year-old lady who developed acute hemorrhagic cystitis, with clots in the urine, tenesmus, and burning, especially at the end of urinating; it came on the day after watching her son's football team play in a snowstorm, 'to the bitter end.' *Chimaphila,* the remedy in this case, scored low in the repertorization; but it did appear in several rubrics, and I probably read it simply because I'd never used it before. This is what Clarke says about it: *"Chimaphila {pipsissewa} is a remedy used by many North American Indians in gravel and urinary disorders. The Eclectics use it in cases of cystitis, strangury, smarting, or burning pains on urination. Vesical tenesmus. Constant desire to urinate. Blood in the urine. The symptoms of* Chimaphila *are worse in damp weather, after washing in cold water, and from sitting on a cold, wet stone."*

That last sentence did it for me. Like most homeopaths, I love to try out remedies that I've never used before. Anyway, I gave her *Chimaphila* 6X, which was all I had of it at the time; and within a few days, her symptoms were essentially gone, although they came back briefly a week later, after making love with her husband. After a few more doses, she completed her recovery.

Maybe the whole point of this is to show that you can often find the remedy, even if it's one you've never used before, just by paying careful attention to those features of the case that seem odd, peculiar, and otherwise important, or simply catch your eye for whatever reason. I'm sure you already know this; but take my word for it, it can stand plenty of repetition.

*A Wound Heals -- After 25 Years**

Almost 30 years after a radical mastectomy for breast cancer, a 70-year-old woman came in seeking remedies to help her close an open, draining wound in her chest. Her long saga began with a local recurrence of her cancer one year post-op, followed by total hysterectomy and extensive X-ray treatments of the chest wall, which resulted in osteomyelitis of the lower ribs on the right side, near the costo-sternal junction. This continued for a full year, even after removal of the affected rib and intensive antibiotic treatment. In the ensuing twenty-five years, her old wound had reopened several times, most recently well over a year before seeing me; although painless and odorless for the most part, it had become a sizeable fistula, oozing a bloody, mucopurulent discharge and requiring constant attention. In view of the extensive bony defect created by the original surgery, further resection was not an option, and she was advised simply to "live with it." Amazingly, her health had remained excellent the whole time.

For the past three years, I have tried every remedy I could think of, including obvious choices like *Calcarea sulph.* and *Silica,* seemingly well-indicated constitutional remedies like *Lycopodium* and *Phosphorus,* and more learned prescriptions like *Radium bromatum.* and *X-Ray* itself; but none of them had the slightest effect on her osteomyelitis, which continued to suppurate as before. About a year ago, I gave her *Gunpowder* 30C, once a day for a few weeks, whereupon the fistula closed over and stopped draining, the scab fell off, and the wound remained clean and dry for the first time in years. Several months later, it reopened and bled a little, but a few doses of *Gunpowder* 200 were enough to help her heal it again; and she has been fine ever since.

* "A Wound Heals -- After 25 Years," ***Homeopathy Today,*** February 2007.

*A Sampling of Animal Cases**

In the following cases, good results were obtained with animal remedies that are less well-known than the usual *Sepia, Lachesis, Apis,* or *Tarentula*.

Snake Remedies.

While *Lachesis* is by far the most familiar of the Ophidians, Mangialavori emphasizes that the other snake remedies should also be considered in animal cases when the main themes of *Lachesis* are prominent:

1) one-sidedness;
2) intolerance of tight clothing;
3) ailments during or after sleep;
4) special affinity for the throat, sinuses, and heart, blood, and blood vessels, with symptoms of constriction, choking, and bleeding and clotting phenomena;
5) ailments from menopause, amenorrhea, or PMS, or those relieved by menstruation, talking, or any discharge;
6) passionate, sexual, and competitive nature; and
7) deadly cunning, deviousness, and psychic ability.

Sharp-Tongued One-Liners.

With a two-year history of amenorrhea, ovarian cysts, and Raynaud's syndrome, a woman of 40 responded well to remedies, but always relapsed after a few months, and eventually new ones had to be found. After two years, her flow was restored, and her Raynaud's had improved a lot; but her periods were still irregular, intermittent, 'stopped up' in the daytime, and fuller and quite painful at night, especially in the right ovary, just as they had been in her twenties, consisting mainly of dark, clotted blood. Two months after *Crotalus horridus* 30C, made from the venom of the Western diamondback rattlesnake, she was much better. With her cramps more manageable, her

* "A Sampling of Animal Cases," ***Homeopathic Links*** (Netherlands) 16:15, Spring 2003.

flow more normal, and her Raynaud's symptoms almost gone, she also felt more positive and energetic in general. Over the next several years her periods were stable for the most part, and she remained quite healthy, apart from minor digestive symptoms for which she came in at rare intervals and did well on other remedies.

After ten years, she came back on the verge of menopause, complaining mostly of feeling depressed and crying all the time, feeling 'aggravated, old, emotional, pale, and washed out', especially before her periods, when her old constipation and right-sided abdominal and lower-back pain were also bothersome. Notwithstanding a good, stable job that she liked and was esteemed and appreciated for, she felt prematurely old and 'used up,' with no lasting accomplishments that she could point to. She also complained of a vague but constant undercurrent of sadness that took on an exaggerated importance because she could find no reason for it.

Looking very snappy in her black leather outfit, she recounted a dream about her sister, a ballet dancer in real life, in which my patient was holding her sister's legs in a headstand and carelessly let go of her, causing a bad fall on her back that left her paralyzed. In part because this admired and talented creature had never done her ill in real life, she castigated herself for feeling envious of the other's success, good fortune, and happy life, and for the repressed wish to harm her, to which the dream bore irrefutable witness.

After a round of *Crotalus horridus* 200, she disappeared for a year and a half, coming back only after a relapse of more or less the same symptoms. Almost forgetting how well she had been for most of that time, she felt weepy and useless again since the Boston Ballet season ended, and with it the opportunity to give freely of her time and energy to something beautiful that she loved and cared about. Although her flow was more normal and her premenstrual symptoms much milder than before, the periods were still regular, and she remained quite emotional and weepy as they approached. Again she accused herself of being 'ungenerous' and 'uncaring,' regretting her predilection for 'sharp-tongued one-liners' that were apt to skewer their unwary victims before she herself realized what she had said. Yet until quite recently, she finally acknowledged, the last remedy had worked 'like a miracle.'

Six weeks after repeating it, she came back excited and hopeful. Although she still felt depressed or sad at times, the episodes were much briefer and less intense, as were the wounding remarks, which were less frequent; and she had even learned to apologize for them at the time. Her stomach and digestive symptoms were almost non-existent. Armed with a vial of the 200 for future use, she still checks in from time to time, every year or two on average.

A Fear of Bleeding to Death.

Attractively and even seductively attired, a 37-year-old housewife and mother of two sought treatment for endometriosis and ovarian cysts, which had recurred repeatedly in spite of four surgical procedures, produced nagging pain in the right groin, and obliged her to sleep on the painful side. Nearly breathless in the telling, she was even more worried about her periods, which gushed out so forcefully that she sometimes feared she would die from the loss of blood.

Ever since the death of her father, she had also suffered panic attacks in theatres, churches, and restaurants, when her heart would pound and force her to leave. In addition, she had lost control of her anger at the children several times to the point that she could easily have hurt them. A lover of animals of all kinds, with a house full of pets of every description, she still had a horror of reptiles that she was anxious to overcome, since both of her kids were excessively fond of snakes.

One month after a dose of *Crotalus cascavella* 200, a South American rattlesnake, there was no major change, except for left ovarian pain in the fourth week that was worse than ever, but with somewhat less bleeding and anxiety. Afraid to wait any longer, I gave *Lycopodium* 200, and after another month she was 'thrilled and amazed' to report that the two largest cysts on the right side had disappeared on her latest ultrasound, leaving only two small ones on the left, for which surgery was unnecessary. Since her periods had also reverted to normal, nothing more was done until her ovarian pain returned two months later, at which point we were uncertain which remedy had acted; so we repeated *Lycopodium* first, with absolutely no effect, and then *Crotalus cascavella* soon after. Within a few days, she was well again. That was more than a year ago, and she has remained well since.

A Second Stroke.

Years after a stroke, for which *Lachesis* had been very helpful, a 75-year-old woman from Maine called when a second one, much more severe, left her with a left hemiparesis that confined her to bed for months, slurred speech, and difficulty swallowing, especially liquids, which choked her and came back out through her nose. She also felt profoundly cold all the time and unable to get warm. This time *Lachesis* failed to improve her speech or swallowing, although her energy and strength revived a little, and as the months passed her recovery was slow and protracted, with little benefit from remedies, until we hit upon *Bothrops lanceolatus*, the venom of the yellow viper or *fer-de-lance,* almost a year later. Within 2 months of a dose of the 200, she was much warmer, stronger, able to walk around, do the dishes, and even swallow milk and soup fairly well, although she still had trouble with water and clear liquids, and her voice remained weak and gravelly.

After repeating the remedy, she continued to improve for the next six months, to our mutual surprise and delight, still avoiding water and speaking little, but no longer slurring her words. After a third dose she felt increasingly positive and optimistic, but her two residual symptoms had not improved much and probably were as good as they were going to get. Although we have since moved on to other remedies, and she continues to recover slowly, we both know that *Bothrops* was the one that turned things around for her and helped her onto a healing path.

Varicose Ulcer.

After years of partly successful homeopathic treatments for hypertension and other complaints, a 69-year-old man first came to see me after a bad fall opened up a large varicose ulcer in his left leg that had not healed in spite of three months' rest and enforced inactivity. His colorful medical history included severe thrombophlebitis of the same leg following an IVP twenty years earlier, which left the whole lower half of the leg blackish, indurated, and chronically swollen, and for which he had been taking Coumadin ever since; but he insisted that it had never really troubled him until now. Since the accident, he complained of stinging pains in the area, especially if he allowed his pants or bedclothes to brush against it, and when lifting the heel to walk or dangling the leg over the arm of a chair.

I gave him the German viper, *Vipera redi* 200, once a week for 3 weeks, and 6 weeks later he reported that the remedy had given him 'a big kick upstairs' in all respects: in addition to the ulcer itself, which had granulated in and scabbed over nicely, a number of aches and pains and several other problems he hadn't even mentioned had also cleared up or at least 'fallen into place.' Even the ugly, black discoloration of long standing had faded to a considerable extent. Because the remedy had acted so beautifully, and he still had a good deal of lower abdominal cramping and gas on waking, I gave him a fourth dose, and repeated the remedy several more times over the following year for whatever ailed him, with splendid results each time.

Headache.

Petite, self-assured, attractive, and well dressed, a 44-year-old business-woman came in for treatment of severe headaches in her temples, especially the left, with nausea and extreme fatigue. They began not long after selling her cosmetics business for a tidy sum, when she learned that the buyers were engaged in unethical practices that went against her core values. Previously ambitious and unsparing of her personal life, she had already benefited a lot from remedies; but now, having accomplished almost everything she had worked for, other facets of her nature were demanding her attention. A lover of dogs and horses, she had recently met a man who lived on a ranch out west and contemplated leaving the area to stay with him after years of hardly dating at all.

Extremely intolerant of wearing anything tight around the neck, she felt as if her whole left side were out of balance and her skin was stretched too tight on her frame. Within two days after a dose of cobra venom, *Naja tripudians* 200, her headaches were gone, and they have not come back for over three years. Since leaving the area to live with her boyfriend, she has consulted me for other complaints and taken other remedies, but has remained quite well.

Insect remedies.

As with the snakes, in this first insect case I was led to the correct prescription because the clinical picture closely resembled that of *Apis melifica,* the honeybee, the most familiar remedy of the group, which helped her quite a bit at first, but failed to cure.

Stiletto-like Pains.

With virtually her entire face disfigured by clusters of itchy, bright-red pustules, a 41-year-old wife and mother came in desperate for relief. In the midst of her third such episode in as many years, what began with a few small lesions had rapidly grown and spread into ever-larger confluent patches that left very little normal skin in between. Worst of all, she was being tormented day and night by nasty stiletto-like pains that were hot, itchy, and stinging, rather like bee bites, as well as worse from heat and better from ice, and that often made her irritable and angry at everyone and everything, especially her husband and children, and unable to concentrate on or even think about anything else.

Repeatedly plagued by impetigo since early childhood, at thirteen she contracted severe chicken pox, followed by another persistent *Staphylococcus i*nfection. In college, she developed eczema with a similar propensity to boil formation that obliged her to resort to antibiotics several times. But her skin didn't flare up really badly until after the death of her father, a talented and attractive man who had been convicted of fraud, done jail time for arson, and finally left home at her mother's insistence when my patient was in her twenties. Ever since the pregnancy and birth of her second son, the outbreaks had become pustular and occurred in crops involving large areas of her face. The boy was three years old at the time I first saw her.

Although happily married to a 'wonderful' husband whom she adored and often fantasized about in sexually explicit dreams, she disliked having intercourse and typically refused his advances. This peculiar state of affairs she traced back to the age of 24, when she aborted his child but vowed to abstain from further sex outside of a fully-committed relationship; that vow had ripened into an aversion that persisted even after they were married, and indeed right up to the present, like an old grudge that for some profound but inscrutable reason she could neither forgive nor set aside.

The first remedy I chose was *Apis mellifica* 200, which worked very well for a time, and even helped to restore her sexual desire briefly, a respite for which both she and her husband were most grateful. But she could tell that the remedy wore off after dental work a few months later, and with her sister and brother-in-law moving in for the last trimester of a high-risk pregnancy, she was too preoccupied with them to travel down from Maine to see me. Indeed, she didn't tell me any of this until coming back over a year later, after her sister had given birth and moved out, when her skin flared up worse than ever, and a self-prescribed course of *Apis* 30C was only slightly beneficial.

When *Tarentula cubensis* 200 also gave no relief, I went back to *Apis* 200, which again helped, but not nearly as much as before. Meanwhile, she had developed a huge, painful boil behind her right ear, her eczema drove her to scratch and tear at her legs for brief periods every day, and large crops of new pustules had appeared that stung as intensely as the time she was attacked by a swarm of yellow-jackets in her teens.

This new bit of history led me to study *Vespa crabro,* the hornet, and I gave her the 200, three doses in 24 hours, followed by one dose weekly for up to two more weeks as needed, with dramatic results. Within 24 hours her whole face was flaming red and hugely swollen, 'as if I'd been stung by ten bees', followed by rapid disappearance of the pain, redness, swelling, and other signs of infection. At her next visit, six weeks later, she reported that her skin looked clearer and felt better than it had in a very long time, and that her libido had been reawakened as well. While it is still too early in her treatment to predict the outcome, I feel confident that her improvement on this remedy will continue for a long time to come.

Ulcerative Colitis.

With a long history of ulcerative colitis, for which I had treated her very successfully with *Staphysagria* at long intervals for the past ten years, a 39-year-old Icelandic woman came back for a relapse that didn't respond to either sulfasalazine or the remedy, which by then she knew very well how to take for herself. With her symptoms felt mostly low down in the rectum, she was passing chunks of tissue along with bright-red blood and pus in her stools. The sensation she described as 'like a hole in there, with something percolating in it!' Peppy and energetic, even 'hyper' to most people, she had lost ten pounds in recent months, and seemed quite worried about it, as was I. My next suggestion, *Mercurius vivus,* worked to some extent, but she had continued bleeding moderate amounts on most days, especially after a large meal.

First coming to the United States as a nanny, she had travelled, lived, and worked in poor, underdeveloped, underserved areas in Africa and Latin America, always teaching school or doing research, never settling down in any one area for too long. With family in Northern Europe, friends in America, a house in Mexico, and a job in Africa, she lived her whole life 'out of two suitcases,' and was currently teaching high school kids for almost no pay in a church school in the Namibian bush. She said that it was like a dream come true, but she was no longer so sure she still wanted it.

A biologist by training, an adventurer by temperament, and a missionary in her zeal for good works, she had dreamed of Africa ever since reading the story of Tarzan as a child; but now, nearing forty, with most of her friends married and having children, she often wondered if she had missed out by letting these opportunities pass her by. With a fierce passion for elephants, 'big, wise, good, strong, and beautiful, the best mothers,' she expected her ideal man to be the strong one, but insisted on being 'the queen, the only one' for him, and certainly would never be willing to share him with other women. However tempted to marry and settle down in one place with a regular 9-to-5 job, she dreaded most of all being 'trapped inside four walls and a mortgage' with a man she couldn't trust and no good means of escape.

A serious alcoholic in the past, she had sworn off liquor years ago, but still went on rampages at times, flying into a rage, picking fights with men twice her size, and even, she boasted, fracturing several noses thus far. In addition, she felt more irritable and aggressive than usual, even with her students, whom she dearly loved most of the time, and hurled such foul abuse at them that one dignified 16-year-old protested, 'Even my mother wouldn't talk to me like that!' The remedy I chose was the Spanish fly, *Cantharis vesicatoria*, and many months after a dose of the 200 she wrote me a letter from the bush:

"Hallelujah! I have started the first black AA group in the country. Please pray for it, since I'm certain that the guy with the pitchfork doesn't want us to succeed. Despite the Angolan civil war across the river, and the AIDS epidemic, our little school scored the

second highest in the country! As for follow-up, Cantharis *works 100%! I have had symptoms only once since returning to Africa, and that due to self-indulgence, a huge meal eaten way too fast. After so many remedies, including African ones, this one did the trick. Thank you!"*

Mammalian Remedies.

Chronic Bronchitis.

Brought in by her grandmother for chronic bronchitis that often lasted all winter, a chubby, red-faced girl of five seemed quite pleasant at first, but sniffled and sulked whenever she felt left out of the history-taking. Raised by her grandmother, both parents had been drug addicts and were murdered when she was a small baby. Described as 'a happy child who got along with everyone,' she constantly blew her nose and hawked up quantities of thick, green mucus from her throat, and still wet the bed at night. When she smiled, I noticed that most of her upper teeth were rudimentary, brown-stained, and broken off in places. Her eyes turned in, alternating from side to side, and she craved salt, milk, and dairy, and was quite allergic to cats.

One month after a round of *Calcarea sulphurica* 200, she was no better, sniffling loudly as she arrived, this time wearing a sweatshirt literally crowded with pictures of dogs of every description. I gave her the remedy made from dogs' milk, *Lac caninum* 1M, and by her third visit she was greatly improved, rarely coughing at all since a bad spell the second night after the remedy, only wetting the bed once every few weeks, and breathing much more easily through her nose. Six months later, I repeated the remedy for the fall season, and that winter was her best to date, with no bronchitis, minimal coughing, and even her residual sinus congestion had subsided to the extent that the grandmother felt no further need of remedies. I haven't seen her for more than three years, but another patient and friend of the family assures me that she is thriving.

Man's best friend.

Constitutionally, *Lac caninum* is often thought of for a character and temperament reminiscent of 'man's best friend,' the animal of whom T. S. Eliot says:

Now dogs pretend they like to fight;
They often bark, more seldom bite;
But yet a dog is, on the whole,

What you would call a simple soul.
The usual Dog about the Town
Is much inclined to play the clown,
And far from showing too much pride,
Is frequently undignified.
He's very easily taken in —
Just chuck him underneath the chin
Or slap his back or shake his paw,
And he will gambol and guffaw.
He's such an easy-going lout,
He'll answer any hail or shout.

Subdued, repressed, and often abused, like dogs and other domesticated species, patients benefited by *Lac caninum* may become angry and aggressive if mistreated or scorned, but ultimately crave the approval and affection of their masters, in part because of a low opinion of themselves.

Migraine Headaches.

Described as a 'saint' by a close friend accompanying her, a 62-year-old librarian looking at least ten years older came in for treatment of migraine headaches, which she had had ever since her teens. Typically precipitated or aggravated by any stress or emotional misunderstanding, they began with the illusion of flashing lights over either eye that soon crossed over to the other side, were followed by sharp, knifelike pain that did the same, were sensitive to both light and noise, and obliged her to go to sleep.

Usually cool or on the chilly side, she reacted poorly to cold wind, and often got headaches before a big storm, as well as feeling nervous and apprehensive from lightning. Freaked by all snakes, she could not wear anything tight around her neck, craved milk and salt, and avoided wine because of her headaches. Cheerful by nature, she was perfectly happy being alone and quiet, and seemed hesitant to speak, but wrote the following description of herself in reply to my questionnaire:

"At one week of age was adopted by a Minister, a wonderful, saintly man, and brought up with older people in a very subdued atmosphere, but with excellent values. Not allowed to play with other children, so remained shy and unsocial. I love children a lot. I'm shy, avoid conflict and disagreement (my husband has an awful temper!) and sleep a lot. I have strong religious views, and all the family attend Church regularly."

Years later I learned that her husband had cruelly and repeatedly beaten and abused her to such an extent that their daughters, both patients of mine, had never forgiven him for it. As yet ignorant of these details, I chose *Lac caninum* 200, and it 'worked like a charm' for half a year, during which time she had very few headaches and was able to abort them with the 12C.

At her next visit, 10 months later, they were back, and she took another dose, followed by a third seven months after that. Ten years passed before she returned, this time for severe bruising from mosquito bites, probably on account of taking anticoagulants for thrombophlebitis. By then her migraines were long gone, although she still had sinus headaches occasionally before a storm, craved salt as always, and had recently noticed a salty taste in her mouth most of the time. Repeating *Lac caninum* 200 a fourth time, she called 2 months later to say that her new problem had also cleared up. That was our last contact, over 4 years ago, but I hear from her family that she has remained in good health.

Asthma.

A 13-year-old boy came in for treatment of asthma, which he had had for three years, since his parents had bought and remodeled an old house full of dust, mold, and crumbling insulation. Limited at first to the autumn months, his condition had actually worsened on regular drug therapy, such that when I saw him he was having severe symptoms all year round in spite of a daily routine of Albuterol, Singulair, and inhaled corticosteroids, plus oral prednisone for two acute flareups in the past year alone.

Tormented by congestion and vain attempts to clear his throat throughout the day, he had a violent fit of coughing as soon as he lay down in bed for the night; it sounded wet and even rattling, but he raised sputum only by vomiting, and the whole process left him hoarse, stridulous, and gasping for breath afterwards. Otherwise he had been and remained in good health, and his parents described him as sensitive, affectionate, and beloved by family and friends alike.

The remedy I chose was *Mephitis* 200, made from the malodorous secretion of the skunk, 3 doses in 24 hours, up to once a week thereafter, and also in water as needed for acute symptoms, up to four times in a day, with vigorous succussion each time. At his first follow-up, 4 weeks later, he reported that he had stopped all his medications within a few days on his own initiative, because they made his symptoms worse, and hadn't taken or needed any since. Although he continued to have symptoms, especially in bed and during and after exercise, they were milder and no longer kept him from practicing karate, skiing with his dad, or sleeping well at night. His peak flows had also risen to about 300 on average, which had been at the very top of his range before.

The main problem was his mother's constant need for reassurance, which was quite understandable in view of his unilateral decision to stop all medications, despite his lung specialist's dire warnings, and without consulting me either. I gave him another dose of the remedy, with instructions to continue using it as needed, up to once a week, as well as in water as before. Six weeks later, he had improved even further, to the point that he seldom coughed or needed to clear his throat at all, had skied for two full days without any symptoms at all, and had achieved even higher peak flows, once reaching 400 and generally averaging around 350.

At our next visit in late spring, 3 months later, he had had some throat symptoms and mild coughing with the flowers in bloom, but refused to take any asthma medications or even measure his peak flows, a procedure which he associated with them. Continuing with the same regimen of *Mephitis* 200 occasionally, and in water as needed in between, he has truly blossomed in the past year and a half, with no symptoms at all for weeks and even months at a time. Recently we moved on to other remedies when he developed a cold with no asthma and a dry cough for which *Mephitis* was totally ineffective, a good sign that this least favorite chapter of his life had finally come to an end.

Force-Feeding.

Treated intermittently and mostly successfully with *Sepia* and other remedies for miscellaneous complaints over a period of years, a divorced woman of 36 first came to see me for the vague but intense discomfort of her colon 'backing up,' such that she couldn't get food down properly at times, rice would stick in her throat, or she would regurgitate the food she had just eaten, especially muffins and pasta. Together with the associated feeling of 'toxins building up' in her body, these symptoms always reminded her of her childhood, when her father tried to force her to eat vegetables and got very angry and abusive if she refused. As a result of this bullying, the experience of eating became unpleasant for her in general, especially during her marriage, when she would have to eat with her husband, although it had been less of an issue since leaving and finally divorcing him.

Even earlier, as an infant, she recalled fighting similar battles over toilet training with her mother, who forced her to sit on the potty for long periods even as a baby, and later shamed her with the standard fable that she had smeared her feces all over the walls as if in protest. Never allowed any privacy for moving her bowels even as an older child, she still feared that someone would come in whenever she went to the toilet. As the family scapegoat, she was punished whenever her siblings got hurt, and for most everything that went wrong in the household; in her teens she decoded the underlying message that anything pleasurable or sexual was automatically filthy, disgusting, or shameful.

Based on this and other information, I gave her *Ambra grisea* 200, made from ambergris, an intestinal secretion of the sperm whale, and did not see or hear from her again for 8 months, during which time she had moved far away to keep as much distance as possible from her ex-husband. By then her symptoms of choking and reflux had lessened considerably, and she felt a 'shift' not only in her digestion and bowels, but above all in her primary symptom of feeling backed up with toxins. Now she was suffering mainly emotionally, with PMS, but along much the same lines, so I repeated *Ambra grisea,* and once again it acted beautifully. In 2 months, she came back looking a bit puffy and overweight, but much calmer and more positive about herself, despite relapsing a bit before her last period. Giving her another dose of the 200, I then lost track of her for another 5-month stretch, through most of which she felt much better, as I found out later, in fact 'settled, balanced, and pretty normal, really!'

Having relapsed again in recent weeks to some extent, she was given *Ambra grisea* 1M, and I've not seen her again in nearly 4 years; but she recently called back to say that she was feeling fine and has not needed or taken the remedy again.

Multiple Fibroadenomas.

With a history of benign fibroadenomas of the breast and four surgeries to remove them, a 46-year-old artist came in in pain from a fifth, seeking relief and a way to prevent them in the future. As big as an egg and growing rapidly, it felt heavy and sore 'like a lump of lead' if she moved too fast, but could no longer be related precisely to her menstrual cycle, ever since her hysterectomy years ago for multiple fibroid tumors of the uterus and ovaries as well.

In addition, she had had chronic back pain since being thrown from a horse in her teens and crushing three lumbar vertebræ, but her fractures all healed nicely, and she never stopped riding, having grown up with horses as a child, still felt mystically drawn to them, and featured them in her paintings as well.

After years of smoking pot in her teens and a major lesbian relationship in her twenties, at 25 she became a born-again Christian, still believed in angels and sensed Christ's presence in the world, but favored Buddhist meditation to dispel her fear that she was really a 'witch' on account of mystical experiences like ESP and soul travel. Nor could she deny the existence of a darker side to her nature, such as robustly hating her ex-husband for neglecting to pay her back for her share of the property once he had persuaded her to sign it all over to him.

But hardest of all to exorcise was the rage she felt at sexually and physically abusive relationships in her family, which had driven her mother and brother insane, and left her and the other children to be cared for by a succession of foster parents when her father moved out. Alone in the woods for long periods of time, she saw herself as an Indian brave riding her pony in the wilderness, not a proper little girl winning ribbons in horse shows, as her grandmother intended. Lean and lanky, with a long, graceful neck, two buck teeth jutting out in front, and a strong craving for lumps of pure cane sugar, even in her physique and constitution she seemed to embody the image and archetype of the horse as a kind of personal totem.

With not much else to go on, I decided to try *Lac equinum* 200, mare's milk, and within 6 weeks neither she nor her gynecologist could palpate the cyst. In some respects the interview itself had had a powerful effect, she felt, especially when she heard herself exaggerating her rage in order to describe it. Since then she had felt much calmer on the whole, substituting fruit for her lumps of sugar, and remaining in good health otherwise. I've not seen her for three years, but she recently phoned to tell me that her cysts and tumors have never come back, and that she has remained in good health and hasn't needed remedies for any reason.

A Case of Palliation.

In conclusion, I can't resist presenting this case, even though several remedies were needed, not all of them animal, and the patient was much too far gone for me to help him in any profound way.

Almost boasting of his long history of emphysema, gastritis, and two-pack-a-day cigarette habit, a much-older-looking man of 56 hobbled in on crutches, daring me to 'SAVE MY TOE!' in a jaunty, almost flippant tone, although his prospects were certainly no laughing matter. Ten days earlier, after stubbing his right fourth toe, it had become ulcerated and then promptly turned gangrenous. By the time I saw it, the tip and under side were swollen and completely black, with severe burning and cutting pains radiating out from it whenever he lifted the foot to walk or tried to dangle it over the side of a chair.

My first remedy was *Vipera redi* 200, three doses in 24 hours, and within a week he was able to walk a little more easily, and the blackened area was much smaller and less painful, although it still hurt a good deal at times, especially in cold air and from going too long without eating. Switching to *Carbo animalis* 200, made from charred oxhide, I saw him again in two weeks, by which time the whole toe appeared normal except for a small black spot on the tip that looked ready to slough off, and it hurt only when covered with a sock or blanket. On that indication I gave him ergot, the rye-fungus, *Secale cornutum* 200, and after 3 more weeks the whole toe and foot were no longer discolored or painful, except for stinging pains and blue discoloration whenever the leg was dangled.

So I came back to *Vipera*, and again the 200 acted beautifully; the toe was indeed saved. But I leveled with him and his wife that gangrene indicated a serious underlying vascular pathology that could itself be fatal, and urged him to come back for constitutional treatment and to remain under close medical supervision. This prudent advice he chose to ignore, since he felt well enough to go back to work, and the toe seemed entirely healed.

In six months, he was back, this time short of breath even at rest, and especially from overeating and hot, humid weather. Despite considerable help from *Carbo vegetabilis* 200, he was soon hospitalized with congestive heart failure, and placed on digitalis, heparin, bronchodilators, diuretics, oxygen, and prednisone, and still developed osteomyelitis with deep bone pains in his bad leg. Calling long distance, he nevertheless continued to insist that he was quite well and in no real danger. On the strength of that I gave him *Arnica* 200, which worked splendidly for a few weeks each time, but I never saw or spoke to him again.

Two years later, his wife called to tell me that he had recently died in his sleep, and that of all his treatments "only the remedies really helped!"

*A 42-Year-Old Man with Bronchiectasis, Among Other Things**

Naturally, we homeopaths love to present cases cured of serious organic pathology with our remedies. Nor can we be blamed for omitting the vastly more numerous cases where our learned prescriptions fail, since "anecdotal evidence" of cured cases, while held in low repute throughout the rest of the profession, is almost the only way that we can teach and learn what our remedies are really like, as well as almost everything else that we know. That is because we do not treat "diseases," of which the patient is but a specimen, but *illnesses*, which are unique expressions of the individuality of the patient, and the remedies have to match or at least approximate that uniqueness as closely as possible.

So this is not simply a case of bronchiectasis, but that of a 42-year-old man who *has* this disease, along with plenty of other things. I should also preface it by saying that his is no "cured" case by any means, nor is it likely to be, and that in addition to bronchiectasis his varied diagnoses and complaints include asthma, allergies, GERD, and a cough of several years' duration, with considerable quantities of sputum, from which *M. kansasii* and *M. szulgai,* two species of atypical mycobacteria, were recently cultured.

His story really began with a prolonged episode of osteomyelitis of the lumbar spine in 2002, which improved substantially after seven weeks of intensive antibiotic treatment, but required changing the formula several times because of abnormal liver enzymes, fever, nausea, and vomiting after Dicloxacillin, Vancomycin, and Cipro. Even so, the osteomyelitis did not subside completely until the cough in effect replaced it several months later. At first rather mild, and without any other signs of illness, in November of 2003 it developed into a severe bronchopneumonia in both lungs that

* "A 42-Year-Old Man with Bronchiectasis, Among Other Things," ***American Journal of Homeopathic Medicine*** 102:78, Summer 2009.

left him with bronchiectasis and an increased susceptibility to these other infections, both of which have continued ever since.

By then, although less severe than it had been at its height, the cough still sounded wet, and produced quantities of thick, greenish-yellow phlegm, often stringy or globular, and with a sweetish taste. Especially productive after breakfast, and to some extent after other meals and from taking a deep breath, it was often accompanied by hawking of the same kind of sputum from his throat, and flu-ish feelings of malaise, especially during and after his frequent colds and acute flare-ups, when all of his symptoms were exacerbated.

In the course of his allopathic treatment, serial CT-scans revealed a number of diffuse, migratory lung infiltrates, and pulmonary function tests indicated a moderate degree of asthma and chronic obstructive pulmonary disease, for which he took Serevent 50 mcg. and QVAR 40 mcg. twice a day, all year round.

One month before seeing me, atypical mycobacteria were identified in his sputum, and he was offered a 12- to 18-month course of antituberculous treatment. But in view of its substantial risk of side effects, with no guarantee of benefit and the likelihood of recurrence in any case, he became intrigued by what he read about homeopathy, and decided to give it a try.

His eventful medical history also included

1) a major car accident at age 7, in which he sustained fractures of the pelvis and both legs;

2) a severe case of chickenpox at 16;

3) migraine headaches with visual aura ever since puberty, which had not bothered him much lately; and

4) intermittent signs and symptoms of GERD for the past several years.

These last consisted not of heartburn, but a dry, scratchy, and often paroxysmal cough on lying down at night, which was aggravated by drinking beer and eating chocolate, forced him to sit erect, and ended in gagging or retching. After obtaining some relief from Omeprazole, he resolved to heal himself naturally, obtained even better results with vegetable juices and apple cider vinegar, and for some time had not needed the drug at all. His family history was notable for lung cancer, malignant brain tumor, and Hodgkin's disease on his mother's side, and emphysema and cancer of unknown type on his father's.

When I first saw him, in October 2007, he complained of inward pressure on his lungs and chest at times, "like someone standing on top of me," but was not short of breath, and exercised daily, strenuously, and almost obsessively to keep fit. In a hoarse, raspy voice, with frequent clearing of his throat, he described himself as a "worrier," a nervous wreck about tests in school, which he always did well on, and a "neat freak," intolerant of a messy desk and incapable of leaving the dishes unwashed overnight, while his wife was of quite the opposite disposition. From feeling at odds and quarreling with her over these and other matters, their affection for each other had rather dimmed of late, but he loved being a father to his 7-year-old son, and he generally liked his work as Senior Editor of a mid-sized publishing firm. He preferred eating small meals often, reacted badly to meat, chocolate, beer, and overeating, and wilted in summer and the hot, humid weather.

I did not interrogate him sufficiently to extract any "vital sensation," and found no striking mental or "strange, rare, and peculiar" symptoms or exotic, little-known remedies to break open the case. What impressed me the most were prosaic things like the quantity and character of the sputum, his strong family history of cancer, and his marked fastidiousness and other traits suggestive of the cancer miasm. I chose *Kali bichromicum* 200, once a week, for up to 3 weeks if necessary, but with instructions to stop after the first or second dose if he noticed a definite improvement by then.

In six weeks he returned for his first follow-up. "Quite good!" was the verdict, which he announced with no little solemnity. Since his asthma and bronchial symptoms were better after the first dose, he never took a second. By the third week, he had cut his drugs in half, from twice daily to once, and the pressure on his chest continued to lessen. His sinus congestion had actually gotten worse, with snoring, which he'd never done before; fits of sneezing and blowing; and culminating in a nasty sinus headache that made him dizzy. Yet by the time I saw him again, the quantity of phlegm was greatly reduced, the snoring had largely subsided, the cough was all but gone, and his peak flows had already improved quite a bit. Naturally, my prescription was to wait.

At his next visit, two months later, he was proud of having stopped all medications soon after our previous visit, while his peak flows had held their own and even attained record levels at times, and the pressure on his chest had disappeared. Even with a brief and relatively mild episode of shortness of breath during a recent cold snap, he experienced no wheezing and needed no drugs to relieve it. Meanwhile, his sinus condition had improved dramatically, his wife no longer complained of his snoring, and he felt generally healthier than in a very long time. There was still some thick phlegm, but it was greatly reduced, and no longer had any color. Perhaps most interesting of all was how much calmer and more relaxed he felt, as his wife was delighted to point out. So we waited some more. I failed to persuade him to go back to the lung specialist and repeat the tests, after he read online that one CT-scan emitted as much radiation as 500 chest X-rays.

That was in January of 2008. I didn't see him again until December, in response to my letter suggesting a return visit. "Great, really," was his qualified assessment this time, citing his clogged sinuses, hawking of thick, whitish phlegm, and frequent, sometimes forceful sneezing, which had bothered him somewhat throughout the fall. Yet he remained drug-free, and his asthma and wheezing were gone. Although he did feel short of breath during spring and fall allergy season, with somewhat lower peak flows, it never happened during exercise. He had had only one cold in all that time, which he attributed to lack of sleep, and with the help of *Kali bichromicum* 12 it subsided much more rapidly than he had expected. The biggest change was the buyout of his firm by a large publishing house, which allowed him to keep his old job, but only by working longer hours, resulting in loss of sleep and the return of some old symptoms from long ago, anxiety at being "rushed," and palpitations in bed at night, both of which were worse from thinking about them. So I gave him a second dose of *Kali bichromicum* 200.

His last visit was in late February 2009, just a month ago, and again he reported a major improvement soon after taking the remedy. By the next day, the sputum was clear and much reduced, and when I saw him it was "90% better, only a touch from time to time." Although he still snored at times, with some nasal congestion in the daytime, he was able to blow it out easily, with minimal blockage, and his postnasal drip was gone. Still he had had no drugs for over a year, his asthma was gone, and his allergies were "hardly an issue." In spite of having been given a raise, he was still working longer hours, feeling rushed, and in need of more sleep, but his anxiety had lessened considerably, even after a valued colleague was let go. The only dream he could remember was a vivid and scary one in which his car was "speeding out of control." At the end of the visit, he thanked me, saying, "It's amazing how well this remedy suits me!" I gave him nothing further.

I need hardly add that he is far from cured. Bronchiectasis typically involves necrosis, scarring, and thickening of the bronchial wall, while mycobacteria are themselves notoriously difficult to get rid of, and his obstinate refusal to undergo more PFT's makes it almost impossible to know for certain that his improvement extends beyond the symptomatic level. Although certainly improved, even his symptoms are by no means gone. I tell his story mainly because he does have an obstinate infection with atypical mycobacteria, in a setting of advanced and quite possibly irreversible structural pathology, to show the degree of improvement that is attainable with familiar homeopathic remedies prescribed in the good old-fashioned way, which is still the way I do it most of the time, notwithstanding all of the valuable improvements of recent years, for which I am also very grateful. In short, we need all the help we can get.

III. Political Statements.

"The Great Malpractice Scandal"

"On Lay Prescribing"

President's Message, 1985

President's Message, 1986

"NCH Goals and Objectives"

"Hospital Ethics Committees"

"Ethics in Homeopathic Practice"

"Who Needs the AIH?"

"To Have and Have Not: Homeopathy in Cuba"

"The AIH Bioterrorism Project," Excerpts

"Advisory on Bird Flu"

*The Great Malpractice Scandal**

As many of you know Dr. Matt Kelly, Dr. Florence Khedroo, and I face immediate dismissal from the Medical Staff of St. Vincent's Hospital for refusing to buy malpractice insurance. All of us have lived and practiced here for a long time and are already well known to many of you. Most of what we have to offer is a lot of education, advice, simple caring, and a minimum of high-risk intervention. We appeal to the people of Santa Fe to persuade the hospital not to take this action against us and our patients.

The hospital claims that its insurance premiums have gone up because of uninsured physicians on the staff, but they have never produced any evidence that this has in fact happened, or that it ever would happen. The truth is exactly the opposite. None of us has ever been sued; yet we are being compelled to underwrite *their* malpractice risk, which is already the talk of the town and growing more serious all the time.

We do not oppose malpractice insurance simply because it costs too much. It costs too much because of the kind of medical practice that it promotes, including the extra diagnostic and treatment procedures that it requires, and the mutual fear and distrust that it engenders between doctors and patients. Malpractice insurance means high-cost, high-tech, high-risk medicine: that's why we want no part of it; and we believe that once you understand how it works, you'll want no part of it either. It sounds like a simple financial scheme to compensate the injured patient without putting the doctor out of business. Physicians are asked to pay a certain annual premium based on their individual malpractice risk, as determined by the company. Their combined premiums, plus the income made from investing them, then constitute a fund out of which all successful malpractice claims can be paid.

Malpractice insurance certainly protects the doctor and the hospital in several important ways. First, it secures their personal and corporate incomes against litigation by guaranteeing that all claims will be paid out of the special fund. Second, it shields them from possible criminal

---

* "The Great Malpractice Scandal," ***The Santa Fe Reporter,*** April 16, 1981.

penalties if they are convicted, and allows them to continue practicing, although their premiums may go up, and they may be required to modify their practices and submit to a period of probation by the company. Third, it is an extremely profitable investment in its own right. The initial outlay is steep, but this is soon made up many times over by the much greater volume of hospitalizations and diagnostic and treatment procedures that are called for and the much higher fees that can be commanded for them. In the case of the physician-owned companies, like Physicians Mutual of New Mexico, the premiums themselves also constitute a tax-free mutual investment fund, which can then generate considerable new income for the company if the amount of successful claims against it can be kept sufficiently small.

It is often said that malpractice insurance also protects patients by guaranteeing that they will receive adequate compensation if they are injured. But the victims of malpractice are people who have already been maimed or killed. The kind of protection they needed was the kind they didn't get, an open, honest communication with their physicians and a clear sharing of responsibility for their own health care. The insurance company is merely a fund to buy off the victim quietly, so that business can go on as usual, and the basic philosophy of medical care that it underwrites will go unexamined and unchanged.

A recent study of a major university hospital found that 36% of all patients admitted there suffered from at least one iatrogenic or doctor-caused complication at some point during their stay, and that 25% of these complications were serious or life-threatening. The authors were also able to show that these risks had nothing to do with the kinds of drugs prescribed or the specific diagnostic or surgical procedures performed, but only with the number of such transactions with the medical system, regardless of their specific content. In other words, the risk of death or serious injury to a patient has much less to do with how well or badly medicine is practiced than simply with *how much* it is practiced.

As the law presently defines it, malpractice is a *mistake,* an act of human error, whether through negligence, incompetence, poor judgment, or simple inadvertence on the part of a physician, resulting in death or serious injury to the patient. Naturally, mistakes will occur in any system, and especially in one where the technology is complex and dangerous to begin with, and requires a high level of skill and training to use it properly.

But the vast majority of malpractice cases are of quite a different type, involving suffering or disability caused by drugs, surgery, and other procedures that are inherently dangerous, even when prescribed and administered on the usual indications and in accordance with commonly accepted standards of the time. In such cases the doctors and hospitals are almost always acquitted, and the victim is left without any compensation whatsoever. Far from protecting the patient, malpractice insurance is one of the most important reasons why the vast majority of such lawsuits are unsuccessful.

Here's a simple example. If a gynecologist performs a hysterectomy and leaves a hemostat in the wound or severs a ureter, that's malpractice, and the patient will probably collect if she survives and can still afford an attorney. But if the surgery is performed competently and the patient dies of an allergic reaction to the anesthetic or from a hospital-acquired infection, her death will be dismissed as simply an unfortunate accident, as indeed it is, and the doctors and the hospital will never have to take responsibility for it.

Why is our present medical system so dangerous? Primarily for two reasons. The first is that our technology is designed primarily to manipulate specific life processes and suppress or control certain isolated abnormalities and mechanical causes or factors of disease, without any coherent or unified vision of human life that could guide or restrain us in its use. The result is a formidable array of deadly biological weapons, each with the power to kill, maim, or create even stronger physiological dependencies than the original illness and thus keep patients trapped within the system.

This is evident in the case of the woman just mentioned, who had her uterus removed, let us suppose, because of a fibroid tumor growing within the muscular wall. We have the technical capability to remove her uterus, but not the deeper understanding of life that would make it a comparatively simple matter to assist her in healing such a basic process. That is why no one could accuse her physician of acting in any way contrary to the state of the art at the present time.

Simply a corollary of the first, the second reason is that our medical technology is by no means freely available to the public, but rather a major industrial commodity, marketed and sold exclusively for the profit of the companies that produce it, the hospitals that administer it, and the doctors who prescribe it. Patients are the ultimate consumer of these goods and services, yet may purchase them only as part of an approved diagnostic and treatment program, in which case it becomes mandatory to purchase them. In this manner, they are reduced to mere specimens of their disease and passive recipients of its treatment, with only nominal power to give or withhold consent, but not to supervise or control the treatment.

Thus in a very real sense, the patient stands alone against the entire medical system, with every reason to be afraid of it, no effective protection against it, and a malpractice suit after the fact as his or her only available recourse. To that extent, the so-called malpractice "crisis" must also be understood as an expression of the growing resentment of patients against the doctors and hospitals upon whom their lives so precariously depend.

For exactly the same reasons, the insurance company is ultimately a threat us all, doctors as well as patients, because by deciding which doctors it will insure and how much it will charge them, which practices it will defend and which it will settle out of court for, this huge for-profit industry has come to exert a decisive and largely destructive influence over how medicine is actually practiced.

As we've already seen, when actually faced with a malpractice suit, the insurance company does not have to prove that the standards of practice observed by its clients are safe or effective, but merely that they exist and are generally known, accepted, and adhered to. Yet our medical practice system is largely a euphemism for a heterogeneous collection of techniques with only a certain methodology to unite them, so that doctors are quite often unable and unwilling to agree on which practices are acceptable and which are not.

In the face of this confusion the insurance companies, particularly the physician-owned companies like Physicians Mutual of New Mexico, have tried to fill the void simply by creating their own standards, loosely based on the record of their member clients in court and their own corporate motives, and then enforcing them by investigation and even intimidation and blackmail of applicant doctors seeking to qualify for malpractice "protection."

The way this is done is quite simple. Instead of being computed from actuarial tables, the malpractice risk of each applicant is determined individually by a lengthy investigation that covers not only the nature of each practice, but even personal and sexual habits, other details regarding their lifestyle, and so forth. So-called "risk factors" could be almost anything from an unsubstantiated rumor of homosexuality or an extramarital love affair to an arrest on narcotics charges that were later dropped, or a tendency to prefer unorthodox methods like megavitamin therapy, biofeedback, or meditation instead of conventional drugs and surgery.

Moreover, the insurance company's threats are apt to be quite persuasive, because physicians understand that what they are buying into is the probability that they will be acquitted of any malpractice charges, provided they adhere fairly strictly to the required standards and guidelines, however expensive or dangerous they may be to the patient, and however repugnant to their physicians.

Under these circumstances, the insurance company is usually able to persuade its applicants to practice in conformity to its standards; in many cases they are simply internalized and projected by the individual doctor without even having to be formulated explicitly. Let us suppose, for example, that a physician is consulted for headache, and it appears to be tension-related. The probability that it could be a brain tumor may be 1% or less; but knowing he could be in big trouble if he missed it, the physician might well decide to hospitalize such a patient, consult a neurologist, and obtain a CAT scan, just to make sure.

In this way he effectively limits his liability by sharing it liberally with his colleagues, while his patient receives an enormous bill, very little useful information, and a treatment that at best merely suppresses the symptom temporarily. For the woman with the fibroid, there is always the suspicion that the tumor could be cancerous, in which case it could have metastasized already, or could even do so later as a result of the surgery. But the gynecologist would want to remove it in any case, because that is what he or she knows how to do, that is the policy recently advocated in the literature, and the insurance company can more easily defend the treatment that everybody else is advocating, whatever the outcome, than either not treating or simply admitting that we do not understand what cancer is, much less how to fix it, which is the plain truth. In this way the insurance company has effectively replaced the critical judgment and moral conscience of the individual physician with the corporate standards of high-cost, high-tech, high-risk medicine.

I myself practice classical homeopathy, using small doses of herbs and other medicines to try to strengthen the natural self-healing capacity of the patient, rather than using large doses of chemicals to suppress individual symptoms; and I also help women to give birth naturally at home, again without the use of drugs or surgery whenever possible.

Six years ago, shortly after coming to Santa Fe, I visited Dr. Harry Ellis, then the President of Physicians Mutual, as well as a past President of the New Mexico Medical Society and a former trustee of St. Vincent's Hospital, to find out if the company would in fact be willing to insure my rather unusual practice. He replied by calling me a quack, and several other even pithier epithets that I will leave unmentioned. This man could dismiss my entire career, my years of evolution as a healer and a student of the natural world, because he had arrogated to himself the authority to decide that what Physicians Mutual believes, and what he and his companions do to their patients, is what passes for medicine, for the real thing, while everything that they can't understand, including a lot of the real healing that goes on in the world, is not. This was my initiation into the fact that Physicians Mutual is not simply a financial institution, but also a kind of medical FBI, designed to enforce a certain Neanderthal conception of what health care is all about.

This, then, is the company that represents more than 95% of all physicians practicing in the state. If such a company were representing Dr. Kelly, Dr. Khedroo, and me, and a suit were brought against us, how could we possibly rely on these people to protect our best interests, let alone those of the patient? How could we prevent them from settling out of court for something we believed we were innocent of, or securing an acquittal for wrongs we did commit, purely on the basis of their own corporate needs?

The simple truth is that malpractice insurance offers us absolutely nothing that we can use, and tries to enforce on us a standard of practice that we cannot accept. We suspect that a lot of our colleagues in town think the same, and that with enough support from you, the public, they might be willing to say so openly. We believe that it is infinitely simpler, safer, and less expensive for everyone if we try to speak openly and honestly to our patients, to be as clear as we can about our own limitations, and thus persuade or allow them to take as much responsibility for their own health care as possible.

Obviously, this may not always be enough. Misunderstandings are bound to happen. But it is clear that malpractice and other forms of iatrogenic illness happen mostly when that communication breaks down, or was insufficient to begin with. The need for malpractice insurance on the present scale is thus a tragic and disgraceful reflection on how far we as physicians have chosen to distance ourselves from our patients. That is why we three prefer to take our chances.

The concept of malpractice insurance arises very naturally out of the view so prevalent today that birth and death, health and disease are essentially technical or professional matters, for which we physicians must take ultimate responsibility because of the superior scientific knowledge that we posses. Once we come to believe that we understand the needs of our patients better than they do themselves, it quickly follows that we alone can heal the patient, and that we can eventually devise purely technical or mechanical solutions to disease and all other human problems.

The incalculable risk to which malpractice insurance does in fact address itself is precisely this added liability that the physician incurs by taking away that ultimate responsibility from the patient and vesting it in our own person, our own ego, our professional competence, so that it then does indeed fall on us to decide if and when the patient lives or dies, recovers or fails to recover.

The three of us who are appealing to you now tend to see most of what we do with our patients in very simple terms. We believe that final responsibility for patient care and for all decisions regarding it must rest with the patient. We believe that life and death, health and disease are likewise natural processes that ultimately belong to the people undergoing them, and that our rôle is simply to assist their own natural healing effort in any way that we can. This is our insurance, and ultimately we believe that there need be and can be no other. We hope that you will help us to continue to serve the hospital and the people of Santa Fe in that spirit.

*On Lay Prescribing**

I would like to speak about lay prescribing, because it is an issue that has divided us in the past and will become even more important as we grow stronger.

The giving of remedies by unlicensed persons has always been an important part of homeopathy, as is evident in the fact that our medicines are readily available to the public without prescription. The law thus clearly recognizes that homeopathic remedies are mostly safe and to that extent suitable for home use, in simple ailments that do not require the services of a doctor, or in remote or emergency situations, when a doctor is not available.

There is also an extensive literature on the subject of lay prescribing, from Hering's classic work, *The Homeopathic Domestic Physician,* to *Homeopathic Medicine at Home,* by our own Maesimund Panos, published just recently. I take it, then, that most of us in the homeopathic family can readily accept 'lay prescribing' in this traditional sense, namely, the giving of remedies to oneself, one's family, and friends without charge and for the simple conditions outlined above.

Indeed, the validity of homeopathy as a system is nowhere better shown than in the fact that it can teach us all something about our health, and that all of us can use it when we are sick. We may well beware of any healing art, however rigorous or beautiful its laws, if its principal effect is simply to create yet another elite corps of physicians, answerable only to themselves.

The problem with lay practice is simply that it has developed to the point that a growing number of people without licenses, and in some cases without proper training or ability, are opening offices, giving out remedies to the public, and charging for their services just as if they were licensed, and that nobody has quite figured out what to say or do about it.

---

* "On Lay Prescribing," ***Homeopathy Today,*** NCH Newsletter, April 1982.

It is easy to see why this has happened. The decline of homeopathic medical education in this country has left us with fewer and fewer doctors trained and experienced in the method, and the public has had no choice but to take care of itself as best it can. Most of our younger physicians have had to learn homeopathy essentially on their own, with nothing more than a brief introductory course, a few books, and a deep personal commitment to continue teaching themselves as they go along.

Under these primitive conditions, homeopathy needs to be kept alive by those who know it best; independent practice would not be necessary if the physicians among us were able and willing to provide the kind of leadership that the public has a right to expect. The fact is that some of our greatest living masters are basically self-taught, like the incomparable George Vithoulkas of Greece, who remains unlicensed in his own country, and that many of the finest practitioners in the U.S. today have likewise risen from the ranks of the public, without formal medical training or licensure of any kind.

Indeed, there are two good reasons why this should be so. The first is that a dedicated lay person does not have to unlearn a lot of orthodox medical training, which is based on pathological diagnosis, or to carry on a medical practice of some sort in the meantime. There is much more time for *materia medica* study, and much less temptation to give in to the demands of a paying patient for an instant cure.

The second reason is simply that you will see a much truer picture of most illnesses in the patient's own home or living situation than is ever possible in a doctor's office or waiting room. That is one reason why my untrained, unlicensed birth assistant so often comes up with the correct remedy when my own more learned prescriptions have failed.

I guess what I'm trying to say is that all of us who love homeopathy are in the same boat, and that, at least for the present, neither the M. D. nor any other degree or license is a guarantee of homeopathic ability. We are all fellow-students on the path, which means that we must all be teachers as well for those just a little way behind. So hopefully we will not feel obliged to obey or disobey if some of us decide that theirs is the only true path. All of us, whatever our training and ability, are going to make mistakes; so we had best be ready to learn from them and be honest enough about our limitations to those who would take remedies from us.

The lay prescriber, however, is legally and morally vulnerable in three basic ways. First, he or she may lack formal training or ability in the basic medical sciences that would permit a proper diagnostic evaluation. Diagnosis can be especially important in homeopathy, precisely because the treatment should *not* be based on it, so that even an experienced physician easily forgets to perform a physical examination or other diagnostic tests, sometimes with unfortunate results.

A second area of liability arises from the fact that even homeopathic remedies are by no means completely innocuous, and under certain circumstances may cause serious harm to the patient. Purely from a legal point of view, both categories of liability could easily be avoided in several ways: by working as a para-professional under the direct supervision of a licensed physican; by requiring that the patient be examined or diagnosed by a physician prior to the treatment, as in South Africa, for example; or by requiring the patient to sign a release consenting to treatment, knowing that the practitioner cannot diagnose or guarantee a curative result, as required by the court in a recent California case.

But the final source of liability cannot be avoided, and it even includes the other two. It is simply the karma of undertaking to heal the sick, a profession inherently fraught with risk for both parties, and invariably exacting severe penalties if its standards are violated. Thus the practice of any healing art by persons without a license or in a manner not regulated by law becomes a possible felony as soon as offices are rented, appointments are made, fees are charged, and so forth, or in other words, as soon as a person represents himself or herself to the public as in any way qualified to diagnose or treat any disease or ailment.

Unlicensed persons may therefore legally prescribe homeopathic remedies on a fee-for-service basis only under the direct supervision of a licensed physician, or in a few isolated jurisdictions, mainly in California, where the courts have explicitly permitted it, and have set forth specific guidelines for it, as above. If the rest of us want to have such treatment made more widely available, it is our responsibility to see to it that such legislation is enacted.

The basic problems of lay prescribing are the same, whether you are doing it professionally, or simply for your friends. First, you need to develop a sense of when to call for help and of the types of ailments that *may* require the services of a physician. I will suggest a few from my experience: *chronic* ailments, especially if present for a year or more, or recurring several times over a longer period; ailments serious enough to threaten loss of life or major organ damage; ailments as yet undiagnosed by the patient; and, finally, any ailment that you have treated unsuccessfully, or that feels too serious or obscure for you to treat by yourself, without medical supervision or assistance.

Second, you need to know when homeopathic treatment is apt to be ineffective or dangerous. The cases that I find the most difficult are those with a long history of suppression with allopathic drugs, especially corticosteroids and anticonvulsants, where abrupt withdrawal may precipitate severe rebound symptoms; and those with very few symptoms and extensive tissue or organ damage. A relatively large number of these cases, particularly in the second group, will prove to be incurable, and high potencies or often-repeated doses of the *simillimum,* especially in the very old, could provoke a serious or even fatal aggravation.

We all know that homeopathy has suffered a great deal of persecution in the past, and it is understandable why today many of us would prefer to remain invisible rather than risk a similar fate in the future. We certainly owe a great debt of gratitude to our elders in the movement, because today our *materia medica* is still protected by law and available to all without restriction. Nor can we doubt that, as we grow stronger and homeopathy becomes once again more widely known, we shall again have to fight for what we believe, just as our elders did.

In any case, the fact is that we live in the midst of a crisis; and we all know, just as the general public knows, that high-tech, high-cost, high-risk medicine is a major part of it. We who are acquainted with the beauty and power of homeopathy cannot just sit idly by and fail to offer it to the public, or be blind to the fact that today, notwithstanding decades of neglect and an underlying philosophy that remains basically mysterious, homeopathy is once again an attractive alternative to doctors and patients alike.

So instead of ostracizing our lay practitioners, as if we were afraid or ashamed of them, I propose rather that we pay them tribute, as an expression of the spirit that has kept the movement alive all these years. And now let us try to provide effective leadership for them, in the form of educational services, professional supervision, and some realistic guidelines for their practice, before somebody gets hurt, and the FDA or the courts or some other governmental agency that knows nothing of homeopathy decides to do it for us.

*President's Message, 1985**

Today I want to speak about "lay practice" as a subspecies of the larger issue, the legal and moral status of homeopathy as a profession, and the qualifications of those who practice it. Until quite recently, the general assumption has been that mainly licensed physicians could practice homeopathy and whatever else according to their conscience, so long as the formal requirements of the corresponding licensing board were met. Presumably the same is true of nurses, dentists, veterinarians, chiropractors, naturopaths, acupuncturists, physician assistants, nurse-practitioners, nurse-midwives, and so on, all of whom are duly licensed and regulated in many states, and therefore may use homeopathic remedies, most of which are protected by law as over-the-counter drugs, within the scope of their respective licenses.

Nowhere in the U.S. are homeopathic practitioners licensed separately, except in Arizona, Nevada, and Connecticut. In Arizona and Nevada, a new law allows homeopathic licensure for MD's, DO's, and other graduates of an "approved" U.S. homeopathic medical school, upon examination by the board; but to date only MD's and DO's have been licensed there, since as yet no such school exists in the United States. In Connecticut, licensure is open only to MD's and DO's.

The recent disciplinary actions of various state medical boards against licensed MD's for practicing homeopathy, chelation, and other alternative therapies may threaten even that basic assumption; and naturopaths, veterinarians, nurses, and dentists have similarly been disciplined or harassed in several states. So one big part of the problem is that even duly licensed health professionals not infrequently get into trouble simply for being themselves, for practicing what they are licensed to practice in their own way.

Moreover, the laws governing the practice of medicine and other health professions are themselves questionable in many cases, simply because *all* people posses the innate power to heal and be healed, with or without

* President's Message, ***Homeopathy Today***, October 1985.

specialized medical training, and *no* law or authority has the right to proscribe or restrict the freedom of its exercise. As one enthusiast put it recently, "We believe the art of healing is inborn. It requires dedication and commitment to develop. It should not be suppressed—whether in a physician or a lay person—by law or ignorance."

We all know people who, through years of study and selfless dedication to homeopathy, have helped many, many people to heal themselves naturally, without drugs or surgery, or to give birth at home in their own way, or simply to find solace in the present moment after years of suffering. Indeed, these are our truest healers: every society creates them, and neither homeopathy nor allopathic medicine could long survive without their quiet, unsung assistance. Certainly history teaches that the greatest healers among us have not been physicians.

But the laws nevertheless must be respected and obeyed, even when we disagree with them. The medical practice acts of most states are sufficiently broad and general that District Attorneys may ignore those practitioners whom they wish to ignore, and prosecute those they wish to prosecute. There is nothing in the letter of the law to prevent them from prosecuting a woman who gave remedies *gratis* to her own son or nephew; but, to my knowledge, such an action has never been brought. Likewise, the law permits prosecution of unlicensed persons practicing para-professionally under the supervision of a physician; but the intent of these laws is clearly directed elsewhere.

Nor does the law make any formal discrimination between a person who is well-trained and experienced in the use of remedies, let us say, and one who is not. As I have said before, what the law regulates is not homeopathy *per se* but the *relationship* between professionals and their clients, whatever specific approach or modality is used, and also the *scope* of that relationship, as set forth by each particular licensing board. In virtually every state, the practice of medicine is interpreted to mean

1) that the individual advertises or claims special qualifications to diagnose or treat illness or disease, and

2) that the individual *earns a living* by doing so, whether by charging regular fees or receiving some other form of compensation.

My most urgent reason for saying all this is as background for the latest series of arrests involving, at last count, no fewer than eleven self-styled "homeopathic physicians" in the state of Florida. Several of these people already hold valid professional licenses: two are licensed acupuncturists, one is a pharmacist and a naturopath, and two hold MD degrees, although one had his license to practice medicine revoked several years ago, and the arrest of the other suggests that his license may also be inactive. But the majority of those arrested have no professional training or experience whatsoever, and the only "licenses" they hold are those issued by the self-styled "Florida State Society of Homeopathic Physicians," the legal status of which is very much what all these trials seem to be about. For these people are not your typically scared, isolated lay practitioner, attempting to create a semi-clandestine professional identity with legal and moral pitfalls on every side. They are right out there in the public eye, advertising themselves as "homeopaths," and commanding hefty fees without shame or hesitation.

One news item that caught my eye was the fact that several of these lay people, when "set up," by investigators from the State Department of Professional Regulation (DPR), were alleged to have performed pelvic examinations, given learned diagnoses, administered injections, and collected fees; whether or not they actually did so, which is the business of the jury to decide, there can be no doubt that, if so, they were indeed practicing medicine according to the standard criteria; and I cannot yet see any possible way that these people could be acquitted in *any* state, even by a jury of their cured patients.

The explanation for all these unorthodox practitioners and their arrest clearly has to do with the historical and political conditions in Florida. A variety of homeopathic practitioners in Florida emphasize the legitimacy of their practices by pointing out that homeopathy is *not* the practice of medicine— that both the state medical board and the state legislature were given the opportunity to regulate homeopathy but chose not to do so. But even if that were true, the idea that persons calling themselves "homeopaths" can establish their own board, and that such licensure gives them the right to perform pelvic examinations, give injections, etc., or in other words to practice medicine, is either very crazy or very stupid, either a blatant *non sequitur,* or a disingenuous word-game, i. e., a scam. Either way, the state and the people have every reason to be concerned about it; and practitioners of this type will get no aid and comfort from me or the National Center for Homeopathy. Maybe some of you feel differently; if so, let the debate continue.

The National Center is dedicated to disseminating information and educating the public about homeopathy. We give courses to professionals and lay people; we desire to extend these courses to all levels of proficiency and experience. But we can't license anyone to practice homeopathy, nor have we any ambition to do so. What we can do is to certify our lay and professional courses, and to adapt them to the needs of the various professionals and para-professionals who want to use remedies, so that their practices can fall within the scope of their respective licenses.

In this way, we can also support and encourage these groups to lobby to expand the scope of the laws themselves, to allow more latitude to practitioners as their experience grows and the public in turn becomes more familiar with homeopathy and other alternatives. Eventually, we expect to provide CME certification for doctors, nurses, dentists, veterinarians, and other established professionals, and to create certified courses for para-professionals in homeopathy, rather like the "barefoot doctors" in China or registered lay homeopaths in India, Britain, or South Africa. By that time we expect that the laws will change to accommodate these new categories.

But for the present, the medical practice laws exist, and ways must be found to work within them, to change them democratically. This is what I really want to speak to you about, because it was precisely the need to heal the doctor-patient relationship that first drove me out of medicine and later helped me to discover homeopathy, and so find my way back into healing work. I left medicine not only because of its content -- suppressive drugs, surgery, etc. -- but above all because of its style or attitude, e.g., "We know what's good for you, better than you do yourself; so sit back and leave the driving to us," and so forth. I chose homeopathy for the same reason that I chose home birth: both accept the wisdom of the patient as the ultimate healer, and therefore the proper judge of the healing relationship. That is why I try not to tell my patients how to live, and only offer alternative ways of looking at illness, and suggest remedies that may help them if they're up for trying them.

The reason I can't support the people in Florida who do pelvic exams without licenses and proclaim themselves as homeopaths without training is not simply or primarily because they are or are not homeopaths, but because they con their patients just as the rest of us were trained to do, with presumption and arrogance. These qualities I find especially objectionable in homeopathy, and, I'm sorry to say, equally widespread in our ranks, whether licensed or otherwise.

I have a friend on Cape Cod who is a nurse and practices homoeopathy in a way of which all of us can be proud, a way that is not at all the practice of medicine. She is essentially a health counselor and advisor: she sees the mother with the sick child, and shows her how to use the Repertory, how to find her own remedy for herself, rather than simply giving it to her. That's what you all do in your study groups; that's what our movement is all about. That is not the practice of medicine, because no claim is being made, and no diagnosis or treatment given.

There is nothing unlawful about helping someone to use natural remedies that are freely available. But the line is a fine one. Many will be tempted or fooled into crossing it, and there is nothing that we can do to protect them. What we can do is simply provide the information, teach people about the remedies, and so to encourage the public to create the kind of health-care system that it needs and wants. To those of you who know a lot about remedies and are impatiently waiting for the opportunity to use them, let me say that your opportunity is already here. All you have to do is to make sure that what you do is not practicing medicine, but rather helping people to heal themselves.

For that opportunity, in a very real sense I envy you, because I'm obliged to earn my living at it, which is quite a different thing, and fraught with karmic pitfalls on every side. People come to me precisely because I'm a physician licensed to diagnose and treat them, prescribe a regimen for them, and to that extent take charge of their lives. And I in turn, like every other practitioner, swell with pride when my chosen remedies work, and feel defeated when they don't. But the role that I covet, aspire to, and sometimes am graced to attain is that of counselor, advisor, teacher, helper, midwife, or nurse, call it what you will, helping people with their process, offering remedies, and leaving plenty of space for their own human response to take over and eventually free itself from me, from the remedies, and indeed from *my* dependence on them, which is at least as formidable as theirs.

This is only possible to the extent that we are all students on the path together, with much to teach and learn from each other; the lore of the remedies is an open book into learning about ourselves and each other. So to those of you who wish to practice homeopathy, to use your knowledge of remedies to help people, I say that the way lies open to you already. It is only when you aspire to practice medicine that the law correctly requires you to qualify for a license, because the practice of medicine is indeed fraught with hazard for physicians and patients alike. Those are the rules of society, like them or not, while the study of remedies is one simple and exemplary way that we can create and follow our own rules, without hindrance or penalty. Let us continue to learn and be worthy of it.

*President's Message, 1986**

The case of the North Carolina Board of Medical Examiners against George Guess, MD, was presented at a formal hearing on Friday, October 18, 1985, in Asheville, North Carolina. It began with the Board interrogating Dr. Guess for nearly four hours about homeopathic and allopathic methods alike. Then two physicians named by the state testified that although Dr. Guess was obviously a competent and a caring physician, his homeopathic practice was widely deviant from normal medical practices in that state.

The attorney for Dr. Guess presented his ample qualifications as a licensed physician; detailed the status and reputation of homeopathic medicines throughout the world, as well as the official recognition of homeopathic remedies by the U.S. Food and Drug Act; and documented the practical success and effectiveness of Dr. Guess' medical practice. For supportive testimony, he called as defense witnesses a Professor of Neurophysiology whose daughter was successfully treated by Dr. Guess after a reputable allergist had failed, and a local internist who knew Dr. Guess, was somewhat familiar with homeopathy, and offered eloquent praise for both.

Other defense witnesses included NCH Vice-President Bill Shevin, MD, who testified to the use of homeopathic remedies in his hospital practice in Connecticut and his role on that state's Board of Homeopathic Medical Examiners; NCH Treasurer Ben Hole, MD, a former Professor of Radiology, who emphasized the widespread recognition of homeopathy throughout the world and the official status of the Homeopathic Pharmacopœia of the United States; and I, who pointed out that state licensing boards were created for the protection of qualified physicians, whatever their school or belief, and that they could not lawfully restrict the practice of medicine to any one particular doctrine of teaching. The Board then recessed the proceedings and set a final hearing for December to hear Dr. Guess' remaining witnesses.

* President's Message, ***Homeopathy Today,*** January 1986.

It seemed as though the Board had already decided against Dr. Guess and homeopathy even before the hearing started. Certainly they were surprised to learn that the homeopathic movement is well established nationwide and in other lands. Whether they are wise enough to change their minds and to drop the case at this point remains to be seen. But their case against Dr. Guess is seriously flawed, in my view, and cannot survive a serious legal challenge, which surely will follow if their final decision goes against him. To be sure, they insisted that homeopathy was not on trial, but only Dr. Guess' failure to conform to the "acceptable and prevailing" standards of practice in North Carolina.

Yet the only specific charge against him in the record is that he uses homeopathic remedies and practices homeopathy. In the second place, the "acceptable and prevailing" standard and the concept of "unprofessional conduct" to which it refers were clearly intended to apply to matters of ethics and morality, rather than to the individual physician's chosen mode or style of practice, which the Board is obliged by law to protect. In the third place, the equation of "acceptable and prevailing" with what most other people happen to be doing or are capable of understanding aligns the Board squarely against anything new of different *per se.*

I must also say that Dr. Guess comported himself throughout as a worthy champion of our movement in particular and of the highest ideals of the medical profession in general. It was an honor and privilege to be associated with him, and to be in a position to take a stand for homeopathy at this critical hour.

*NCH Goals and Objectives: How Can It All Be Done?**

The primary goal of the NCH is promotion of the homeopathic concept nationwide at all levels, through education and public information, through the use of the media, and through political change.

The problem of the NCH is that this growing interest and excitement has arisen largely out of the self-care movement, and involves primarily nurses, nurse-practitioners, physician assistants, acupuncturists, midwives, chiropractors, naturopaths, psychotherapists, and other health professionals and lay people, whereas in the past the NCH has always supported primarily the education and training of physicians. The NCH has therefore been relatively inhospitable to the full implications of the self-care concept, while the bulk of homeopathic patients, students, and consumers have not felt strongly motivated to join the NCH, and have generally not been listened to when they have joined.

The result is that homeopathy remains essentially a private language, elegant and beautiful, to be sure, but intelligible only to those taking the trouble to learn it, so that even its most spectacular "cures" produce many referrals, but no new concept that captures the public imagination, and no organizational structure to channel its successes into broader awareness of the method and its point of view.

The NCH can best solve this problem by assisting and making use of the energy that is already out there, by empowering the local groups of patients, students, and consumers of homeopathy, to help them network, and to give them a voice in the homeopathic movement. This means that the primary goal of the NCH, the education of the public, can best be achieved at the grassroots level as part of the self-care movement, based on the single-remedy concept, i.e., as an organized effort to complete what is already happening spontaneously.

---

* "NCH Goals and Objectives: How Can It All Be Done?" Unpublished lecture presented at the NCH Annual Conference, May 1987.

A good case in point is the formation of the Mid-Atlantic Regional Study Group (MARSG), a loose coalition of several study groups in the D. C., Maryland, Virginia, and West Virginia area, which arose quite spontaneously, without any encouragement or support from the NCH, started to meet on a regular basis, put out a newsletter, and began speaking out on issues of general concern to the homeopathic community. They invited prospective and incumbent NCH Board members to declare themselves on the issues, and in the 1986 election succeeded in electing one Board member instead of another candidate with excellent qualifications and wider name recognition. Moreover, when another incumbent Board member resigned, the MARSG proposed the replacement whom I later selected. Thus in a very short time the MARSG demonstrated the existence and value of a new and powerful constituency of NCH membership, both present and future.

Similar constituencies exist elsewhere, in areas where homeopathic interest is established or growing; but for the most part they either have not joined the NCH, or have not yet formed themselves into politically articulate groups taking an active interest in our future. In Massachusetts, for example, where homeopathy has experienced a tremendous resurgence in the past few years, our present roster lists only 31 members. Our experience nationwide likewise continues to be that the great majority of our patients, as well as members of the various study groups and buyers of homeopathic products, do not join the NCH even when they identify with our concerns, as in the George Guess case, when they responded magnificently to our appeals.

The obvious practical task facing the NCH is thus simply to help organize all of this energy and enthusiasm for homeopathy into an effective and articulate network or infrastructure capable of translating homeopathic concepts into the ordinary language of everyday life. Furthermore, this must be accomplished primarily at the local and regional level. The NCH's small centralized bureaucracy is straining its meager resources to "catch up" with what is happening out in the communities. Once the local groups realize that their goals are essentially the same as ours on the national level, then "they" will become "us," and they will make their voices heard in the NCH, just as the MARSG has done.

The NCH must therefore devise effective strategies for empowering homeopathic patients, study groups, and consumers in each locality to network together, in effect constituting a branch office of the NCH at the local level. At the moment, it makes most sense for the study group to be the nucleus, because these will be the people most highly motivated to work for homeopathy and best qualified to spread it. So what we would like to initiate is a series of incentives for study groups to encourage their members to join the NCH: these might include special bulk membership rates for ten members or more, and similar bulk discounts on books, kits, and seminars for large orders made through the study group, in exchange for volunteer help provided by study group members.

The NCH could then designate a person or persons to be its local representatives in each locality, and supply them with updated lists of new, lapsed, and old NCH members to make contact with. The NCH and its local representatives might then encourage homeopathic practitioners and educators to provide lists of their patients and students, while health food stores, bookstores, and pharmacies could be asked to provide both NCH and local information to customers buying homeopathic books and remedies. Calls to the NCH office for referrals and information could also be sent on to the local group that would be best able to answer them.

Thus empowered, the study groups would almost certainly become a major force in the development of homeopathy in their localities, and would naturally want to network with other groups in the same state, as well as eventually on a regional and national basis. The NCH would then become essentially the federation of all these groups, each one semi-autonomous, with its own individual character, while the NCH central office could provide help in the form of instructors, instructional materials, news, and information to them all. A mass-based membership organization such as I am proposing would then in turn create the basis for a powerful organization of homeopathic nurses, potentially our largest and most influential professional grouping, and would thus tend to create the demand that would attract more physicians and other health professionals as well.

Once again, our emphasis must remain on self-care and the single remedy, because these are the concepts that can educate the public and bring homeopathy into the language, as is already happening. Homeopathy at this level must be seen not as an "alternative" to conventional medicine, but as something complementary to it, as our friend Prince Charles has suggested; this idea dovetails perfectly with the overall direction of the nursing movement in the US, training free-standing nurse-practitioners to treat "functional" ailments and free up the doctors' time for serious organic pathology.

The emphasis on self-care and the single remedy will also naturally promote smoother, more co-operative relationships with other consumer groups in the self-care movement, as well as more wholesome relationships with health professionals generally, based on self-care and taking responsibility for one's own health, rather than simply the practice of medicine. These same eminently practical issues will automatically put the old questions of potency and repetition and single or multiple remedies in proper perspective, as fitting subjects for learned debate by serious professionals, rather than ongoing sources of antagonism and dissension. Finally, they will tend to generate new research models, not only for homeopathy, but for energy medicine as a whole, based on the evolution of the bioenergetic "totality of symptoms," the total health picture as it evolves over time.

*Hospital Ethics Committees: The Healing Function**

As a GP with no prior experience of Hospital Ethics Committees, I came to the Miami Seminar[1] rather like a journalist investigating a political movement, and was repeatedly impressed by the sheer magnitude of the phenomenon, the more or less simultaneous appearance of such institutions almost everywhere, typically on a voluntary basis and without financial support or official backing. Clearly there was powerful magic at work somewhere within a medical system in critical condition nearly everywhere else.

Even more striking was the practical success of many Hospital Ethics Committees in resolving major ethical dilemmas, in which contradictory viewpoints often seemed equally compelling, equally unacceptable, or both, and in spite of the fact that they generally lack the power or authority to enforce their recommendations. This high degree of effectiveness under such adverse circumstances likewise suggests both a powerful need and a reliable mechanism for satisfying it.

Furthermore, the analytic description of what Ethics Committees do once they are formed -- self-education, policymaking, case review, and consultation – cannot account for the dynamism that created them in the first place. Still less can ethical principles themselves account for it. For even when these are familiar and clear enough in the abstract to be generally accepted and agreed upon, their application in specific cases is still likely to be problematic, controversial, and evocative of strong passions on every side.

With these general concerns in mind, I wondered if there were not some logically prior and more generic function that underlies whatever these committees do, and might help us to understand why they are so necessary and so effective. It is clear that the development of elaborate biotechnologies has created troubling dilemmas regarding the allocation

---

* "Hospital Ethics Committees: the Healing Function," ***Hospital Ethics Committee Forum*** 1:309, January 1990.

of scarce resources (e.g., artificial or donor kidneys). It is also true that Ethics Committees often succeed in resolving disputes voluntarily because all parties know that unpleasant and expensive litigation will likely follow if they fail.

But these socioeconomic explanations also fall short, since reducing difficult ethical questions to more narrowly technical ones overlooks large parts of what Committees actually accomplish. One hypothesis that suggested itself seemed at first like a mere platitude, but then reminded me of Bertrand Russell's taunt that "the point of philosophy is to start with something so simple as not to seem worth stating, and to end with something so paradoxical that no one will believe it."[2]

I'm thinking of two cases presented at the Miami Seminar. The first was that of an incompetent elderly patient, seriously but not terminally ill, whose personal wishes were unknown, and whose next of kin appeared confused and ambivalent about what would be an appropriate disposition or level of care for her;[3] the physician asked the Committee for ethical guidance well in advance of any actual conflict. There was nothing remarkable or controversial about what the Committee *did,* or about the Durable Power of Attorney statute that it relied upon. What was impressive was simply the fact that such a Committee *existed,* that it represented all the major players in the hospital community, and that both the physician and the family saw fit to consult it and to abide by its recommendations.

In that sense the Committee performed a basic "healing" function within the hospital that was implicit in whatever it did, including the principles that it invoked and the procedures that it developed and followed. What was healing was the *process* that the Committee helped set in motion, as much as the substance or content of its deliberations.

The second case was that of another seriously but not terminally ill patient who wished to discontinue further treatment, with the full support of his family. The medical staff, on the other hand, wanted to continue aggressive treatment as long as it held out a reasonable hope of recovery, since the patient would almost surely die without it.[4] In principle, both claims seemed genuine and compelling; and again the Committee actually did very little, beyond carrying out some additional discovery at first. It was helpful mainly by *being there,* by providing a supportive atmosphere and helping the parties communicate and work out their differences in an amicable way. The diversity of its membership encompassed a broad spectrum of ethical views and facilitated an informal reconciliation without the need of a more elaborate or formal proceeding. What I am suggesting is that Ethics Committees perform an authentic healing function within the hospital community and indeed for the medical system as a whole.

The same conclusion can be arrived at from the opposite direction, by asking what happens when the Committees are not consulted and more coercive tactics resorted to. This was the tragic fate of Angela C, who was hospitalized in her 26th week of pregnancy with a rapidly growing tumor and was given only a few more days to live. Counsel for the hospital immediately requested a judicial opinion, and the District Judge came to the bedside, flanked by attorneys appointed for the patient and the fetus. Against the clearly stated wishes of the patient, her family, and her attending physician that she be allowed to die, the Judge ordered that a Caesarean section be performed in an attempt to "save" the fetus, arguing that Angela's terminal condition nullified her legal right to refuse this obviously cruel and indeed lethal treatment.[5]

In retrospect, it seems obvious that the Committee could have worked out a more humane solution had it been asked to, just as such committees often succeed in the worst circumstances, simply because the alternatives are so ghastly. A similar lesson was provided by the Linares case, in which a Chicago hospital continued to maintain an irreversibly brain-damaged child on full life support, against the clearly stated wishes of the family and the medical opinion of the physicians and nurses involved in his care. Facing a long, expensive, and possibly futile court action as his only available recourse, the father tearfully disconnected his own son's respirator while holding off the doctors and nurses at gunpoint.[6]

Once again, an Ethics Committee might well have averted this confrontation if the hospital authorities had seen fit to provide one, and their error is evident in the fact that the District Attorney eventually dropped all charges against the father, Rudy Linares, who had become something of a folk hero, while the hospital came to be regarded as the villain for refusing to honor the family's wishes for their child.

In addition, the Committee's educational and policy-making activities comprise the furthest possible extension of its healing function. Participants at the Miami Seminar gave inspiring reports of concerned hospital and community groups collaborating to formulate policies on AIDS, informed consent, and other controversial issues, or at least to discuss them as openly and thoroughly as possible.[7]

Even where formal agreement is not possible, Ethics Committees can nevertheless identify problems before they arise and articulate the sense of the community that would be needed to resolve them. One such Committee had actually chosen to limit itself to education, arguing that by leading public discussion of ethical issues they had created an atmosphere of trust and collaboration that had clearly prevented many potentially serious cases.[8] This was truly a commitment to ask questions, and be guided by the values of those directly involved as much as by any preformed solution, however rigorous or logical. At this level, healing work resembles the art of jurisprudence, which also must be applied uniquely each time, and depends on learned analogy to be applicable to other cases past and future.

In conclusion, it should be pointed out that the spectacular achievements of Ethics Committees are applicable only in highly specialized and unusual situations. By the time patients get to the ICU, become incompetent, and have to be maintained on artificial life support, highly unpalatable choices have to be made that should have been foreseen and might have been prevented long before. The technical question of whether to employ or discontinue artificial life support, for example, merely illustrates the prior human question of how doctors can know and honor the needs and wishes of their patients. These complex ethical dilemmas will seldom arise if healing relationships can be established before hospitalization and technical dependency are required.

The extraordinary success of such committees in healing the medical system thus poses the more basic challenge of healing the doctor-patient relationship itself, before the technical imperatives of the system pre-empt all but the most drastic and difficult choices. I therefore propose that we form similar committees *outside the hospital,* to help doctors and patients articulate their concerns and resolve their differences on a voluntary basis. Through frank and open discussion, they could begin to develop ethical standards for what doctors and patients have a right to expect from each other, and thus to prevent the kinds of misunderstanding that so often lead to tragedy.

Actual disputes between doctors and patients could then be settled by mediation and arbitration, based on the ethics of human relationships, rather than by costly and prolonged legal combat, based on the technical outcome. What is needed is not any specific method or content, but only a shared commitment to genuine healing, so well exemplified by Hospital Ethics Committees as both an ethical imperative and a practical criterion for the medical system as a whole.

NOTES.

1. Seminar, "Hospital Ethics Committees," University of Connecticut School of Medicine, Prof. Stuart Spicker and Dr. Thomasine Kushner, Directors, Miami, 1990.
2. Russell B., The Philosophy of Logical Atomism," in *Logic and Knowledge,* Allen and Unwin, London, 1968, p. 192.
3. Rues, L., et al., unpublished case report.
4. Koch K., unpublished case report
5. Annas G., "She's Going to Die: The case of Angela C," *Hastings Center Report,* February/ March 1988, pp. 23-25.
6. "Hospital Blamed for Failing to Aid Parents," *American Medical News,* May 12, 1989.
7. Perkel R., "Ethical Issues in HIV and AIDS," unpublished discussion paper.
8. MacDonald J., The Ethics of Giving Placebos," unpublished discussion paper.

*Ethics in Homeopathic Practice**

Those of us who learned classical homeopathy in the '70's and have continued to practice it in the United States can take pride in the altogether improbable revival now in full bloom all around us. When I took the NCH Millersville course in 1974, my teachers tended to be old and saintly, and most either did not need or were no longer able to make a living from homeopathy alone. Without the experience or example of the lost generation in between, it was difficult to imagine how the method could survive much longer.

Today, thanks to the vitality of the alternative health and self-care movements and the glaring deficiencies of high-cost, high-tech, high-risk medicine, homeopathy has risen again, phoenix-like, as if from its own ashes. As this conference will attest, the United States currently produces more and better-trained homeopaths than at any time since its golden age over a century ago. But this newfound visibility has also exposed and even highlighted several important political and ethical issues that have largely been ignored or swept under the rug since the long years of decline:

1) the advertising of homeopathic remedies for baldness, impotence, and the like, often using outlandish "New Age" slogans, and in some cases made by obscure manufacturers in defiance of the industry's minimal self- policing efforts;

2) the use of electro-diagnostic and other experimental devices, often illegal or unlicensed for commercial use, by unlicensed or poorly-trained practitioners, or in circumstances where informed consent has not been obtained or even clearly formulated; and

3) malpractice suits and various disciplinary actions against homeopathic physicians, sometimes involving disregard of basic duties to patients or standards of care required of all medical doctors, whatever their philosophy.

In all of these areas, those of us who practice homeopathy or produce homeopathic remedies for sale are obliged to regulate ourselves more

---

* "Ethics in Homeopathic Practice," ***Journal of the AIH*** 86:238, Winter 1993-94.

effectively, or face the consequences of having the government or a generally hostile medical establishment do it for us.

1.

My subject today is limited to ethical rules and standards for the profession, i.e., to how homeopathic practitioners can and should be expected to behave with our patients, colleagues, and students, and with interested third parties such as employers, schools, insurance companies, courts of law, and the media.

In preparation for this talk, I looked at several codes of medical ethics both ancient and modern, including two recently developed for homeopathic organizations.[1] Their remarkable similarity was serendipitous proof that the basic moral questions have not changed that much since the earliest times. Consider, for example, the following passage from the Hippocratic Oath:

> Into whatever houses I enter, I will help the sick and abstain from all intentional wrongdoing and harm, especially from abusing the bodies of man or woman, bond or free. And whatsoever I shall see or hear in the course of my profession, if it be what should not be published abroad, I will never divulge, holding such things to be holy secrets.[2]

Thus by the fifth century B. C., in words that are still valid today, the medical profession had already assumed both legal and moral responsibility for two inescapable realities of the healing relationship:

1) the inherently unequal power of all healers over the sick people in our care, implying an obligation not to harm or abuse them that would not need to be sworn were we not also humanly at risk of transgressing it; and

2) the need of the sick to feel safe enough to trust and confide gives us privileged access to their inner world, and thus imposes further duties of confidentiality and discretion in its exercise.

On the other hand, the historical background for and specific formulation of such codes tend to vary widely over time and from one culture to another.

The Hippocratic Oath, for example, is a classic rite of initiation into a secret society, both self-perpetuating and jealously protective of its "trade secrets," in which membership is handed down from father to son and master to apprentice, according to rules not subject to outside scrutiny:

> I swear by Apollo that I will carry out this oath and indenture: to hold my teacher in this art as equal to my parents, to make him partner to my livelihood, to consider his family as my own, to teach them the art, if they want to learn it, without fee or indenture, and to teach it also to my own sons, the sons of my teacher, and to indentured pupils who have taken the physician's oath, *but to nobody else.* If I am faithful to this oath, may I enjoy good fortune and the esteem of all men for my life and art; but, should I transgress it, may the reverse be my lot![3]

Although important elements of this ancient guild mentality remain well-entrenched in the medical profession even today, the Oath no longer fits the modern requirements of a liberal profession or an open, democratic society, and has officially been dropped by most leading American medical schools.

An even more obvious example of historical change is the transformation of medical ethics into a separate clinical specialty, on account of our unsettling technical capacity for keeping patients alive when they are no longer competent to make important decisions for themselves.[4]

In any case, formulating a code of ethics for homeopathic practitioners is especially problematic for several reasons. First, there is as yet no separate homeopathic profession as such, recognized by law and characterized by uniform standards of education and training. Homeopathy today is practiced by health professionals of all types, including physicians, nurses, midwives, acupuncturists, naturopaths, chiropractors, psychologists, and veterinarians, each subject to the rules and jurisdictions of their respective licensing boards, as well as by lay prescribers, homeopathic educators, and counselors, who practice without statutory protection of any kind. Under these circumstances, it is difficult to imagine any code sufficiently uniform and rigorous to enforce meaningful discipline, yet flexible enough to accommodate such a wide range of needs and experience.

An even more basic problem is the lack of consensus about the definition of homeopathy itself. In the two hundred years since Hahnemann's first experiments, a bewildering array of methods, philosophies, and technological applications have claimed legitimate descent from some aspect of his work, with many of them still in enough seeming or actual conflict to keep the family divided and unwilling or unable to agree about fundamentals. Indeed, as a fledgling bio-energetic science homeopathy is growing and evolving so rapidly that it might well be an enormous mistake even to *try* to define it too rigidly or exclusively at this point.[5]

But by far the most important dilemma is one that homeopathy shares with law, medicine, and all the learned professions, namely, that it deals with individuals in unique situations, so that its rules and standards must be adaptable enough to do justice to the infinite variety inherent in human nature itself. This final objection was raised against the AMA Code of Medical Ethics of 1847, in words that still ring true today:

> A physician is not a member of a guild or corporation, the rules of which he must comply with in order to retain his membership therein, but a member of a liberal profession, the rules of which are the unwritten law of humanity, and the special requirements of which must vary much according to the peculiarities of his environment. The physician is a free man: he has ceased to recognize paternal interference with his judgment; he wears the livery of no employer; he acknowledges the restrictions of no trade union.
>
> If as an individual he chooses to abdicate his dignity and put himself under a yoke, he has the right to do it, but [not] to require that others shall follow his example. No one can question the right of any association establishing specific rules of conduct for its members, if it chooses, and requiring conformity to these rules as requisite to membership. But as for myself, I am not able to accept [them] as the sole and authoritative guide by which my professional conduct must be fixed, not to cause me to recognize in any man or set of men the right to bring me to the bar for judgment. I welcome this code as a treatise on the moral aspects of medical life, of value for reference and counsel; but for my decision as to what my action in any given case may be, I hold myself responsible to my own conscience alone.[6]

Our self-protective concern for morality as a deeply personal or even a private matter suggests that we should limit our search to general principles, guidelines, and prohibitions rather than specific, detailed, and rigid rules of conduct. But first we need to ask ourselves why we need or indeed if we can tolerate a code of ethics at all.

Our need to police ourselves is really a call to arms against the historical fact that most of the policing has long since been given over to others. In other words, we need a homeopathic code of ethics primarily to help us come together, to constitute a profession that does not yet exist. Such a code would enable us to suspend for the moment our legitimate differences as to methods and practices and affirm what we all have in common, namely, a patient-centered philosophy of healing and the healing relationship that the medical profession is in stark need of at the moment. The germ of such a philosophy is already evident in these aphorisms of Paracelsus, written three centuries before Hahnemann:

> The art of healing comes from Nature, not the physician . . .
> Every illness has its own remedy within itself . . .
> A man could not be born alive and healthy were there not already a Physician hidden in him.[7]

Their major implications are readily summarized as follows:

Healing implies wholeness.

As a concerted response of the entire organism, healing implies a totality, a deeper integration than can be defined and measured by any assemblage of parts.

All healing is self-healing.

As a basic property of all living organisms, spontaneous healing is going on all the time, such that the role of physicians and other healers is to assist the natural process, never to interfere with or substitute for it.

Healing applies only to individuals.

Always possible, never certain, healing pertains to individuals in unique situations and is therefore inescapably an art, and cannot be reduced to a mere technique or procedure, however scientific its foundation.[8]

With the addition of the Law of Similars, the totality of symptoms, and the Laws of Cure, homeopathy systematizes this holistic viewpoint into a coherent philosophy in which health and illness are natural life processes defined in relation to the lived experience of our patients and therefore amenable to their active participation at every point.

In sum, the ethical core of homeopathy and indeed of all the healing professions lies in our relationships with our patients, whatever methods we choose to practice on their behalf. Insofar as we expect to achieve recognition as a legitimate profession and to exercise leadership in the health care system, we owe it to ourselves and our patients alike to agree about how we intend to conduct ourselves and to what standards we are ready to hold ourselves accountable.

2.

With these general considerations in mind, I will try to identify some of the basic ethical issues that the homeopathic profession needs to address, and discuss the unique implications of the homeopathic viewpoint for each of them, whichever particular formulations of them are eventually agreed upon. As sources I will consider four contemporary ethical codes of conduct from among those already cited, including two for physicians and two for homeopaths:

1) *the AMA Code of Ethics* as revised in 1957 and 1980;

2) *the World Medical Association's Declaration of Geneva of 1949,* which serves as an addendum to the codes of ethics of its member states;

3) *the British Society of Homeopaths' Code of Ethics and Practice,* updated 1992; and

4) *the provisional Code of Professional Ethics* drafted 1992 by Harry Swope on behalf *of the Council on Homeopathic Certification.*[9]

Standards of Practice.

All four codes agree on the responsibility of the profession and its members to maintain high standards of knowledge and technical proficiency through rigorous training, certification, and ongoing self-education. While primary responsibility for upholding such standards remains with the individual practitioner, both the AMA and the Society of Homeopaths reserve the right to hear and investigate complaints of incompetence against their members, and to take remedial and/or disciplinary action if necessary.

Notwithstanding major differences as to how to measure, supervise, and enforce them, the existence of standards of practice and of continuing education requirements clearly and explicitly affirms both the right of all patients to competent health care and the obligation of all healing professions to provide it. Even continuing disagreements about the definition of homeopathy cannot and should not be used as an excuse to justify less than the highest possible standard for each discipline, appropriately formulated in its own fashion.

Honesty and Truth-Telling.

Another theme common to all four codes cited is the fundamental commitment of all physicians and healers to honesty and truth-telling in dealing with patients, students, and interested third panics such as relatives, employers, schools, courts, insurance companies, and the media. With all due regard for confidentiality, an equally important value (see below), and for those rare instances when a part of the truth should best be concealed for the patient's sake,[10] physicians and healers of every stripe owe their patients the following duties:

1) to give true and accurate information and advice, to the limits of their expertise;
2) to consult with or refer to other more qualified practitioners when those limits are exceeded;
3) to give true and accurate reports to interested third parties when requested by the patient or required by law or ethical necessity, as in preventing a serious crime; and
4) to report all research and clinical findings truthfully and with appropriate documentation.

Once again, both the AMA and the Society of Homeopaths, as certifying bodies, specify the further obligation of their members to report unethical conduct by their colleagues, and to establish formal procedures for investigating and adjudicating such complaints. (See below.)

As a philosophy of self-healing, homeopathy promises a deeper fidelity to the lived experience of the patient than is possible in conventional medicine, and its ethical standards should likewise extend beyond honesty and truth-telling to encouraging patients to participate in and assume responsibility for their care insofar as possible.

Confidentiality, Informed Consent, and Patients' Rights.

The right of every patient to confidentiality within the limits set by law encompasses the larger issues of respect for the autonomy and rights of patients at the time of their maximum vulnerability, and the crucial role of physicians and healers as advocates for them. Thus, in addition to protecting clients' privacy, all of the codes cited require practitioners to obtain informed consent based on full disclosure before performing any experimental, diagnostic, or treatment procedure, and to conduct themselves in a seemly and dignified manner in accordance with commonly accepted professional standards.

Both the AMA and the Society of Homeopaths explicitly prohibit any kind of sexual contact with patients or students. But once again, the self-care model also allows and encourages homeopathy to go much further on behalf of the patient and indeed to assume a leadership role within the health-care system as a whole. The CHC code is the clearest and most ambitious in this respect, emphasizing the rights of patients to be accompanied by an advocate or chaperone if desired, to refuse treatment, to participate actively in all health-care decisions, and to continue to receive respectful care even when the practitioner's advice is not followed.

Personally, I would like to see all of these provisions codified in a Patient Bill of Rights, introduced by some kind of general statement like the following:

> Health, illness, birth, and death are inalienable life experiences belonging wholly to the people undergoing them. Nobody else has the right to manipulate or control them, or any part of the body involved in them, without their explicit request or that of somebody authorized by them to act in their behalf.[11]

The Duties of the Patient.

One important matter omitted from all the codes is simply the reciprocal of the above, that physicians and healers also have certain rights within the relationship, and even positive duties owed them by their patient, much as in any contract, intentional violation of or refusal to discharge them being grounds for renegotiation or even termination in some cases. Among the duties of patients I would include:

1) being as well-informed as circumstances permit about their illness and what they can do to assist in their own healing work;

2) knowing and observing reasonable rules and policies governing services offered, appointments, payments, and availability after hours, and honoring all agreements freely entered into; and, above all,

3) taking responsibility for making their needs and wishes known and for giving feedback and constructive criticism when they feel unheard or dissatisfied.[12]

Once again, the more we give to a relationship, the more we are entitled to ask from it in return. Our allopathic brethren might well strive for the level of trust and compliance that most homeopaths routinely earn from their patients.

Duties to Colleagues, the Profession, and the Public.

In this broad category belong general prohibitions against speaking disrespectfully of colleagues or soliciting their patients, advertising publicly for a cure of any disease, and splitting fees or accepting contingency fees or "kickbacks." It also includes the obligation of all professionals to obey the laws of state and country, to observe the customary rules and standards of their respective professions, and to work toward lawful change on behalf of their patients. Finally, it affirms the duty of all practitioners to provide an adequate standard of care to the indigent, and continuity of care to all patients, insofar as possible. In all these respects, it upholds the integrity and honor of the profession as a positive example and constructive force within the community.

Once again, homeopathy could easily go a step further, as in the CHC code, which urges practitioners to assist their colleagues both in study and practice, and to provide collegiality and fellowship as well.

3.

Enforcement: Complaint Procedures, Adjudication, and Due Process.

The four codes cited above differ widely in their approach to enforcement of standards, in much the same way as do the histories of the organizations that created them. Thus the Declaration of Geneva, promulgated by the World Medical Association in 1928, was intended as a contemporary version of the Hippocratic Oath that modern physicians could more easily subscribe to. As an addendum to the pre-existing codes of its member states, it makes no mention of enforcement, leaving it up to each nation to interpret its principles in its own way. The AMA Codes, on the other hand, as official policy of the most powerful medical society on earth, are full of solemn moral pronouncements and quasi-judicial procedures, albeit in practice often "more honour'd in the breach than th' observance."[13]

On the homeopathic side, the CHC Code, a draft proposal for a profession still in its childhood, quite properly shies away from disciplinary matters, and leaves final responsibility with the individual practitioner. Thanks to strict and uniform requirements of training and experience for membership, the British Society of Homeopaths can give real teeth to its disciplinary procedures, yet remain eminently fair and humane to those charged, preferring informal discussions wherever possible.

In this country, the homeopathic profession will at some point also want and need to articulate meaningful standards of conduct, the effectiveness of which likewise presupposes a voluntary but formal agreement by all members to abide by them. The only remaining questions are *how,* in what manner, and under what circumstances? Here again, homeopathy's inherently patient-centered approach offers several important opportunities for creative innovation.

To my mind, the most unethical aspect of American medicine lies in its disempowerment of the patient, who stands alone and defenseless against the system, with compelling reasons to fear it, no effective check against it, and no option for dealing with it but to tread cautiously and bring a malpractice suit after the fact for actual damages done.[14] The so-called "malpractice crisis" boils down to the insurrection of patients against that powerlessness, and the guts of it is the adversarial relationship now prevailing between doctors and patients at every level.[15]

Homeopathy, midwifery, and other patient-centered philosophies are uniquely qualified to offer to the healing professions a model of client relationships that is life-affirming, makes sense, and has already worked for us for a long time. The least that we can do is to "walk our talk," to hold ourselves and be willing to be held accountable to what we say we believe.

The key to the success of the SOH code or any other is the degree to which membership in the profession is something desirable and therefore worthy of protection. Once these values are internalized by the practitioner, most ethical disputes can be worked out informally or even prevented before the fact; and the few that require formal adjudication should be amenable to resolution fairly and in a way that does credit to the profession.

Our best assurance that this will happen is simply to include our patients in these deliberations at every step, from the actual complaint and hearing process all the way back to the formulation of the code itself. Homeopaths very much need to know at first hand the sorts of complaints our patients have had with us in the past and are having with us now, just as much as the health-care system needs to know that it can and must trust the folks on the "receiving" end to know what is best for them.

Claims of either client or professional could then be referred to local *ad hoc* or standing ethics committees representing both groups and perhaps other community leaders as well, such as clergy, social workers, etc., to try to settle disputes informally through mediation, in much the same way that Hospital Ethics Committees already do.[16]

When these efforts fail, as sometimes they must, either party could appeal to the Ethics Committee of the profession as a whole, with similarly broad community representation and a similar predilection for non-adversarial solutions. The courts and professional licensing boards would still be available for disciplinary or legal action if necessary.

But no mechanism can work well unless homeopaths, patients, and other community members are willing to trust one another to work together to bring about a peaceful solution. They cannot substitute for disciplinary or legal action when important code violations and acts of negligence have occurred. But they could go a long way toward creating non-adversarial settings in which broad-based public participation could help to resolve genuine ethical disputes and misunderstandings between healers and patients before irreversible harm has been done.

With models of this type in place, the homeopathic profession will be in a much better position to stand up and be counted without having to agree on or give moral weight to what by comparison are simply matters of technique, very much open to experiment and debate, and certainly not worth killing or dying for.

Homeopaths using electro-diagnostic machines, for example, need only obtain genuinely informed consent from the patient, based on full disclosure of the experimental nature of the device. In short, I submit that the role of an Ethics Committee for homeopaths should not be to define what homeopathy is, or which method or doctrine we must adhere to, but simply how to relate to our patients and to the society at large. In this way, homeopathy has a lot of very important things to offer to the healing and medical professions right now, without waiting for them to embrace the still partly esoteric truths that we all love so dearly, things that they sorely need, and thus earn for itself the credit it should have had all along.

NOTES.

1. "The Oath of Hippocrates," reprinted in Reiser, Dyck, and Curran, eds., *Ethics in Medicine,* MIT Press, Cambridge, 1977, p. 5; the AMA *Code of Medical Ethics,* 1847, ibid., pp. 29-34; the World Medical Association Declaration of Geneva, 1949, ibid., pp. 37-38; the AMA *Principles of Medical Ethics,* 1957, ibid., pp. 38-39; the AMA *Code of Medical Ethics* and *Current Opinions on Medical Ethics,* AMA, Chicago, 1992; Society of Homeopaths, Ltd., *Code of Ethics and Practice,* UK, 1992; and Swope, H., "Code of Ethics for Homeopathy," Council on Homeopathic Certification, 1992 (unpublished draft).
2. "The Oath of Hippocrates," in Reiser, et al., op. cit., p. 5.
3. Ibid.
4. Cf. Moskowitz, R., "Whose Life Is It, Anyway? Some Thoughts on the Doctor- Patient Relationship," *Chrysalis* 6:103, Swedenborg Foundation, 1991.
5. Cf. Moskowitz, "Poverty in the Midst of Plenty: American Homeopathy in 1987," address to the National Center for Homeopathy Annual Conference, Chicago, 1987 (NCH audiocassette).
6. Pilcher, L., "Codes of Medical Ethics," in Reiser, op. cit., pp. 34-36, *passim.*
7. P. A. T. B. von Hohenheim, *Selected Writings of Paracelsus,* J. Jacobi, ed., N. Guterman, trans., Bollingen Series XXVIII, Pantheon, New York, 1958, pp. 50, 76, *passim.*
8. Cf. Moskowitz, "Hospital Ethics Committees: the Healing Function," *Hospital Ethics Committee Forum* 1:309, January 1990.
9. Reiser, op. cit., pp. 37-39; AMA, op. cit., 1992; Society of Homeopaths, op. cit.; and Swope, op. cit.
10. "Informed Consent," AMA, op. cit., pp. 106-107.
11. Cf. Moskowitz, *Chrysalis,* op. cit., pp. 106-107.
12. Cf. Moskowitz, "Some Thoughts on the Malpractice Crisis," *British Homeopathic Journal* 77:25, January 1988, and Haire, D., "The Pregnant Patient's Responsibilities," International Childbirth Education Association (ICEA), Minneapolis.

13. Shakespeare, *Hamlet,* I, iv., 17.
14. Cf. Moskowitz, *British Homeopathic Journal,* op. cit., p. 23.
15. Ibid.
16. Cf. Moskowitz, *Hospital Ethics Committee Forum,* op. cit.

*Who Needs the AIH? A Brief Pep Talk**

Today I want to reflect on our organization itself, because it is caught in a complex dilemma that threatens its future. On the one hand, American homeopathy is now growing more rapidly than it has for decades, such that the goals we set ourselves in the 1970's and '80's are in the process of being realized. In the Boston area, for example, two new stores specialize in homeopathic remedies, books and supplies, and advertise that fact in the window for all to see. This growing success at the retail level I take to mean that the infrastructure required for homeopathy to grow and achieve its potential is already in place, thanks in no small part to what all of you have done and are continuing to do.

On the other hand, while seeking to represent over two thousand physicians who use homeopathy in their practices, the AIH has little more than a hundred members, and no money to pay for our speakers today, let alone such basic priorities as research, political action, or legal defense. Still wholly dependent on the volunteer efforts of our officers and Board Members, we continue to survive more or less by the seat of our pants. "Poverty in the midst of plenty" is the phrase that comes to mind, often applied to diabetes in my medical-school years, but no less applicable here.[1]

From the opposite direction, we are vulnerable to charges of "elitism" from our non-MD colleagues, who could add quality and quantity to our ranks and see only anachronism in an organization for physicians and osteopaths only.[2] Since the community of homeopathic practitioners also encompasses naturopaths, chiropractors, nurse-practitioners, physician-assistants, nurses, acupuncturists, psychotherapists, midwives, and lay educators and counselors, many of them more diligent students and more capable prescribers than I will ever be, they have every right to question why they too should not be included.

These twin riddles prompt me to ask if we really need an AIH and what its priorities should be. After all, we already have the National

---

* "Who Needs the AIH? A Brief Pep Talk," *Journal of the AIH* 87:193, Winter 1994-95.

Center for Homeopathy, representing professionals and lay people, and the Homeopathic Community Council, which is working to create a legitimate homeopathic profession with uniform standards of conduct, practice, and accreditation for everyone, as most of us seem to want. So who needs the AIH, and what is the point of such an organization in 1994? These are my questions for today.

I ask them with some urgency, because the inadequacies of the allopathic model have created a historic opportunity for homeopathy that it would be a shame to waste, however painful and scary it will be to discard the precious cloak of invisibility that has allowed us to operate freely through our long years of decline. Yet at the same time, if we speak out rashly without first healing our own internal divisions, we shall once again most likely find ourselves embattled and overmatched as in years gone by.

I would like to suggest one simple answer that comes straight from our history. As licensed physicians, MD's and DO's, AIH members have the special privilege and obligation to address our non-homeopathic colleagues as equals within the medical profession about health and illness and related topics of general interest. Our common education and training also provide us with a "bully pulpit" from which to participate in the national health-care debate by presenting our knowledge and experience to a public increasingly receptive to what we have to say. If homeopaths genuinely want and expect to play a role in the health care system of the future, they could scarcely do better than to support the AIH in this unique and indispensable role.

Under these circumstances, among our chief purposes and priorities as an organization must be to communicate what all homeopaths know and experience in a way that can be understood by any reasonably literate person, i. e., to create a common language of health and illness that will become part of the contemporary idiom of our culture. Without such a language, our practices will doubtless continue to generate a large number of referrals, as they have always done, and thus to grow and thrive in the future. But the general public and our professional colleagues will remain as mystified as ever by the private language that we use to communicate amongst ourselves, elegant and beautiful to be sure, but still accessible only to those taking the trouble to learn it.

Speaking a common language with our colleagues in a spirit of dialogue must not be confused with simply "working within the system," which means agreeing to speak the technical language now prevailing, from which our own deepest scientific and ethical instincts have been systematically excluded. Even for us to tell what we know, a new, more inclusive idiom will be required, envisioning a new science in which our own values will be fully represented and faithfully expressed. Indeed, I believe that how we think and feel about health and illness is our most timely and valuable contribution at present, especially to those who may never accept or follow the detailed and still partly esoteric rigmarole of what we actually "do" with our patients, let alone how our infinitesimal doses actually "work."

Let me try to be as specific as I can about this. Consider the homeopathic *materia medica,* perhaps our greatest contribution to the profession, which comprises not only detailed accounts of specific remedies but also the nature of medicinal substances in general. To us, each remedy consists of a unique totality of responses, not merely one or two that we desire to manipulate or control in a purely technical sense. Conducted with the aid of healthy human volunteers, homeopathic drug "provings" offer a purely experimental method both elegant and harmless for verifying and amplifying the data of folk medicine, and ultimately for investigating all the medicines of the earth, both known and unknown.[3] The same concept spills over into toxicology, since poisons are also by definition medicinal, by virtue of their power to alter human health, whether they occur naturally in animals, minerals, or plants, or are produced by industrial or metabolic degradation.[4]

In both areas we can and should make common cause with other physicians, to conduct collaborative provings of penicillin, for example, which however misused is certainly one of the great medicines of human history.[5] Every homeopath understands that for penicillin to be effective in the treatment of human illness, it must first be a medicine for human beings, with a distinctive totality of symptoms all its own; that we could use it far more intelligently on the basis of such knowledge; and that even its well-known antibiotic action cannot be properly understood without it.

This is the bare bones of what we have to offer the medical profession, not to mention related fields like ethnobotany, pharmacology, and toxicology as well. Indeed, the totality of the symptoms, the total health-picture of the individual over time, is the basic concept that ties together everything I want to talk about today, because it stands for just about everything that our orthodox medical training was designed to circumvent, discredit, or leave out.

On the most basic level, it explains how we look at out patients and diagnose their illnesses. Consider, for example, the pneumatic otoscope, which makes it possible to detect minute amounts of fluid behind the eardrum, but in the clinical setting inevitably encourages over-diagnosis and over-treatment of "otitis media" in asymptomatic or only mildly symptomatic children.[6] This is the false precision of substituting a ready-to-hand technical abnormality for the laborious task of observing the totality of symptoms in a living patient, a simple non-reductionist message that the public is more than ever receptive to and that homeopaths are perfectly and uniquely situated to articulate.

Although in practice our unique method of treatment claims most of our attention, I will not say much about it here other than to call attention to our reliance on "infinitesimal" doses, which presupposes a radically different concept of medicinal action and indeed of causality in general. The amazing effectiveness of highly dilute remedies means that drugs need not be used to force the organism to achieve a certain preconceived result, that the proper rôle of medicines is simply to empower it to finish the healing work it has already begun and has no choice but to continue.

Similarly, instead of continuing the treatment all the way to the end, the homeopath stops the remedy as soon as it begins to act and does not repeat it for as long as the action lasts, allowing patients to finish the job themselves. In other words, successful homeopathic treatment does not attempt to control or oppose the symptoms with superior force, but only to promote self-healing, and thus reintroduces self-care as the basic model for all healing work and indeed of the doctor-patient relationship itself. Whether or not they understand or accept it, this elementary truth still resonates enough with doctors and patient alike to serve as a basis for real dialogue and health debate.

The totality of symptoms also sheds valuable light on long-term management and prognosis by offering practical criteria for assessing improvement, worsening, and the effect of treatment. These are serious problems for allopathic medicine, which relies almost exclusively on rigid and disembodied technical or laboratory measurements. Thus patients taking cholesterol-lowering drugs have been found to die younger overall than their controls, but many years later and most often of non-cardiac causes, while the leukemia patient who becomes psychotic after chemotherapy, even though the CBC and bone marrow are "in remission," is certainly no better off than before.[7] In this same vein, many HMO's and managed-care plans are learning that case reports and even statistical studies are ambiguous and misleading apart from some overall assessment of the patients' own lived experience and quality of life, including how they feel and function according to their own individual and community standards. Here again, homeopathy merely reinstates the age-old test of common sense that biomedical science has been at such pains to dispense with, and doctors, patients, and indeed the health-care system as a whole stand greatly to benefit from and be grateful for bringing it back.

Finally, the totality of symptoms has equally important contributions to make in the area of medical research. It is hard to find enough words of praise and admiration for the efforts of Jennifer Jacobs and others, who have succeeded for the first time in publishing randomized, controlled studies of classical homeopathic treatment in mainstream American medical journals, a truly heroic achievement.[8] But we also need to create a new kind of research, based on a very different model, to display more faithfully the subtler degree of causal influence that we see in our practices and more of the flavor of what self-healing and indeed everyday life are mostly about.

This means finding an alternative to the double-blind model, which measures the extent to which a drug can surpass the patient's unaided healing capacity and could thereby be said to cure almost militarily, as if by superior force. Such a quantitative design is misleading for us, because remedies work more *qualitatively* by virtue of their special or overall "fit," such that our cured patients truly feel that they have healed *themselves* and indeed might perhaps have done so without our help. In that sense, homeopathic remedies rightly appear to be working on the placebo or "control" side of the equation, such that even when their effect shows through to some extent, it does so more indirectly and obliquely than in the clinical setting.

Indeed, I believe that not only homeopathy but also the medical profession as a whole needs another experimental method based on the milder and more "optional" forms of causality that we are likely to see in everyday life, that do not act by brute force but rather by the force of "persuasion" in patients already attuned to them, much as an enzymatic catalyst facilitates a chemical reaction that already "wants" to happen, and fits with only a few chemical substrates and no others. Subtler influences of this type are likely to be drowned out by the kind of heavy artillery that is required for success in a double-blind experiment.

Having suggested some of the choicer morsels that homeopaths can offer to the public, I would now like to ask you all what we need to offer *ourselves* and also to prospective members, for the AIH to grow and to sustain its work in the future. I stipulate only that it be something that we all want and need, something that will help homeopaths of every stripe and persuasion to come together with a strong voice as a unified profession.

Apart from certification and licensure, which I've already touched on, most of the issues that divide us and keep us apart are disagreements about methodology -- "highs" and "lows;" "unicists" and "pluralists;" adherents of this or that charismatic teacher; dowsers, electrodiagnosticians, and practitioners of radioesthesia, who are in a class by themselves; and doubtless many more, as yet unclassified -- many of them dating back to Hahnemann himself. As I have said before, the movement is evolving so rapidly that we shouldn't really expect to agree about technical matters or even want to try to define homeopathy too rigidly at this point.[9]

Whether MD's or not, professional or layperson, what properly unites us all, I submit, is not rigid adherence to any doctrine or guru or technique, but rather the basic ethics that govern or should govern our relationships to our patients or clients, call them what you will. Indeed I would argue that one of our most valuable contributions to the health professions will be in this area. Much like the treatment itself, the alliance that we can offer to our patients is not a compulsory or exclusive one: we do not "own" them, and they are free to disregard our advice and even to take remedies on their own. Even if they accept what we have to offer, they know or should know that ultimately they must do the healing, and hence that they are the ones in charge.

Perhaps I am naïve to think so, but I would like to believe that all of us can come together on how we relate to our patients and the standards that we are willing to be held accountable for. Far from suggesting that matters of technique are uninteresting or unimportant, I hope that we will not be afraid to disagree about them, even hotly if necessary; but to my mind they are hardly the sorts of things that are worth killing or dying for, or even causing undue pain or dissension for their sake.

One need only look at MacRepertory or RADAR to realize that the homeopathy of 20 years hence will likely be as different from what it is today as the latter is from what it was when I first studied it 20 years ago. Yet we still use and honor the same old texts and will surely continue to do so, so that you need have no fear about the principles that inspired them going out of date.

In short, we live in exciting times. In America the future of homeopathy seems wide open, yet full of perils both old and knew, both known and unknown. Our patients are there, the infrastructure is in place, and the public is waiting to hear from us on all the issues of the day; yet our little organization is still nascent, almost embryonic, and the same forces that almost destroyed us before are more powerful and nasty than ever. So we have a lot of work to do. Keep it up!

NOTES.

1. Moskowitz, R., "Poverty in the Midst of Plenty: American Homeopathy in 1987," Address to the NCH Annual Conference, Chicago, May 1987, NCH audiotape.
2. Herrick, N., "Homeopathic Grand Rounds," *Journal of the AIH* 86:171, Autumn 1993, final paragraph.
3. Moskowitz, *Homeopathic Medicines for Pregnancy and Childbirth,* North Atlantic Books, Berkeley, 1992, pp.4-5.
4. Ibid., p.5.
5. Moskowitz, "Homeopathic Reasoning," *Homeotherapy* 6:137, September-October 1980.
6. Moskowitz, "Childhood Ear Infections," *Journal of the AIH* 87:137, Autumn 1994.
7. Moskowitz, "Some Thoughts on the Malpractice Crisis," *British Homeopathic Journal* 77:20, January 1988.
8. Jacobs, J., et al., "Treatment of Acute Childhood Diarrhea with Homeopathic Medicine," *Pediatrics* 93:719, May9, 1994.
9. Moskowitz, "Ethics in Homeopathic Practice," *Journal of the AIH* 86:238, Winter 1993-94.

*To Have and Have Not: Homeopathy in Cuba**

In February I had the good fortune to teach homeopathy to a group of Cuban MD's in Havana. The five-day seminar was the brainchild of Nancy Kelly, President and founder of Homeopaths Without Borders (USA), and Rogelio Fernandez Argüelles, a Cuban pharmacist who had created the first homeopathy courses in his country. Building on earlier visits by Latin American homeopaths, Nancy hoped that bringing the pooled experience, material resources, and global perspective of *norteamericano* prescribers to an underserved population might also contribute to improved Cuban-American relations in the future. This improbable fantasy actually came to pass nine months later, ironically at the precise moment when politicians in both countries were fanning the flames of national pride over the body and future of a six-year-old boy.

I will pass over the bureaucratic hassles and logistic impediments to my *getting* to Cuba, because they would require an article in themselves, and in any case are no more nor less than what every American has to put up with as a result of our trade embargo, a mere inconvenience when compared to the serious privation it imposes on all Cubans in our name. Under such adverse circumstances, my wife, my daughter, and I could not help feeling acutely aware of our own involuntary complicity in their misfortune as we toured their country in a style that few of them could afford.

Given the history of repeated U.S. invasions of the island dating back to 1898, and our continuing interference in her internal affairs ever since, we were repeatedly surprised by the warmth, openness, hospitality, and delight that were showered on us by almost everyone we met as soon as we announced that we were from the States. Not only do most people have one or several relatives living here, but most cars on the street are classic model Chevys and Fords from the 'Fifties, typically held together with duct tape and baling wire, while kids on every corner play baseball or stickball, just as I did at their age, and the only money tourists can use is US dollars,

---

* "To Have and Have Not: Homeopathy in Cuba," ***Journal of the AIH*** 93:59, Summer 2000.

which we had to carry around in fat wads of cash like *mafiosi,* since U.S. credit cards and travelers cheques were non-negotiable. The supreme irony of Cuba today is that, even after forty years of Communist rule, it feels so much like a down-at-heel province of the United States, like a wayward son who longs to come home again, only to be locked out by unforgiving parents still irate and determined to teach him a lesson.

The seminar, which I taught with John Millar, a Canadian naturopath, was conducted at "La Dependiente," a huge, sprawling general hospital in a run-down neighborhood of Havana, and was attended by anywhere between 20 and 35 physicians, depending on the day. One of the most beautiful cities in the world, with spacious boulevards and colonial architecture as elegant as that of New Orleans or Buenos Aires, Havana is literally and visibly crumbling into dust, having deteriorated to the point that my heart ached at the virtual impossibility of ever restoring it, given that it would cost untold billions at this point and would have to be redone street by street and brick by brick.

An equally glaring disparity in the Cuban scene is its famed medical system, which dispenses good quality care to everyone without charge, boasts more well-trained doctors per capita than any other country in the world, and attracts patients from all over the Caribbean and Latin America, yet pays its physicians a top salary of $30 per month, like all other workers, and since the fall of the Soviet Union has been woefully and perpetually short of drugs, needles, syringes, gloves, bandages, and even soap and toilet paper, not to mention the foreign exchange needed to buy them. Needless to say, the carton of medical supplies I brought from America, though but a token of what is needed, was hugely appreciated and immediately pressed into service.

As I always do, I began the seminar by asking the Cuban doctors how they had come to homeopathy, what issues and problems they were having in their own study and practice, and what topics they wanted us to cover. I was surprised to learn that their interest in the subject arose not out of disenchantment with allopathic medicine, as was true for me and most of my colleagues in North America, but rather from the dire shortage of medicines and of foreign exchange to buy them following the fall of the Soviet Union and the abrupt severance of Russian economic support.

These considerations undoubtedly account for the fact that interest in homeopathy did not resurface in Cuba until the early 1990s, that the

Castro regime has blessed or at least not actively opposed the experiment, and that the homeopaths I met were all "regular" physicians who wore lab coats, worked in hospitals, and dispensed antibiotics, but were open to homeopathy, acupuncture, or whatever else could help their patients, with the sole proviso that it be credible scientifically and supported by up-to-date experimental research.

Hence the urgent e-mails we received prior to our departure, pleading with us not to bring the *Organon* or discuss theoretical or historical issues, which occasioned some skepticism on my part about the depth of their commitment to quality homeopathy, and even, I confess, a bit of elitist snobbery about upholding the purity of our sacred and immutable truths. In any case, all of these holier-than-thou assumptions and misgivings evaporated in the first few seconds of our meeting. In the flesh, our Cuban students were not only serious, intelligent, competent, well-trained professionals, but also thoroughly involved in every aspect of the method, eager to learn anything we could teach them, and indeed in several respects already miles ahead of us.

To give just two examples, our host, René Guarnaluse Arce, M. D., had begun to manufacture liquid attenuations from scratch in the hospital pharmacy, while other students in the class had designed or were conducting or participating in large clinical trials of homeopathic treatment for such common diseases as allergic rhinitis, sinusitis, asthma, chronic bronchitis, and emphysema. In spite of being re-introduced to the subject less than ten years ago, the Cuban medical system has already graduated five hundred diplomates in homeopathy from approved certificate programs out of a total population of ten million, including several in every province and in most large towns. Whatever its motivation, this degree of official government backing has created a more hopeful prospect for the present and immediate future of homeopathy in Cuba than in most other countries I have knowledge of.

In addition to a pulmonologist, an endocrinologist, an immunologist, a toxicologist, a senior gastroenterologist, a few pediatricians, an OB-GYN, a psychiatrist or two, and representatives of other specialties, the class also included family physicians and a pharmacist from the hospital, who told me excitedly of recent neuro-physiological investigations of a spider venom that had demonstrated lytic effects on the myelin sheath. So many of them were actively engaged in clinical or basic research on some aspect of homeopathy that we later devoted a whole morning to experimental work, at which time they reported on the studies they were involved or interested in, while I raised some general issues of method, proposed an alternative to the usual double-blind model, and reported on some of the current research being conducted in the US and Europe.

Facilitated by the excellent and lively translations of Dr. Guarnaluse Arce and Kim Sikorski-Orozco, M. D., an experienced Mexican homeopath who had come all the way from Guadalajara to help, John and I taught freestyle, each in our own way, he on the nitty-gritty of prescribing, case analysis, and repertorization, I covering broad areas of pregnancy, childbirth, and pediatrics to demonstrate the range and flexibility of the method as a vehicle for both primary and specialty care. As is often the case in teaching, however, the highlights of the course, the parts that were most stimulating and memorable both for them and for us, tended to come from unplanned tangents and digressions, typically in response to their questions about issues in their practices.

Thus an asthma case that John presented occasioned a long disquisition on that disease, which is perhaps even commoner in Cuba than it is here, while a passing reference I made to families of remedies provoked intense curiosity and excitement about the mineral, animal, and plant kingdoms and subgroups, and later about miasms as well, all of them subjects that they had never heard of before. Repeatedly I was charmed by the openness and almost childlike receptivity of these seasoned veterans, who though steeped in the modern scientific attitude, yet strained to copy down every word and nuance of these most parlous and controversial topics in homeopathy. For this and many other reasons it was a great joy to have the opportunity both to teach and learn from them, and I would especially like to thank Nancy Kelly and Homeopaths Without Borders for being there and making this experience possible.

AIH Bioterrorism Project, Excerpts*

Introduction.

The AIH Bioterrorism Project arose more or less spontaneously after the attacks on the World Trade Center and the Pentagon in September 2001, followed soon after by the sickening and death of several individuals coming into contact with weapons-grade anthrax that had been mailed to CBS Television News and several Democratic Congressional leaders. While the perpetrator of these crimes has never been identified, we soon learned that the material had been manufactured in our own U.S. Army Biological Warfare Laboratories, and that even the tiny amounts contained in these few envelopes was enough to infect and kill many people.

Fear swept the country as millions realized that the Government is essentially powerless to stop a biological attack from a determined enemy and as unprepared for large-scale biological warfare as for airliners used as explosive weapons, or indeed for serious terrorist attacks generally. The universal outrage, shock, and disbelief were further compounded when we learned that the major producer and supplier of biological weapons was and still is none other than our own government, and that whatever capacity Iraq, Al Qaeda, and other hostile forces and terrorist groups now possess very likely originated in our own laboratories or those of our Russian former competitors.

Like our allopathic colleagues, homeopathic physicians all over the country were beset with more or less frantic calls from our patients seeking advice about how to protect themselves from anthrax, smallpox, and other potential bioweapons; and I wrote and distributed brief advisories on anthrax and smallpox, as did many other practitioners.

In the wake of these events, given the clear and suddenly omnipresent threat of biological attack, the exemplary record of homeopathy in treating epidemic diseases gives the American Institute

* "AIH Bioterrorism Project," ***American Journal of Homeopathic Medicine*** 96:94, Summer 2003.

the opportunity and the obligation to acquaint our own patients, the medical community, and the public at large with a valuable additional service of which they may well be unaware. We have no intention of recommending homeopathic medicines as a substitute for or alternative to conventional prophylaxis with suitable vaccines or treatment with antibiotics and other medications as required. We simply offer these gentler methods of proven safety and effectiveness under the following special and limited circumstances:

1) when an actual attack is suspected or imminent, and the known risk of conventional vaccines may outweigh the uncertain risk of exposure, or no effective vaccine is available;

2) shortly after an attack, for persons already exposed or at high risk of exposure who are as yet asymptomatic, or for early or incipient cases of disease, for whom conventional treatment is not yet available or has proven injurious in the past;

3) for more advanced or desperate cases, when conventional treatment has failed or caused serious adverse reactions that make it impossible to continue with it, or as an adjunct to such treatment;

4) for individuals with known sensitivity to or intolerance of conventional vaccines or medications, or both, or those who refuse to take them for any reason; and

5) for individuals who have suffered major or minor adverse reactions to vaccines or medications.

One further problem with relying on conventional vaccines for prophylaxis is the process of weaponization, which typically involves deliberate alteration of the microbial genome to render vaccines less protective against it. Because the suitability of homeopathic medicines is based on the total symptom-picture of the patient rather than the antigenicity of the causative organism, they should be equally effective under these conditions.

In December 2002, Jennifer Jacobs, M.D., M.P.H., the AIH President, appointed a five-member Committee (Drs. Mitch Fleisher, Jackie Wilson, Bob Schore, Bernardo Merizalde, and myself as Chairperson) to study how and to what extent homeopathic medicines might prove effective for prophylaxis and treatment of anthrax, smallpox, plague, tularemia, and botulism, the five principal biological agents, in the situations outlined above, and to publish a report in this journal and as press releases to the medical community and the media.

Assigning each of my colleagues to research and report on one or two of the five major diseases, with myself as coördinator and general editor, I defined our common task as follows:

1) to summarize the pertinent medical facts (epidemiology, pathology, signs and symptoms, clinical course, conventional treatment, prophylaxis, etc.) for each disease; and

2) to consider for each disease when, which, and to what extent homeopathic remedies might be used in any or all of the situations described above.

Our mission is simply to inform and reassure the public, by showing how these diseases actually behave and what practical measures may safely be taken to combat them, both preventively, in advance of an actual attack, and once such an attack is in progress. The information and advice that we offer will hopefully provide a useful antidote to the atmosphere of dread and uncertainty that is what acts of terror are mainly designed to accomplish. Biological agents are complex, sensitive organisms that are all quite difficult to prepare, easily decompose with improper handling, prolonged storage, or dissemination under suboptimal conditions, and are equally dangerous to their handlers. A determined enemy could kill at least as many people in an even shorter time with nerve gas or other chcmicals, which are much simpler and cheaper to make, far more stable over time, and more reliable to use. But however unlikely it may be that biological weapons will actually be used on a mass scale, they remain formidable as threats precisely to the extent that we imagine we have good reason to fear that they will be. Insofar as they convince us to limit and restrict our lives for fear of them, those who wish us ill will already have accomplished a huge piece of their work . . .

Anthrax: Postscript.

Anthrax is primarily a disease of herbivores such as sheep and cattle, and in nature occurs most often in the cutaneous form, from direct contact with spores in wool or hides. After a short incubation period, it begins as a "malignant pustule" or boil that promptly turns black or necrotic: hence the name "anthrax," which simply means "coal-black," like anthracite. This tendency to produce gangrene or necrosis is characteristic of the disease in all its forms. In susceptible individuals, the disease can progress into a sepsis or blood infection, again with local or more generalized tissue destruction and hemorrhagic phenomena.

The spores may also be inhaled directly into the lungs, in which case the illness begins, after a shorter incubation period of up to three to five days, with flu- like symptoms, but then rapidly evolves into a hemorrhagic pneumonia and septicemia known as "wool-sorter's disease, with a fatality rate of 50-80%, even with the best of treatment. In this aerosolized form it can also be used as a weapon, although the disease is not contagious from patient to patient, so that each victim must be targeted individually. To infect large populations thus requires highly advanced scientific and technical capabilities that might be acquired by a determined enemy with sufficient resources, but seems excessively elaborate, impractical, and expensive for most real-life situations.

Widely touted as the most effective antibiotic for the inhaled form, Cipro has been stockpiled by many hospitals and concerned individuals just in case, but the cheaper and even more potent Levaquin is actually preferred by many authorities. For large-scale prophylaxis during the incubation period, Doxycycline is probably the first-line drug of choice. But even when given intravenously in massive doses, no drug will act fast enough to stop the inhaled form consistently.

Currently required for members of the U.S. military, the one available vaccine has itself been linked with a whole spectrum of disabling chronic illnesses in veterans of the first Gulf War that have contributed significantly to the legendary if ill-defined complex of ailments familiarly known as "Gulf War syndrome." Despite systematic attempts by several Administrations to downplay these reports, hundreds of American military personnel have already been discharged in recent years for refusing to be vaccinated. In sworn Congressional testimony, one former Air Force Colonel, a highly-decorated pilot of many years' experience, has documented substandard conditions and practices in the laboratory preparing the vaccine, which hopefully will not be made more widely available any time soon.

Both the extreme rapidity with which pulmonary anthrax typically develops and its high fatality rate despite the best antibiotic treatment creates a unique and valuable niche for homeopathic prophylaxis and treatment at every stage of the disease. As described in Allen's *Materia Medica of the Nosodes,* the homeopathic remedy *Anthracinum* is prepared from the spleen of infected sheep and was introduced into homeopathy by the veterinarian Lux, a student and colleague of Hering, as early as 1830. It quickly proved its worth not only preventively but also for curing the disease in numerous outbreaks among livestock in the nineteenth century.

While I don't recommend using it for long-term prophylaxis in advance of an actual attack, it should prove very effective if given as soon as possible afterwards, since the incubation period is so short. In this situation, I would suggest taking *Anthracinum* 30 twice daily, for three to four days, and then two doses a week for two or three more weeks, or until the emergency subsides, whichever comes first. If it is not generally available for this application on an over-the-counter basis. it should at least be liberally provided to licensed homeopathic physicians and health professionals and dispensed under their supervision.

For the treatment of frank pulmonary or septic anthrax, intensive antibiotic treatment will clearly be needed, but its extremely high mortality rate makes it imperative to offer homeopathic remedies adjunctively as well. In the early flu-like stage, typhoid remedies like *Bryonia, Baptisia,* and *Rhus toxicodendron* are apt to prove useful, while in the advanced septicemic phase some of the remedies most often cited by Vermeulen and others include *Arsenicum album* and *iodatum, Carbo vegetabilis, Carbolic. acid., Crotalus horridus Echinacea, Lachesis, Mercurius, Phosphorus, Pyrogenium, Secale, Silica,* and *Sulphur.* To these I would add *Scolopendra* and *Tarentula cubensis,* based on Dr. Wilson's research, as well as *Vipera,* my own suggestion, since it is replete with blackish discolorations and gangrenous phenomena, while adding the obvious caveat that other remedies are certain to be needed in individual cases.

As with most epidemic diseases, the *genus epidemicus* or specific remedy corresponding to the majority of cases for that outbreak will be apparent once twenty or so individuals have been treated successfully, after which it should be given out on a large scale to people nearby who are in imminent danger of exposure, as well as to others already exposed but not yet sick, and to those with early or incipient cases. Unfortunately, this tried-and-true method will be of limited value with anthrax, which attacks most of its victims more or less simultaneously, apart from a brief warning period for those living downwind of the attack, and those who weeks or months later come into contact with anthrax spores which have fallen on or in proximity to the skin and clothing.

Because the spores remain thermostable for long periods of time and thus capable of re-aerosolizing and being inhaled hours or days later, simple preventive measures such as scrubbing of clothes, bedding, and exposed skin with soap and water and disinfection of contaminated surfaces with solvents are also imperative. Further research will also hopefully determine the conditions under which spores germinate in the lungs, and thereby lead to safe and effective methods of forestalling or at least inhibiting that process . . .

Smallpox: Foreword.

Of the five main biological warfare agents, smallpox stands alone in two important respects. First, it is by far the best known, with a long and notorious history in Western culture, having played an important role in the Spanish conquest of Mexico, and even been deliberately used as a bioweapon in the form of infected blankets traded by American settlers to decimate the native tribes whose lands they coveted. Like other such weapons, it turned back on the attackers with impersonal savagery, generating deadly epidemics in Europe, the United States, and all over the world, such that it became one of the most dreaded scourges of mankind, while its distant cousin cowpox or vaccinia provided the first effective vaccine, and also lent its name to the general concept of "vaccination," which has since become indispensable to modern medicine in its epic and indeed interminable warfare against infectious diseases of every kind.

Second, while quite contagious and thus capable of propagating itself to large populations far away from the initial target area, it is considerably less so than plague, and has a much longer incubation period, like measles or chickenpox, which gives more time for effective preventive and treatment strategies to be deployed. The absence of any effective antiviral treatment, the well-documented hazards of the cowpox vaccine, and the long, consistently successful track record of homeopathic medicines for prophylaxis and treatment at every stage of the illness all conspire to make this monograph by far the longest and most detailed of the five . . .

Plague: Postscript.

Plague is potentially the deadliest of all bioweapons, in that it combines the virulence and extreme rapidity of action of anthrax with the infectivity of smallpox or tularemia and thus the ability to spread to larger populations outside the immediate target area. Since the weaponized material would be inhaled directly into the lungs, the most virulent pneumonic form would be the main threat, and its brief incubation period of two or three days would allow no time for a vaccine to take effect, even if there were one, and very little for effective treatment of any kind.

If treatment is delayed more than eighteen hours after the onset of symptoms, the case fatality rate increases dramatically: the interval from onset of symptoms to death averages only two to four days. In addition to this fulminating pneumonia, the pathology of severe cases includes sepsis, hemorrhagic shock, renal failure, and necrosis or gangrene of vital organs or peripheral tissues.

Personally, I doubt that plague will be used in a biological attack in the foreseeable future, for two reasons. First, the bacillus is so virulent and dangerous to its handlers that many of the early investigators came down with the disease and died of it. This might not deter a suicidal fanatic, but could make the planners of an attack think twice about the feasibility of getting it safely to the target area and carrying out the attack effectively. Second, only the United States and the former Soviet Union possessed the resources, the will, and the technical capacity to weaponize this stuff. For terrorists to use it, they would have to buy or steal it from us or the Russians and then figure out how to use it: certainly not impossible, but difficult enough to deter almost anyone . . .

Tularemia: Postscript.

Although tularemia acquired naturally from rodents and rabbits can usually be treated effectively with antibiotics if caught early enough in its various localized forms, its principal threat as a bioweapon lies in the extent to which the weaponization process can aerosolize and disseminate it in a form and particle size capable of being inhaled directly into the pulmonary alveoli and thereby producing pneumonia and sepsis, i.e., its most deadly typhoidal form, largely bypassing the usual subcutaneous and lymphatic routes. In this respect it is exactly analogous to the plague, and indeed is properly thought of as a cheaper, more abundant, and only slightly less deadly version of the latter, the main differences being that it cannot be transmitted from one human victim to another, but on the other hand is much less well known, more varied in its clinical presentations, and therefore more difficult to recognize.

Evidently tularemia was first studied and possibly used by the Japanese in Manchuria during World War II. A Soviet microbiologist who defected to the West claimed that large-scale outbreaks on the Russian front may also have been intentional and resulted in tens of thousands of deaths among German and Russian troops alike. Moral considerations aside, this possibility underscores the other major problem with biological and chemical weapons generally, their ability to turn on their users and attack them with equally devastating effect.

This is particularly true of tularemia because of its extreme infectivity, in which it again rivals the plague: one expert has said that ten to fifty bacilli are sufficient to cause disease if they are inhaled or injected hypodermically. In the late 1960's, the U.S. military stockpiled large quantities of virulent material, and by the early 1990's the Russians had done the same, having developed new strains resistant to all antibiotics and vaccines, according to the same Soviet informant. In 1969, WHO experts reported that 50 kg. of virulent organisms aerosolized and dispersed over a metropolitan area of 5,000,000 inhabitants could result in about 250,000 incapacitating casualties and perhaps 20,000 deaths. Like the plague, it is also very dangerous to laboratory workers handling the organism.

There is no mention of remedies or treatment for tularemia in the homeopathic literature. But its general resemblance to the plague bacteriologically and clinically, with tender, swollen lymph nodes, pneumonia, sepsis, hemorrhages, gangrene, etc., suggests that, in addition to the remedies cited by Dr. Merizalde, the others listed under plague might do good service as well. The nosode *Tularemia* probably exists somewhere, and could be of use in the event of an attack; but I've not yet seen or even heard of it.

As with the plague and anthrax, the main application for homeopathic remedies is likely to be for prophylaxis, based on the *genus epidemicus,* and also as an adjunct to antibiotic treatment for advanced cases. The main antibiotics favored for treatment are exactly the same as for plague:

streptomycin, gentamicin, chloramphenicol, and various tetracyclines, with doxycycline the probable drug of choice for large-scale prophylaxis. Cipro has also shown promise *in vitro.* But if the weaponized strains have indeed been altered for maximum resistance to drugs and vaccines, then homeopathic treatment based on the total symptom picture could easily become the principal treatment modality for this seriously underrated disease.

*Advisory on Bird Flu**

The threat of a global epidemic of avian influenza depends on the convergence of several interrelated factors:

1) the appearance of virulent strains in Asian domestic fowl (chickens, ducks, geese), with occasional spread to their human handlers and a high fatality rate in humans, approaching 50% in some series;

2) its rapid transmission across Eurasia by migratory birds;

3) the proven ability of influenza viruses to produce mutant strains capable of human-to-human transmission, causing worldwide epidemics in the past;

4) their short incubation period (2-3 days at most), which spreads them more rapidly than large-scale preventive measures can easily contain;

5) the limited effectiveness of standard antiviral drugs against them;

6) the difficulty of creating a new vaccine every year with enough specificity to be effective, of producing it in sufficient quantity for large populations, and of distributing it in time to do any good; and

7) the lack of adequate hospital beds, trained personnel, and outpatient facilities to administer vaccines and other preventive measures and to treat severe cases on a nationwide or global scale.

This special Advisory is meant to address this important but still purely hypothetical threat. It is not a plea or recommendation that people choose homeopathic treatment in lieu of standard public health measures or effective vaccines when they become available. It is intended solely to inform the public and medical community about a simple method for the prevention and treatment of epidemic diseases that is safe and inexpensive and has repeatedly proven its worth in the past. It calls for a modest three-level strategy that lies well within the capability of any region, state, or locale acting on its own, without any need for Federal assistance or the quota of unwanted surveillance and red tape that often comes with it.

---

* "Advisory on Bird Flu," ***American Journal of Homeopathic Medicine*** 99:16, Spring 2006.

Level 1: *Prevention in advance of the outbreak.*

The first level is prevention in advance of the outbreak, or in its earliest stages, when the first documented or reported cases appear in the vicinity. If the specific vaccine is unavailable in sufficient quantity, either of two common homeopathic medicines may offer significant protection for a period of weeks or months, and may be taken with perfect safety by anyone.

The first is called *Influenzinum,* the remedy or nosode prepared from the virus itself, and may be taken in the 30C or 30th centesimal dilution, 3 doses within a 24-hour period (waking, bedtime, waking), repeated weekly until the outbreak passes. Although the notorious mutability of the virus limits the efficacy of any medicine previously prepared, even from the deadly 1918 strain that is still in common use, this nosode has maintained a good track record in the regular annual epidemics since then.

For bird flu in particular, an even better alternative might be the medicine prepared from duck heart and liver, because ducks are one of the main reservoirs of the most virulent strains, and the medicine has nothing to do with the microbiology of the virus, but only with the reaction of its animal host to it. It is available over-the-counter from several different manufacturers under various trade names, such as *Oscillococcinum* (Boiron Labs), and may be taken in the 200C dilution, on roughly the same schedule as the nosode. It has proven to be highly effective in preventing influenza if begun at or before the time of exposure, and also works quite well for incipient cases if given early enough.

Level 2: *Preventive treatment in the early stages of the disease.*

Once the disease has broken out in the vicinity, homeopathic physicians are trained to examine each case individually and to prescribe the one medicine that coincides most nearly with the unique symptom-picture of that patient as a whole. In the case of epidemic diseases, once 15 or 20 patients are treated in this fashion, one medicine will have proven to be extremely beneficial to perhaps 75% of them, both in alleviating the intensity of the symptoms and in speeding the recovery and thus shortening the course of the illness. Once identified as the basic medicine or *genus epidemicus* for the outbreak as a whole, it may then be given out prophylactically to everyone at the time of exposure, or even beforehand when the disease is nearby. It will also do great service in treating early or incipient cases.

Level 3: *Individualized treatment of advanced or complicated cases.*

For the remaining 25% or so who do not respond to the *genus epidemicus,* other equally beneficial medicines will be identifiable by a trained homeopathic physician, based on further individualization of the total symptom-picture, as above. Some of the more severe cases will require hospitalization and allopathic treatment as well.

Long experience with outbreaks of smallpox, cholera, scarlet fever, typhoid fever, and other epidemic diseases at a time when antibiotics and vaccines were not yet available has shown this simple method to be highly effective, in both treating people who are already sick and preventing the spread and reducing the severity of the disease in others in its path. It is inexpensive and admirably safe, involving the use of simple home remedies that are available to anyone without a prescription, freeing the physician to focus on the more advanced and complicated cases. As part of an overall public health strategy, it could be of great benefit whenever and wherever standard vaccines and allopathic medications are not available.

IV. Reviews.

Ullman & Cummings, *Everybody's Guide to Homeopathic Medicines*

Catherine Coulter, *Portraits of Homeopathic Medicines,* vol. 2

The LIGA in Washington: the Scientific Sessions

Larry Dossey, *Beyond Illness*

George Vithoulkas, *A New Model of Health and Disease*

George Vithoulkas, *Materia Medica Viva,* vol. 1

Harris Coulter, *The Controlled Clinical Trial: an Analysis*

Roger Morrison, *Desktop Companion to Physical Pathology*

Julian Winston, *The Faces of Homeopathy*

Coulter & Ramakrishnan, *A Homeopathic Approach to Cancer*

Julian Winston, *The Heritage of Homeopathic Literature*

Isaac Golden, *Vaccination and Homeoprophylaxis*

Dana Ullman, *The Homeopathic Revolution*

Massimo Mangialavori, *PRAXIS: Method of Complexity*

Catherine Coulter, *The Power of Vision: Life of Samuel Hahnemann*

Prafull & Ambrish Vijayakar, *Predictive Homeopathy*

Karl Robinson, *Small Doses, Big Results*

Dana Ullman and Stephen Cummings, *Everybody's Guide to Homeopathic Medicines**

This book is a jewel and a marvel, in addition to filling an important practical need. Books describing the use of homeopathic remedies in first aid, the treatment of injuries, and simple domestic ailments are as old as homeopathy itself, going back to Hering's ever-reliable *The Homeopathic Domestic Physician.* Hahnemann insisted that homeopaths learn to speak the language of the patient, not only the technical jargon of the medical schools; and the self-care movement in homeopathy flourished in frontier America, where doctors were scarce and self-reliance was a matter of pride and simple necessity. Literally dozens of homeopathic domestic manuals were turned out in the 19th Century, many of high quality.

I am happy to report that today the genre is still very much alive and well on the American scene. Most recently, Maisie Panos and Jane Heimlich's classic, *Homeopathic Medicine at Home,* has succeeded in presenting domestic homeopathy to a broad contemporary audience in a simple and practical way. So you may well ask, do we need another book so soon on more or less the same subject?

Certainly someone wishing to buy just one book could do almost equally well \with either one. But homeopathic books are rather like a fine potato chip in that very few people who have tasted it will want to stop with just one. The Panos and Heimlich book is very much a digest of Maisie's long and legendary experience. It is appropriately chatty, anecdotal, warm, and human, brimming over with a beloved doctor's practical wisdom and a mother's healing touch. Large sections of it could be read with pleasure by a healthy person without any particular need or inclination to give or take remedies.

This latest book, on the other hand, is a systematic attempt to place homeopathy squarely within the mainstream of the new consumer health and self-care movements. It is a book of homeopathy, to be sure,

* Book Review: Ullman and Cummings, *Everybody's Guide to Homeopathic Medicines,* ***Homeopathy Today,*** March, 1985.

and a very good one at that; but it is also a primer of self-care, tackling in detail such thorny questions as how far a lay person can or should go without needing to call a doctor. These are the real-life issues that the folks out there raising their kids are having to wrestle with when they get excited by the idea of homeopathy but can't find a Maisie Panos to guide them.

The authors are certainly well-qualified for the task. Stephen Cummings, a Family Nurse Practitioner in Berkeley, California, is a long time student of homeopathy, and former editor of the fine *Journal of Homeopathic Practice.* A prominent writer, lecturer, health educator, and consumer advocate, Dana Ullman is a gifted and indefatigable promoter of homeopathy and media personality, the proprietor of Homeopathic Educational Services, and formerly a skilled lay practitioner himself.

The main body of the book is organized into three parts of greatly unequal length, the second or middle section being by far the longest. The first part is a concise and well-presented overview of the history, philosophy, and method of homeopathy, including a sample of acute case-taking. The third part is a detailed *materia medica,* likewise economical but very thorough, perhaps even a little more so than the average reader with no previous training or experience could be expected to master right away, and extremely reliable throughout.

But the real heart and soul of the book is Part Two, comprising over two-thirds of the whole, which is devoted to various ailments and complaints, featuring chapters such as 'Fever and Influenza,' 'Earache,' 'Sore Throat,' and the like. Each chapter begins with a general discussion that includes brief descriptions of the clinical and diagnostic possibilities, including typical complications. The chapter on earaches, for example, also includes essential information about how to recognize or suspect otitis media as well as complications like mastoiditis and meningitis. These short descriptions are often quite beautiful: clearly written, succinct, and almost impossible to find elsewhere. Taken together they give the basic outline of such differential diagnosis and triage of the various complaints as a parent, family member, or friend would be called upon to make.

I found them to be uniformly accurate, up-to-date, and written in a simple, non-technical style that any reader of average intelligence could easily follow. This is a notable achievement in itself. Following each major complaint are some brief remarks under the heading 'General Home Care,' including simple suggestions regarding diet, regimen, etc., and then a differential diagnosis or detailed *materia medica* of homeopathic remedies most commonly indicated for that complaint. These descriptions are also quite detailed, generally a good deal more so than in the Panos book, and very well done.

This part of the book also fulfills an important need for those readers who "cut their teeth" on Maisie's book and are ready for something more. For a total beginner, on the other hand, the simple charts in the Panos book are a little easier to use, while the more experienced prescriber will soon want an adequate repertory, which neither book has. The final section of each chapter is entitled 'Beyond Home Care,' and tries to spell out the danger signals that would warrant professional help, and how quickly to seek it as well. This invaluable information is likewise skillfully presented, as well as highly professional and up-to-date.

In my view, this book succeeds brilliantly in adapting classical homeopathy to the needs of the modern self-care movement. The format and type of the book are a pleasure to look at and easy to read. The text is very well written, in a simple, informal, and highly readable style. The brief introduction by a Professor of Medicine at Georgetown University Medical School shows that homeopathy is at last beginning to arouse the curiosity and interest of the medical world at large.

Naturally, there are a few areas that could have received more emphasis, notably pregnancy, birth, infancy, and women's health. Also the complex arrangement of the topics and sub-topics within each chapter makes the book rather cumbersome to use at times. But what the book does cover, it covers superbly well. In our own practice in the Boston area, we carry and sell it alongside the Panos book, tending to recommend the latter for beginners, and the former for serious students who are actively involved in a study group, already using a kit, and looking for more detailed information. So there seems to be a wonderful complementarity between them, after all; and our literature is greatly enriched by having both available. The authors deserve our warmest thanks and congratulations; and their book deserves, above all, to be read, used, and savored.

Catherine Coulter, *Portraits of Homeopathic Medicines, Vol. 2**

Catherine Coulter' s second volume of remedy portraits begins with the polychrests *Nux vomica, Silica,* and *Ignatia.* The next hundred pages are occupied with the nosodes, *Psorinum, Medorrhinum, Tuberculinum, Syphilinum, Carcinosin,* and the general concept of such remedies made from disease-products. The book ends with *"Staphasagria* and Indignation," a treatise on comparative *materia medica.* Ms. Coulter's methodology is the same as in her first volume, and her marvelous knowledge of remedies and of human nature are conveyed in the same elegant prose that graces everything she writes.

But the attentive reader will nevertheless perceive a major difference in the subject matter, which perhaps explains why she chose these remedies to write about in the first place. The contrast is rather subtle at first, and is evident mostly in retrospect, in her selective re-emphasis of certain general aspects of *materia medica* study, which previously she only touched upon. Her introduction, for example, promptly reminds us of the *duality* of remedies, their ability to encompass divergent and even apparently contradictory attributes, which follows from the Laws of Similars itself, from the very definition of a "remedy" as a power of provoking and relieving the same set of symptoms, according to the dosage and the sensitivity of the patient.

Another important subtext is the peculiar nature of homeopathic thinking, which identifies a "keynote" or characteristic symptom and then recognizes an analogous version of it in seemingly remote areas of functioning, establishing it as a "general symptom" that cuts across the boundary between "mind" and "body," for example, and thus becomes predicable of the organism as a whole, i.e., purely energetically. A beautiful example is *Silica's* "albinism of the spirit," in Elizabeth Wright-Hubbard's phrase, an extension of the delicate, pale complexion, a physiognomic

* Book Review: Catherine Coulter, *Portraits of Homeopathic Medicines,* Volume 2, ***Homeopathy Today,*** April 1989.

characteristic, into the mental and emotional realm, a broadening and deepening of the original concept, yet based on and in turn eliciting still further clinical observations.

A striking kinship thus connects the original, more limited version of the symptom, as encountered in the first patients and older texts, with this ever-broadening and deepening recognition of the "remedy" as the composite of all the patients who have ever taken or been affected by it in either fashion. This bidirectional process of widening the range of the symptom by locating its "essence" in more and more analogies, whether generic or specific, is precisely the manner in which our knowledge of *materia medica* is built up; and the mental agility required to travel back and forth between various dimensions of our nature -- animal, vegetable, mineral, human, divine -- and be equally at home in all of them is a lot of what it takes to be a Kent or Vithoulkas, a Whitmont or a Coulter.

Another application is the chronic extension of what originated as an acute symptom, as when *Arnica,* the classic remedy for blunt trauma to the soft tissues, is also used in a sense "constitutionally" for patients whose various ailments appeared to originate from a similar blow. This is the "never well since . . ." concept, which also generalizes and extends the range of the remedies well beyond their original, more concrete or immediate application and eventually leads to the deeper levels of chronic disease, with which the latter part of the book is occupied.

All of these themes take us beyond the idea of the totality of symptoms as a simple collection of unrelated characteristics, and into the patient's inner dynamic, through which one symptom or totality develops and changes into another, involving other layers of functioning not previously apparent.

Thus *Nux vomica* and *Ignatia,* while clearly "polychrest" remedies of wide application and recognizable style, are distinguished chiefly by these developmental themes -- duality or contradictoriness, generalization from the particular application to the essential meaning, and "never well since" or "stuckness" at the acute level prolonging itself into the chronic dimension -- rather than by the striking keynotes or modalities of *Sulphur* or *Lycopodium, Pulsatilla* or *Sepia, Arsenicum* or *Lachesis.* The recognition of *Nux* or *Ignatia* in a patient thus requires a different sort of mentality, involving the perception of personal growth or change, of pathology as transformation, which adds to our understanding of the other remedies as well.

The chapter on *Silica* is one of the finest and most satisfying pieces of *materia medica* writing that I have ever read. That is partly because the totality of *Silica* is somewhat more difficult to recognize, lacking the more spectacular or flashy characteristics of other polychrests, and because her portrait helps to fill in the gaps in my own understanding. Even more striking is her artistic use of imagery, as in her chapter subheadings, "The Grain of Sand," "The Stalk of Wheat," "The Mouse," and "The Cricket." By following these simple archetypes from the animal, vegetable, and mineral kingdoms into the human world of intention and meaning, she is able to show how these various aspects of our nature come together to create a physiology which is thoroughly alive. The discussion of *Silica* concludes with an appendix on the problem of vaccinations, again foreshadowing the larger issue of the miasmatic or chronic-disease structure of the race.

As presented here, the nosodes are both distinctive and important remedies in their own right, and investigational tools into deeper levels of psycho-physical integration. Inherently more difficult to understand and use than the typical polychrests of the first volume, they are derived from the products of actual *diseases* (the scabies vesicle, gonorrheal discharge, syphilitic chancre, tuberculous lung, etc.), which are defined primarily by pathological abnormalities in the tissues rather than the totality of *symptoms* that they can elicit or cure. Yet they are prepared and studied in the same way as all other remedies, with provings, clinical verifications, and characteristic totalities built on them.

In any case, they always have seemed rather shadowy and elusive in character, much more closely tied to what Dr. Eizayaga has called the "lesional" level, the anatomical pathology that medical doctors are so attached to, and thus to certain more or less speculative inferences about the overall lesional pattern and the corresponding "miasmatic structure" or "terrain," allegedly predisposing to illnesses of a certain type.

These are, of course, precisely the sorts of hypotheses that give scientifically trained doctors fits, and that help to maintain homeopathy in its comfortable exile beyond the pale of what passes for science these days. But they do correspond to the deeper reality that chronic diseases often persist and worsen, despite temporary or brilliant cures according to the totality of symptoms, that these patterns are often observable in families, and that it is indeed possible to describe, classify, and ultimately treat them. Nor are these obscure and difficult topics any more suspect from the point of view of conventional science than simply bending the literal truth of mechanical causality into metaphor and archetype, as all classical homeopaths habitually do without shame or hesitation.

In any case, the nosode chapters are necessarily somewhat briefer and sketchier than the others, impressionistic and more difficult to grasp as a whole: that's just how it is. In my view, the chapter on *Psorinum* is by far the best of these, not least because the Hahnemannian notion of "psora" still seems like such a wastebasket of loose ends. Using her customary art and skill, Ms. Coulter somehow manages to pull together her experiences with this oddest of nosodes, prepared from a scabies vesicle, into a coherent and recognizable remedy picture that illuminates the classical literature but also goes beyond it. Her wonderful idea of "ineradicability" (e.g., the great *unwashable,* not simply unwashed, like *Sulphur)* and its extensions into the mental sphere -- "despair of recovery" -- and the special application of defective reaction and multiple allergies, is a brilliant piece of imaginative scholarship that cannot fail to delight and instruct the *aficionado* even more than the novice, and the experienced student most of all.

Her words repeatedly stimulated the thought that perhaps the salient features of the nosodes can be more difficult to recognize at first, or until apparently well-indicated remedies fail to act or hold, because they correspond to the deeper characterological levels of integration, rather than simply to the "personality," or the more superficial aspect, i. e., what appears most striking on the surface. The polychrests of the first volume might thus be easier to recognize because they encompass both levels and indeed demonstrate the evolution of one into the other.

To me, the chapter on *Medorrhinum* is rather less satisfying, because it does not make an effective imaginative connection with the known pathology of gonorrhea and thus remains largely impressionistic, even fragmentary, although it is just as well-written and as much of a pleasure to read as the others. The same reservation is applicable to the remaining nosodes as well, but it is less a criticism than an acknowledgement of the difficulty of working in this field. *Tuberculinum,* for example, is similarly innocent of pathology in the medical sense, but the portrait hangs together better, and is more satisfying and instructive as a result, while *Syphilinum* and *Carcinosin* are admittedly sketchy, and tend to stay as close as possible to the previous literature.

The final chapter, "*Staphysagria* and Indignation," is an experiment in comparative *materia medica,* a *genre* already familiar to many of her readers. For the goal of all remedy study, identifying and recognizing the peculiar characteristics of each remedy, means learning how to distinguish it from all others, and especially from those that most closely resemble it. The well-known fastidiousness of *Arsenicum,* for example, is quite different from that of *Natrum muriaticum, Nux vomica, or Thuja;* the keynote is simply a word, a broad analogy between a number of diverse and even competing styles. "*Staphysagria* and Indignation" is really a treatise on this particular keynote, having the twin purposes of illuminating the psychophysical dynamic of *Staphysagria,* a fascinating and important remedy in its own right, and at the same time exploring the basic human and biological importance of that symptom through its many varieties.

It is not entirely satisfactory, in that it skips back and forth a good deal between well-worn aspects of several remedies, using a speculative scheme that is questionable in itself. But the great thing about it is the experiment, and of course the vintage Coulter prose. I loved the book; by turns, I found myself amused, surprised, moved, provoked, and enlightened by it. It is a book that will grow on you as you re-read it, and you gain more experience, just as many of the remedies she discusses are best appreciated on the rebound from other remedies that didn't work quite as well as we hoped. Above all, it highlights the dual nature of *materia medica* study, with its parallel sources that are reciprocally nourishing, the lore of medicinal substances as an integral part of the greater study of human life.

*The LIGA in Washington: The Scientific Sessions**

The recent LIGA Congress in Washington presented a fascinating microcosm of world homeopathy in action. It was an opportunity to meet colleagues and friends from all over the world, and to learn from some of the greatest homeopathic physicians alive today. Yet it also exposed many of the same divisions and rivalries that have plagued homeopathy ever since Hahnemann himself and continue to undercut its message.

The hotel accommodations were pleasant and tasteful, the service reliable, and the commercial exhibits, although few in number, were interesting and often of high quality. Among those I especially liked were the old homeopathic books of Bill Kirtsos of Chatham, NY, and the MacRepertory software program developed by David Warkentin. The principal remedy manufacturers were there, as well as several other book dealers. Others seen in attendance were the British Society of Homeopaths and the Northern College of Homeopathic Medicine, two first-rate training programs for lay homeopaths in the UK.

The International League of Homeopathic Physicians, or LIGA, was formed in the 1920's by a small group of homeopathic physicians from several different countries; and membership as well as attendance at its conferences remains open only to licensed physicians, dentists, veterinarians, pharmacists and scientists engaged in relevant research. Honorary Associate Memberships are occasionally awarded to lay or unlicensed supporters of homeopathy who financially or in some other way have made a significant contribution to the movement. The attendees included 43 licensed physicians from the United States, an impressive testimonial to the renaissance of homeopathy in this country in recent years, long after having championed it before the world.

---

* "The LIGA in Washington: the Scientific Sessions," ***Homeopathy Today,*** July/August 1987.

What follows is essentially a travelogue of my own impressions and prejudices. I didn't see or hear everything and haven't reported on all that I did attend; I've concentrated on papers that were provocative or of special interest to me, and have doubtless neglected others of equal or greater worth.

The session opened with welcoming remarks by our own Drs. Sandra Chase, Jennifer Jacobs, and Jackie Wilson, followed by a brief concert with singers and musicians from the Washington Opera, and a delightful slide show by Julian Winston that highlighted the development of homeopathy in America. The AIH then awarded a special medal to Dr. Maisie Panos, Honorary Chairperson of the Congress, in honor of her long and dedicated service and mentorship to the younger generation of homeopathic physicians.

The first day was taken up with papers concerning theory and philosophy. After a few lectures of broad, general import, I was particularly taken by one from Prof. Denis Demarque of the University of Bordeaux, entitled "Hahnemann, Follower of Pasteur," beginning with a scholarly exegesis of the term "miasm" in the plays of Molière and the pages of Hahnemann's *Chronic Diseases.* In the latter work, Hahnemann refers to cholera as a "living miasm, imperceptible to the senses," and contagious and transmissible to others, i. e., a *microorganism,* anticipating Pasteur and Koch, pioneers of the germ theory several decades later.

Demarque's point was to demonstrate that the Hahnemannian idea of miasm is wholly that of a material substance, and thus has nothing to do with the "spiritualist" emendations put upon it by subsequent writers such as Kent, J. H. Allen, and other Swedenborgians. This seeming tension between "scientific" and "vitalistic" or metaphysical hypotheses was already evident in Hahnemann's own writings, and still persists today, with each side quoting apposite scriptural passages from the master. Demarque then proposed updating the miasm concept by adopting the term "infectious agent," as proposed by Künzli and Pierre Schmidt, and concluded with an assessment of the three chronic miasms in the light of modern research.

Another delightful paper from the French delegation was presented by Dr. Alain Horvilleur, entitled "Twenty Years of Practice," and including a number of pithy aphorisms covering a gamut of clinical subjects, ranging from how he became a homeopath to how he practices now. (He uses a *big* computer to cross-reference those giant rubrics in Boenninghausen!) He also spoke of the *art* of homeopathy, defining the "seasoned" homeopath not as the one who knows the most remedies, but the one who knows how to ask the right *questions,* to facilitate the self-healing process in the patient. He urged all homeopaths not to make a "fetish" of Hahnemann, but indeed to "kill the father," in the modern Freudian sense, and, ultimately to "embellish his memory," presumably by attaining our own independent judgment based on his principles.

Describing his conversion to the method of Boenninghausen, he then wondered if the modern concept of miasm as a possibly inherited "terrain" or predisposition to a certain type of illness might not precede and thus even eclipse Demarque's more materialistic concept of the infectious agent as a specific *etiology.* Finally, now that the three great Hahnemannian miasms appear to be all but inundated by the weight of all the petrochemicals, X-rays, and the other toxic influences of our time, culminating in AIDS, he wondered, "what next?"

The esteemed Dr. Künzli then gave a paper on "The Hierarchy of Symptoms," based upon Hahnemann's own instructions as to their priority, which I found magisterial but dry, at times hard to follow, and in any case offering nothing new or unfamiliar to the classically-trained American homeopath. What bowled me over, however, was his new *Repertorium Generale,* recently published by Barthel of West Germany, and on sale for a cool $290.00. Beginning with Kent's *Repertory,* Künzli daily and painstakingly, over a period of forty years, added rubrics and remedies from Allen, Hering, Boenninghausen, Yingling, Gentry, and others, carefully noting the source in each case. This heroic labor went on until at last he *rested,* saw that it was good, and delivered it for publication. Homeopathy has always depended unduly for its growth and its voluminous literature on the labors of such saints, particularly those blessed with the same obsessive-compulsive attention to detail that our method seems to require. I'd say that this book is worth every penny of what it costs, except for the bright orange cover, which I found rather disconcerting.

Roger Morrison, M. D., of the Hahnemann Clinic then presented a lucid and comprehensive summary of the views of George Vithoulkas on the significance of acute diseases appearing at various times during the course of chronic or "constitutional" treatment. Taken together with the papers by Drs. Schore, Nossaman, and others, it showed that American homeopathy could certainly give a good account of itself on the world stage.

The afternoon session was largely taken up with papers concerning the assigned philosophical topic for the Conference, namely, paragraph 5 of the *Organon,* i.e., the concept of the "exciting cause," or *causa occasionalis,* and the general subject of etiology. I was especially taken with the three consecutive papers given by Dr. Jutta Gneiger and other members of the Vienna school, currently headed by the venerable Dr. Dorcsi, who has particularly emphasized the importance of such etiological factors in his teaching. All of the papers originating from this school were intelligent, well-organized, and capably presented.

Tuesday morning I spent in a separate auditorium listening to those talks assigned to the "satellite" program as not pertinent to the specified theme of the main conference, which on that day was the *materia medica* of *Colocynthis* and *Staphysagria.* Presented by F. J. Master of India, the first talk I heard recounted the tale of a patient gravely ill after a stroke caused by a ruptured cerebral aneurysm buried deep in the brain, making surgery impossible. The patient was in a deep coma, with hemiplegia and violent hiccough. Dr. Master first gave *Arnica* 10M by inhalation every 2-3 hours, a general prescription for severe head injury, meanwhile obtaining a history from the family and observing a pattern of tremors on the opposite side. His second prescription was *Veratrum alb.* 50M by inhalation every 3 hours, followed by *Hyoscyamus* 10M and 50M likewise, as the patient began showing signs of mental activity -- mainly, delirium -- and responding to painful stimuli. Gradually, the rigidity lessened, the spinal fluid cleared, and the patient regained consciousness and the ability to speak. He was discharged from the hospital in about three months, after which *Bothrops 200* and *Calc. fluor. 30* were also given. The patient did not make a full recovery, but I love to hear of cases like this, that show the beneficial action of remedies in seriously-ill or hospitalized patients, such as I seldom have the opportunity to see or the skill to help. Perhaps we should rotate our physician-trainees through a busy Indian hospital for a year or two until such times as we can arrange it in this country.

I also very much enjoyed a talk by Dr. Prakash Vakil, another Indian physician, entitled "The Tongue Does Not Lie," which summarized some of his experience with and favorite tips on tongue diagnosis. What really intrigued me was the fantasy, for which I take full responsibility, of Dr. Vakil manning an outpatient dispensary somewhere, teeming with sick humanity, seeing hundreds of patients a day, and having to dispense remedies on the spot without the luxury of spending two hours with them. "Tongue diagnosis" was evidently part of the ritual he had developed to be present for each patient to whatever extent he could in the few minutes at his disposal. What could easily have seemed to some as mere pathological prescribing impressed me as rather another species of missionary sainthood that I clearly wanted to believe produced excellent results for many of his patients.

Fuller Royal, M. D., of our own Nevada Clinic then gave a refreshingly irreverent talk explaining some of the many uses of electro-diagnostic machines and what I propose to call "experimental homeopathy" in general, i.e., the use of homeopathic concepts and remedies in new ways not yet proved or officially approved by anybody. He presented a wonderful case of an elderly patient taking 12 different drugs, a veteran of two bypass operations, in whom the machine diagnosed an energy disturbance in one wisdom tooth, and whose clinical condition improved dramatically and immediately after the its removal. He used the case to highlight what he somewhat disconcertingly described as the principal advantage of the method, namely that there is no need to *talk* to the patient; the machine could give its own bioelectrical reading quite independently.

From his experience, he estimated that about 30% of all patients will show some evidence of environmental pollution, toxicity, or sensitivity to some chemicals at exposure levels well below their EPA thresholds. Inasmuch as every good classical homeopath has dozens of cases where the totality of symptoms seems to be defective, or where the seemingly well-indicated remedy doesn't act, it would make a lot of sense to invite them to hook up to such a machine and see what hidden mysteries could be revealed.

I believe that electro-diagnostic machines represent an exciting and important advance in energy medicine technology. They already have made the effort to combine the databases of acupuncture and homeopathy, and they have infinite applications to the study of some of our most difficult patients, for whom the classical method alone seems inadequate.

Wednesday's scientific assembly was given over to clinical cases, many of a serious nature. These are the ones that doctors love, especially when hospitalized with dangerous lesions, incriminating laboratory tests, and whatever else serves to remind us that we too are physicians trained and licensed to treat the sick, no less than our allopathic brethren. And these are the heavy-duty pathological cases that we hope and expect one day to try our mettle against.

So, as might be expected, Wednesday was also the day when a good deal of professional disagreement, most of the fireworks, and also some really splendid work, were presented for all to see. One notable example was Dr. Diwan Harish Chand of New Delhi, official Physician to the Prime Minister of India, who presented three hospital cases, two of them on dialysis with chronic renal failure.

The first case was that of a 33 year-old man with intestinal obstruction; at the time of hospitalization he had been vomiting for two days without passing any stool or flatus, and also without urinating. X-rays showed multiple distended bowel loops. *Plumbum met.* 200 was given every 2-4 hours, largely on pathological grounds, and the patient passed flatus within two hours and several large bowel movements soon after that. Three days later, he relapsed somewhat, and the dose was repeated. He has remained well ever since, about 3 years. This tale reminded me of some classic articles by Harvey Farrington on that favorite subject of homeopaths everywhere, "Cases Saved from the Surgeon's Knife."

The second was a man of 50 who developed renal failure in the course of a flu-like illness, and had been on dialysis for about 6 months; his chief symptom was nausea at the sight of garbage. *Arsenicum album* was prescribed, in the 6C, 30C, and 200C, 1 dose of each on the first day; and after the following day he never needed another dialysis treatment. After one year his shunt was removed, and he has been entirely well since, more than 6 months so far. Previously he had spent thousands of dollars on allopathic treatment until homeopathy was given, with lifesaving results and at minimal cost. Someday, he prophesied, insurance companies will be the ones to make homeopathy's case.

His final patient was a 54 year-old man with chronic renal failure, nephrotic syndrome, and encephalopathy. *Opium* 30 was given every 4-6 hours for 16 doses. Within 2 days he was fully conscious, and within a week he felt "100 times better." He has remained well for over two years, and has required no further dialysis treatments. It is noteworthy that Dr. Chand's results were obtained with the single remedy in medium potency and infrequent dose, i. e., with nothing but good, old-fashioned *skill.*

I will briefly summarize some of the cases presented by other speakers, to give some idea of their range and seriousness. Dr. A. U. Ramakrishnan presented several cases of hemorrhagic disorders, including a boy of nine with congenital hemophilia, who was seen during a prolonged episode of bleeding following a tooth extraction; his clotting time was about one hour. He was given *Arnica* 200 every 5 minutes for 10 doses, followed by *Phosphorus* 200, 1M, and 10M in ascending order, once a month for six months. There has been no bleeding for 3 years, and all his tests remain normal.

Another was a girl of 17 with idiopathic thrombocytopenic purpura and a history of spontaneous bleeding episodes since early childhood. She was given *Phosphoric. acid.* 200 initially, then *Kali carb.* constitutionally and *Ceanothus* 3X daily for 6 months to reduce the spleen. There were no further bleeding episodes; the patient has since married and given birth with no complications.

Next in line was Professor Eizayaga of Argentina, who presented four cases of severe organic pathology cured or greatly improved following his method of pathological prescribing using the low dilutions first. One was a baby girl of 6 months, nursing, with severe bronchiolitis, and congenitally blind from degenerative lesions in the retinas. She was given *Phosphorus,* which covered both the lesional and the characteristic symptoms of the case, the 6C and later the 30C. There was "complete recovery" in 3 months, with cure of the retinal lesions and restoration of vision.

During the question period, Dr. Peter Fisher, Editor of the *British Homeopathic Journal,* challenged Dr. Eizayaga to define what he meant by "cure," and got him to admit that he meant *clinically* cured, and histologically *arrested.* Dr. Cesar Cremonini, representing a rival school in Argentina, insisted that it is *always* necessary to treat the patient, even in these serious "organic" cases; and a heated exchange ensued between them, in which points of doctrine were debated and much self-righteousness was displayed on both sides, chiefly in what they *agreed upon,* namely,

1) that the test of a "true" homeopathic physician is the willingness and ability to treat and cure these heavy-duty cases, and

2) the implication, derived from Hahnemann's own life and works, that homeopathy represents a sacred, revealed truth, a creed eminently worth living and dying for.

But by far the most moving of all the case reports was the one presented by Dr. David Flores Toledo of Mexico, that of a 10-year-old girl who developed viral meningitis with convulsions during an attack of suppurative otitis media. What gave special poignancy to her story was that the ENT consultant had pronounced the case hopeless without strong allopathic drugs, and that the girl was Dr. Flores' own daughter, who kept begging him to cure her with remedies. After studying the case, he prescribed *Nitric. acid.,* which had no effect; eventually he prepared an autonosode from her own ear discharge, potentized it up to a 36C, put one drop in 60 ml. of distilled water, and gave her one teaspoon, whereupon the convulsions stopped immediately, and the girl developed a fever for the first time. Eventually he found the simillimum in *Calcarea silicata,* although the "cure" took two months and the girl was left with a 50% hearing loss on the affected side. The illness occurred in 1973; the child is now a medical student in Mexico.

The senior Dr. Wadia of India, who taught at our summer courses on several occasions, concluded the afternoon with two splendid cases of postoperative urinary retention in which *Staphysagria* acted curatively.

On Thursday, several research papers were presented, including one by Dr. Lawrence Badgley of the United States, on a test which he has developed for selecting remedies in AIDS cases, with promising results. Dr. Chase has summarized the Assembly Meeting which followed, about which I can only add that the shouting and blustering which took place there ended the Congress on a note of wild and reckless disorder that left the American delegation more or less speechless with disappointment and disbelief.

Larry Dossey, M. D., *Beyond Illness**

This is a wise and wonderful book. It follows in the footsteps of Dr. Dossey's first book, *Space, Time, and Medicine,* in which the physicochemical model of human functioning is shown to break down in attempting to explain the lived experience of patients without mental and emotional categories, i. e., without elements of *meaning.* The present volume recognizes the fundamental importance of spiritual categories in healing, and attempts to develop a metaphysic capable of accommodating them within that experience.

It is therefore a sort of dialogue between great sages old and new, Eastern and Western, with some wonderful quotes, and the more narrowly reductionist viewpoint of modern "scientific" medicine, still largely prevailing. Best of all, the moderators of the discussion are some of Dr. Dossey's own patients, who are partial only to getting well, living, dying, or whatever else seems to be happening to them.

The book also has considerable literary merit, not least on account of these splendid clinical parables. One involves the paradox of a man fatally and unrepentantly ill, yet mentally and spiritually healthy in the highest sense, while another describes a man who remains profoundly ill without diagnosable pathology until at last he suffers his heart attack and dies, exulting in that unity of mind and body which had eluded him throughout his life.

Other tales demonstrate the inadequacy of various related mythologies of the physicochemical viewpoint, e.g., of death as "the enemy," and of "real disease" as objectively fixed in the tissues and therefore recalcitrant to mental or spiritual influence. Several demonstrate remarkable self-healing in the face of serious or life-threatening illness, while another describes an illness involving a suicidal *refusal* to be healed, and another shows dying in full awareness as the truest and most profound healing of a young child.

The metaphysical exploration that attempts to connect and even "explain" these stories is rather less satisfactory, grappling with some

---

* Book Review: Larry Dossey, *Beyond Illness,* ***Chrysalis,*** Journal of the Swedenborg Foundation, Spring 1989.

of the same issues that have engaged and puzzled philosophers since the beginnings of human thought, and opening some doors and indeed Pandora's boxes that are not so easy to close again. If illness and health are not just the presence or absence of diagnosable pathology, for example, then how *are* we to understand them? Dr. Dossey seems to want to take us *beyond* them, into the spiritual realm beyond linear space and time and the discursive separation of subject and object, in company with the great spiritual traditions of the past and the new physics of the present century.

In comparison with the reductionism of modern medicine, this clearly represents a wise and humane step, a practical prescription offering much solace for physician and patient alike. But as an explanatory principle that seeks to account for the variety of clinical experience, simply leaping into "spirit" as if by magic tends to prove both too much and too little. Too much, because it still neglects to consider those purely energetic phenomena which, while defined largely on the physical level (e.g., an illness or aggravation mainly on one side of the body, during certain hours of the day, or in certain types of weather), nevertheless need not involve diagnosable pathology nor salient psychospiritual conflicts. These are precisely the distinctive data of acupuncture, homeopathy, and other species of what is sometimes called "energy medicine."

Upping the ante by diving straight into the spiritual realm overlooks the existence of these energetic phenomena, and therefore, by implication, ignores the legitimacy of those therapeutic approaches that do address them. In this way, Dossey ultimately restores more or less intact the conceptual structure of allopathic medicine that he previously refuted so well, simply by making *an exception* to it, by adding in the extra or special category of the psycho-spiritual world and thus ultimately reinstating the old dualism in a new guise.

On the other side, it also proves too little; in bypassing the whole vast realm of bioenergetic phenomena, he seriously misinterprets and underestimates the thrust of the holistic health movement, of which he is himself an important spokesman, and at least implicitly dismissing alternative medicine as a facile species of pop psycho-spiritualism, a reductionism of the opposite kind. While nominally open to and tolerant of all forms of healing, including those that he doesn't understand, he doesn't specifically discuss or evidently take seriously the contributions of cranial osteopathy, acupuncture, homeopathy, and the other bioenergetic therapies.

Nevertheless, the book remains an extremely thoughtful and valuable exploration of what for most physicians remains forbidden or unfamiliar territory. It deserves to be widely read and talked about by doctors and patients alike, and hopefully it will lead to further contributions from the same author.

George Vithoulkas, *A New Model of Health and Disease**

I had two strong incentives to take my time with this book. The first is my esteem for its author, whom I consider to be one of the finest homeopaths who have ever lived, and whose dedication to and mastery of every aspect of our art continue to teach and inspire me as they did when I first met him long ago. The second is his stated purpose to develop a practical philosophy, not just for homeopathy, but for the whole of medicine, which, as he says, is urgently needed at this critical juncture in human and indeed in planetary history.

For both reasons, before examining the content of his argument, I need to say a few words about his *style.* By that I do not mean his vigorous but sometimes rough-hewn English prose, which has greatly benefited from the capable editing of George Guess and others. Nor is this the place to explore the curious enigma underlying all his books — that he chooses to write them in a foreign tongue and thereby conceal no small part of himself behind the considerable technical difficulties of editing, transcribing, and even at times of "ghost-writing." What I really mean by "style" in this instance is the spiritual heart or "essence" of the work, which does indeed shine through all of these intermediations and even colors the proto-scientific model he proposes. It is already fully evident on the first page of the Foreword, wherein he seeks to apologize for his sometimes harshly critical tone:

> The book is written to show that established medicine has failed in its mission to prevent or cure disease [and] is responsible for a degeneration of health of worldwide dimension due to the excessive use of powerful chemical drugs. I sense a rapidly approaching planetary catastrophe; the style of writing reflects the urgency I feel about this problem.

Already we can sense the radical difference in attitude and perspective from his earlier book, *The Science of Homeopathy: A Modern Textbook,* which

---

* Book Review: George Vithoulkas, *A New Model of Health and Disease,* ***Homeopathy Today,*** January 1993.

presents much the same model of health and illness "from the inside," so to speak, as a straightforward exposition of homeopathy, in admirably clear and economical English, without any of these heavy polemics or sharp edges. In the present work, his purpose is much larger and more pressing: to offer homeopathic ideas to the general public without any prior exposure or prerequisite, apart from the overpowering sense of the inadequacy of the medical model, now widely felt even within the profession itself. He further implores the reader not to reproach him for an often grim and even frightening book that gives little enjoyment or pleasure to read, because his purpose is rather to catalyze historical change.

On the other hand, this special pleading obliges us to judge his work not only on the conceptual merits of the model he proposes, which are considerable, but also on its effectiveness in persuading the general public, which I fear will fall well short of his ambition. In this respect, as in many others, *A New Model of Health and Disease* is strongly reminiscent of Hahnemann himself, whose own fundamentalist convictions and moral absolutism in defense of them brooked no opposition even from his own followers, let alone from the medical profession at large. Which is too bad, since Vithoulkas himself is well aware that

> . . . the task I have undertaken is tremendously difficult, and thus my attempt is by no means complete or final, [but] only a suggestion of the direction in which medical thinking should proceed.

It is this Hahnemannian dilemma as to its *stance*, it seems to me, that is the real problem with the book, far more than its occasional *non sequiturs* or its sometimes opaque literary style. A basic incompatibility between its difficult and complex scientific task and the evangelical certitude of its actual pronouncements often infuriates me at precisely those moments when I want to agree most strongly, and makes it arduous and tedious work to extract and ponder the considerable number of good and estimable things that lie scattered throughout like uncut diamonds in rough and unforgiving ground.

By no means the least of these are the research data cited in the text, indicating how epidemiology and other basic sciences can be used to support a more holistic viewpoint at least as well as orthodox medical science. Thus, for example, he documents plausible relationships between antibiotic treatment for nonspecific urethritis and subsequent development of chronic prostatitis, and between repeated courses of antibiotics for sexually transmitted diseases and AIDS. While falling well short of "proof" in the usual sense, these and many other citations provide strong and sometimes compelling support for his general theoretical position. For this his research staff deserves a sizeable measure of gratitude and praise, as does the theory which inspired and directed them.

The twin purposes of the book are, first, to show how modern chemical medicine is not only inadequate to cure or prevent chronic disease, but also itself a major contributor to the progressive degeneration of human health on the planet; and, second, to develop a new and more inclusive model for diagnosis and treatment, incorporating the more holistic perspectives of acupuncture, herbalism, homeopathy, and various psycho-spiritual disciplines. In both respects, it goes a good deal further than *The Science of Homeopathy,* a textbook for serious students already committed to such a viewpoint, which is expository and optimistic throughout. *A New Model of Health and Disease* aspires to reach beyond the small circle of the already converted, to preach to the heathen, as it were, and accordingly invokes the spectre of AIDS and even worse plagues to come as both logical consequence and apocalyptic punishment.

Insofar as we take the book seriously, therefore, it is imperative, first of all, to judge how well or badly he succeeds in his indictment. In the second place, he seeks to reintroduce the basic concepts of homeopathy, chiefly the vital force and the totality of symptoms, as part of a general philosophy of health and illness for the general public that requires no prior exposure or commitment to either the elegant private language or the elaborate methodology that homeopathy has already developed. This task is even more ambitious and important than the first, and therefore also deserves to be evaluated separately on its own merits.

The importance of both questions obliges me to write a somewhat longer and more detailed review than usual. Most of all, I honor the heroic *attempt* of such a book, quite apart from how cogently it has persuaded me or how successful it will be in persuading the public. Despite its inherent difficulties and the shortcomings already referred to, the book does go a long way toward persuading me, especially on a second reading, and is therefore well worth studying carefully, although I cannot promise you a pleasant experience, much less a "good read" for summer vacation or night table.

Clearly addressed to a growing awareness in the American public, his major critical thesis is that prolonged and repeated suppression of acute diseases with antibiotics, vaccinations, and other powerful drugs tends to confuse and weaken the immune system, thus rendering it more susceptible to the deeper chronic ailments of our time. Here again, echoes of Hahnemann fulminating against allopathic drugging are audible throughout. Refuting the conventional wisdom that longevity is attributable to the level of medical care, he cites some interesting studies that life expectancy is comparatively low and actually declining in the U.S. and other countries relying primarily on high-tech medicine, while rising rapidly and often superior in less-developed areas such as Greece or Latin America, with much poorer standards of care. Other studies document the growth of antibiotic resistance through the need for ever-larger doses and the growing number of exotic, resistant bacterial and fungal infections acquired in the hospital.

The key subtext, of course, is that killing bacteria, like the suppression of isolated symptoms, is meaningless and dangerous without the underlying standard of the health and well-being of the patient as a whole — the Hahnemannian "totality of symptoms" — which "*the Model*" (written with a capital M and usually italicized) is intended to elucidate. So far, so good. But unfortunately, his analysis of the philosophical basis of chemical medicine often degenerates into crude polemics against the greed of the drug industry, etc., all true enough but falling well short of the tough-minded critique and systematic indictment that we were promised.

In Chapter 3, "Preliminary Ideas," he finally switches over into the affirmative mode, introducing three fundamental assumptions. The first is a bioenergetic criterion of health and illness, prior to any abstract "disease entities" or categories, and modeled on his familiar three-tiered version of Hahnemann's "vital force." The second is the unattainable ideal of "absolute health" as the ultimate reference point against which all individuals can be measured by the degree and kind of their departures from it. The third is the individuality of the patient, the unique, underlying predisposition or susceptibility to certain kinds of illness, as the indispensable basis, both theoretical and practical, of all legitimate healing work.

For myself, I confess, I fail to see how individuals with unique and ever-changing needs can or should be held to absolute standards of health that are unattainable on principle, yet comparable enough for quantitative assessment. But in this and other sections to follow, Vithoulkas displays his rare and precious gift of expressing in simple language ideas so basic as to resist conceptualization altogether, thus coming close to fulfilling Bertrand Russell's whimsical definition of philosophy, "to start with something so simple as not to seem worth stating, and to end with something so paradoxical that no one will believe it."

In Chapter 4, he begins laying out the principles of "the Model" itself as a series of quasi-mathematical postulates written in a dense, almost oracular style, followed by a longer interpretive section in more everyday language. Two examples follow:

> Man lives in the universe as an integral part of it. The individual actually exists in and copes with the environment through his capacity to exchange energy with it.

> All evidence permits us to assume that there is not only a possibility, but a necessity under certain circumstances for the organism to "unite" or "dissociate" the complex energy fields of the mental-emotional planes or parts thereof, and the fields of the physical body.

Together with their elucidations, these aphorisms constitute the main body of the text, are written in bold type for special emphasis, and numbered and arranged in logical sequence, again, exactly like the paragraphs in Hahnemann's *Organon.* They range in tone all the way from simple tautologies to abstruse and highly technical passages with all the opaque lucidity of an engineering manual. As in Euclid's *Elements* or Spinoza's *Ethics,* each aphorism is built on all that preceded it, and the systematic interconnectedness of the whole becomes fully apparent only as the whole sequence unfolds, thus generating a lot of conceptual power, but also requiring some critical distance on the part of the reader to resist being swept away by it.

Thus, for example, he provides some clearly-written and useful digressions on the three bioenergetic levels or planes, illustrating the separateness of each with simple examples. So engaging are these that readers untrained in philosophy might easily miss the fact that he has simply *postulated* the separate existence of the mental-spiritual, emotional-intuitive, and physical-organic dimensions of experience, thus disposing in a few sentences of some of the knottiest questions in the history of human thought. Here again, as in many other places, he comes off sounding more simplistic than any empirical evidence could possibly justify, or indeed than he himself probably intended. He simply accepts uncritically the data of "common sense" or "ordinary experience," whatever that means, and instantly inflates them into universal truths of supreme ontological power. It is precisely to the extent that we want to agree with him that more theoretical sophistication seems imperative.

His discussion of the spiritual and moral dimension as the "highest" function of the mental and intellectual plane seemed especially tantalizing in this respect. Despite some examples of how pure intellect can be used unethically — with lawyers and politicians ranking high on the list — he discreetly omits any but the most bland and general formulations of ethical or moral precepts that even lawyers and politicians might solemnly avow. At least the principle of wholeness is very aptly illustrated, although perhaps not as clearly as in *The Science of Homeopathy.*

Likewise, he rightly points out that Western education all but ignores the emotional level, in which he includes "psychic" and "intuitive" realms, and forcefully insists that its special data, i.e., *feelings,* be included in the model. But in the next breath, having documented higher suicide rates and allopathic drug usage in the developed and ex-Communist countries than he undeveloped world, he gratuitously assumes that the former is attributable and indeed proportional to the latter. Well, it's *possible,* I'll allow, but I'm afraid that this particular *non seauitur* is too blatant to persuade even a dyed-in-the-wool homeopath like me, let alone those rednecks and yahoos he seems to have in mind for his main audience.

Later in the same chapter, he introduces the concept of ranking or the hierarchical importance of symptoms, both within the same level and from one level to another. Once again, he simply *postulates* such a rank order, citing his many years of clinical experience, including the reappearance of suppressed symptoms according to Hering's Laws, in support of it. Finally, he concludes that the three levels must be separate "entities," based on the similarly postulated "fact" that they *appear* to have distinct "vibrational frequencies" and "informational patterns," i.e., capacities for receiving and responding to different types of stimuli.

For me, these middle chapters carry most of the philosophical or conceptual weight of the book, seeking to articulate basic principles in a quasi-scientific language that, as in all philosophy, must essentially be invented as he goes along, resulting in a motley brew concocted from roughly equal parts of quantum physics, holistic medicine, and ordinary language. I would call it an important and indeed a heroic experiment, not entirely successful perhaps, with plenty of strange things in it, and certainly not to everyone's taste, but supremely worth doing, therefore laudable simply for being attempted, and all the more so however and to whatever extent it can help others to do the same.

In Chapter 5, for example, he turns conventional medicine on its head, much as Hahnemann did, by using a standard of *health* rather than disease -- first in general, then for each of the three levels -- and thus reintroducing the vital force and the totality of symptoms as the only possible starting points for a genuine bioenergetic medicine. He might have helped his readers along here by showing how and why the orthodox view allowed or even helped these concepts to "fall through the cracks," so to speak.

Chapters 6 through 14 complete the central core of the book, wherein he deduces one principle after another from these few basic postulates, much as Hahnemann derived the whole of homeopathy from the vital force and the Law of Similars. Although I have some reservations about his definitions of physical, mental, and emotional health, for example, I'll leave these and other more technical problems -- dissociation between levels, entropy, etc. -- for readers to address in their own fashion. As I've said before, don't expect anything cute or facile here. What you get is what might be called "philosophy in the trenches," a lot of tough spadework trying to crank out a new technical language for a bioenergetic science that is still in its infancy. Not easy to write, and about as much fun to read as an instruction manual for computer software.

We might well pray for him to make it a little easier or more intelligible sometimes, but it isn't entirely his fault. The grand finale is, of course, the promised hypothesis on AIDS, which I won't give away, although it should be no mystery to anyone who's managed to come this far. Let it suffice for the moment to say that it's interesting, provocative, and even clinically useful to some extent, and that the mainstay of scientific prophylaxis and treatment turns out to be homeopathy, in case you haven't guessed. In short, I don't think the last word has been spoken on this subject; and I don't see how his hypothesis is going to help me as a practitioner in treating my AIDS patients.

But my main problem with this book is not that it falls short of solving the eternal riddles of health and disease, which have always been with us and are certain to persist long after we're both gone. It is rather with his messianic vision of homeopathy as the savior of mankind, like that of Kent and Hahnemann before him, which breathes a spirit of certitude and intolerance quite at variance with the scientific spirit and not so very different from that of the ruling orthodoxy he rightly deplores. Those willing to follow him through this difficult and uncharted terrain will not have made the journey in vain. But as for me, I'm waiting for his *materia medica.*

George Vithoulkas, *Materia Medica Viva, Vol. 1**

This is the one we've been waiting for, at least the first installment of it, and it's splendid, although seeing the finished product also helps me understand why it took the author so many years to get it out, and why, alas, he'll never finish it. I do not hesitate to say that George Vithoulkas is one of the greatest homeopaths who have ever lived, and I daresay that few who have heard him or studied with him over the years would disagree. In particular, the incomparable depth and breadth of his understanding of remedies, coupled with his rare gift for discovering their relevance to the issues of contemporary life, have opened up new dimensions of *materia medica* study only dimly hinted at before him.

His recognition of distinctive remedy "essences" or themes capable of organic development over time yields not only masses of new information, but also a whole new way of "seeing" patients that nobody else has articulated so clearly or applied in such a systematic fashion. And, not least, his inspiration of a whole generation of classical homeopaths throughout the world has made it possible to create a thoroughly contemporary *materia medica,* to build upon the contributions of the older masters a more inclusive and relevant literature for our own time.

At least since the mid-'70's, many of his students have been asking him to write down for posterity and in a more systematic fashion the tantalizing bits of *materia medica* he presents at his seminars. At first such requests made little headway against his evasive, almost mystical preference for personal, face-to-face transmission. In 1982, for example, I offered to transcribe more or less *verbatim* several remedy-pictures from his seminar in Alonissos, only interpolating in a few places where my notes were sketchy or his meaning seemed unclear. Some months later he wrote back that what he had presented to us was only a part of the truth and that therefore he

---

* Book Review: George Vithoulkas, *Materia Medica Viva,* Volume 1, ***Journal of the AIH*** 86:257, Winter 1993-94.

could not subscribe to any finite, written rendition of it. But this Platonic riddle of how to give permanent written form to living truths inevitably partial, incomplete, and evolving is precisely the challenge of the writer's art, never to be mastered by reasoning alone. In vain I tried to reassure him that all we needed was such relative truth as he had already given us in good measure.

By the mid-'80's. with several pirated versions of his aptly-named "Stolen Essences" already in wide circulation, he reluctantly decided to produce a *materia medica* after all, and enlisted the help of George Guess, Paul Herscu, and others on the project. I assumed that what he had in mind was simply a more complete version of his lecture notes past and future, including small remedies not yet covered, with enough keynotes and particulars to locate and trace out the essential themes in his characteristic style. A brief introduction would have sufficed to explain how living *materia medica* pictures must always necessarily continue to grow, develop, and be retouched in the light of new information and experience.

But what Volume 1 gives us is much more than this, indeed so much more that I fear his own unique and indispensable contribution will be obscured by if not buried under the weighty scholarly apparatus that he has created to substantiate it, almost all of which is already available in other texts. Possibly to refute both Künzli's charge that his essences are overly mentalized and Eizayaga's that they are "illuminist" fantasies of his own imagination, he has been almost obsessively careful to locate them in and even wherever possible derive them from the earlier compilations of great authorities now safely deceased. Above all, perhaps to appease his own scruples against partiality and impermanence, he has piled on as much detailed information about each remedy as possible, resulting in a reference of encyclopedic proportions, worthy of comparison with Clarke's monumental *Dictionary.*

Thus each remedy portrait begins with its botanical name or chemical composition, geographical distribution, toxicological information, and actual cases of overdose or poisoning where possible. To be sure, Vithoulkas' conception of the remedy as a whole is presented in a section entitled "The Essential Features," with the familiar flavor and style of his seminar presentations. The next, entitled "Generalities and Keynotes," lists more specific and detailed characteristics, both generals and particulars, in the traditional sequence of Kent's *Repertory.* Concluding with a summary of clinical applications, remedy relationships, and other technical details such as dosage, wherever possible he adds a number of cured cases from the older literature, compiled by Paul Herscu, but omitting his own cases, presumably in order to publish them separately at a later date.

This editorial decision is most disappointing, since it is primarily through his own clinical experience, his own unique way of understanding patients, that his profoundly enriched and often strikingly original remedy interpretations are developed and constructed. Based on older, more limited conceptions, the cases seldom give any hint of the evolution in the master's own thought. I have no wish to sound ungrateful, because what we do have is truly magnificent, indeed far beyond anything I imagined, namely, an authoritative reference text of the homeopathic *pharmacopoeia* that will undoubtedly last for generations, embodying George's own vision of what a comprehensive *materia medica* should look like.

Yet it is this same obsession for permanence and completeness that will almost certainly prevent him from ever finishing it. Volume 1, with over 250 pages of text, covers 26 remedies, beginning with *Abelmoschus* and ending with *Ambrosia,* not even halfway through the A's. At this rate, even if all ten projected volumes are actually published, we can expect to be left hanging somewhere between *Fraxinus* and *Gambogia.* Vithoulkas himself is very candid and realistic about the prodigious efforts required to complete such a project. At the end of his Introduction, he appeals to homeopathic prescribers all over the world to contribute their own cases to a collective *materia medica* under his editorship, in much the same way that Kent's magnificent *Repertory* was assembled by the old master's students under his supervision. But does that mean that the publication of subsequent volumes will be delayed still further until his students are prepared to take up the challenge?

Personally, I prefer to hope that, with limited time and energy at his disposal, he will concentrate on setting down his own unique experience of as many remedies as possible in a more personal style, more in the spirit, say, of Nash's *Leaders,* rather than squandering so much of himself on details already available elsewhere. Delegating his students to compile toxicological data, particular symptoms, and other reference material would indeed free him to concentrate on "Essential Features" and whatever leading

"Generalities and Keynotes" and case vignettes from his own experience he would need to finish his own singular contribution in his own lifetime. In future years, his students would then be ideally positioned to move on to still other remedies that Vithoulkas himself had insufficient experience with to write about.

For the present, we can learn some useful things about his methodology, and indeed about *Materia medica* study in general, by comparing what Vithoulkas says about the remedies with what was already available to him in the literature. In some cases, such as *Alumina silicata* or *Ailanthus,* the details are taken almost entirely from other sources, which he is usually careful to acknowledge. With these remedies, most of them much less well-known, his own originality lies mainly in their arrangement and relative emphasis, and thus as always in his own clinical experience, his ability to discern the same patterns or themes in ever broader and deeper applications, until the themes themselves are transformed. Under these circumstances, the high degree of congruence between his and the older accounts is actually very reassuring.

In other cases, such as *Aethusa* or *Allium sativa,* new themes have been added, and whole new areas of clinical exploration opened up, such that what had long been regarded as small remedies of very limited applications have been greatly enriched and upgraded in status by adding a significant chronic dimension. Even for relatively familiar ones like *Alumina* and *Agaricus,* a wealth of living detail has been added, often with characteristic vignettes and typical phrasings, which are of great help to the student. Vithoulkas' incomparable experience and understanding of remedies is evident on every page, and will delight the serious reader, whether novice or expert. The book is also handsomely produced, well-edited, and generally readable, thorough, and scholarly in tone. Unfortunately, it is also very expensive, and the thought of having to shell out a hefty sum for each of for nine more volumes seems quite daunting. A paperback Indian edition is thus both mandatory and inevitable; and an abridged version, including the "Essential Features" and "Generalities and Keynotes," without the particulars, cases, toxicology, etc., seems like a good idea. But in any format, no serious student will want to miss it.

Harris Coulter, Ph. D.
*The Controlled Clinical Trial: An Analysis**

Harris Coulter is already well known to many homeopathic readers, both for *Divided Legacy* and other scholarly works of medical history, and for *DPT: A Shot in the Dark* and various journalistic writings of a polemical type. In this book, the heat of his passion is perfectly tempered with the keen edge of his critical faculties, and the result is a masterpiece.

Once again, his righteous anger is reserved for the sacred cow that gives no milk and is dangerous to health -- in this case, the "double-blind" model of clinical research that has held sway over the profession for the past 40 years or so. Like the heroic *ronin* of Japanese legend, he prefers to exploit the inner weaknesses of his bigger and stronger opponents to defeat them, without any recourse to homeopathy or any assumptions other than the writings of the medical profession itself.

Although readily discernible in the text, holistic concepts like the totality of symptoms and the Laws of Cure arc redefined purely in allopathic terms, thereby preserving both his objectivity as a historian and the sharp edge of his analysis. Even the individuality of the patient is never merely assumed or postulated, yet becomes the starting-point and true protagonist of his work, as the great obstacle of human variability that the double-blind method was originally intended but in the end fails to overcome.

The book is, first of all, a splendid history of the double-blind technique, from its origins in the 1930's to its perhaps overly hasty acceptance by the medical establishment in the '50's and '60's, and its current usefulness to the major drug firms, who alone have the resources to follow the method when necessary, and the influence to circumvent it when possible. This evolution is ably and thoroughly documented in the author's characteristically direct, forceful, and yet lucid and elegant style.

---

* Book Review: Harris Coulter, *The Controlled Clinical Trial: An Analysis*, ***Journal of the*** *AIH* 86:254, Winter 1993-94.

But I value the book even more as philosophy of science, for its systematic analysis of the weaknesses of the methodology itself. In logical sequence, it begins with the basic assumptions:

1) the need to overcome human variability, which may well be neither possible nor even desirable (Chapter 1);

2) the concept of the "Disease Entity," which is fraught with insoluble ambiguities at every level (Chapter 2); and

3) the requirements of homogeneity and generalizability, or representative-ness of the sample, which turn out to work against each other (cf. the "therapeutic paradox," Chapter 3).

Then he proceeds to the actual design and conduct of such studies, in stepwise fashion:

4) sample size, randomization, and stratification, the last two designed to make the sample more generalizable and homogeneous, respectively, thus reintroducing the paradox of 3) above (Chapter 4);

5) defining "cure," thus reintroducing the ambiguities of 2) above (Chapter 5);

6) the procedure or conduct of the trial, in which true blinding is often inconvenient or impossible, and data thus actually falsified (Chapter 6); and

7) statistical analysis of the results, in which any design flaws or improper procedures are likely to be compounded still further (Chapter 7).

Entitled "The Clinical Trial: For or Against," Chapter 8 is the last and longest, summarizing the whole argument in a completely different way. Beginning with the official mythology of the method as presented by physicians to the public, namely,

1) that the procedure is scientific,

2) that the practice accords with the theory,

3) that it is the only reliable way to discover valid new forms of treatment, and

4) that its results largely determine how medicine is practiced, he then demolishes each one in detail, as physicians often do when speaking privately amongst themselves.

The result of this final *tour de force* is an astonishing, brilliant, point-for-point refutation of both the theory and the practice of the "randomized" or "controlled" clinical trial, in which each component of the official myth is turned into its opposite, i. e.,

1) that the method is unscientific in almost every sense;

2) that it is rarely, if ever, conducted as the theory stipulates;

3) that it is not the only way, or even a very useful one, to develop new treatments; and

4) that its results are often ignored by practicing physicians.

In short, this book is Harris Coulter at his mordant best, dissolving away medical cant, myth, and outright chicanery through his characteristic blend of careful scholarship, well-reasoned argument, and elegant but forceful style. I am especially grateful to him for being willing to do the hard work and sustained mental effort to address and think through what for most people is not even a problem. Although he does briefly and tantalizingly allude to "orphan drug" research as a possible alternative model, somehow based on "idiosyncrasy," he does not spell out what it might look like, or suggest other ways to conduct medical research in a more holistic way. But that, I suppose, is my particular hobby horse, not his, and would require further concepts from the vitalist tradition which fall completely outside his more limited purpose here.

I suppose that the book will not suit everyone, perhaps not even a lot of homeopaths. For one thing, it takes a lot of hard, critical thinking to get through it, and the end result is simply a deeper conviction of what many of us already know, or should know. Why, then, should they bother to read it? Apart from the pleasure of following a good mind at work, let me suggest another more practical reason. If the double-blind model is indeed fatally flawed in concept and execution, as I truly believe it to be, then we and our friends in Washington had better think twice before jumping though all those hoops to design our own research in accordance with it. If only people will read it and live it, as I did, this book could help us let go of trying to join the club by doing what passes for science these days, and work together to develop an experimental method for our science that will make plain what we know and thereby create a better standard for the profession as a whole.

Roger Morrison, M. D.,
*Desktop Companion to Physical Pathology**

This is a book that took some courage to write and badly needed to be written. Although wholly contemporary in feeling and style, it speaks to the dilemma of busy homeopathic physicians in every time and place: how to keep doing good quality work under pressure of time, reputation, and ever more difficult and demanding cases to come up with creditable prescriptions for without delay. It is perhaps a measure of the extent to which our own practices have grown and prospered in recent years that homeopaths today are seeing more and more patients with serious organic pathology, many of them chronically dependent on powerful allopathic drugs, who need and want the unique kind of help we can offer and can in fact make use of it. Now as in the past, we overworked GP's in the trenches have always had recourse to compilations that summarize our collective experience with different pathological entities, including practical "tips" on the remedies most frequently indicated for each and how to differentiate them.

In addition to manuals for first aid and self-care, like Hering's *Domestic Physician*, Panos' *Homeopathic Medicine at Home,* and specialized monographs on particular organs and organ systems, like Roberts' *Rheumatic Remedies* or Guernsey's *Obstetrics,* our literature has always included texts of therapeutics for the busy professional, like Jahr's *Forty Years' Practice,* Dewey's *Practical Homeopathic Therapeutics,* and Lilienthal's *Homeopathic Therapeutics*, classics of the genre that I myself have sampled more often than I might care to admit at a fancy case conference.

Dr. Morrison's book is clearly and unapologetically of this lineage, and will undoubtedly gladden the hearts of practicing homeopaths both new and old. Like the other titles I've mentioned, it also should and probably will revive legitimate questions about the classical method *per se* that were

* Book Review: Roger Morrison, *Desktop Guide to Physical Pathology,* **Homeopathy Today,** April 1999.

already raised by Hahnemann himself and have generated controversy from the very beginning. With everyone from the master on down insisting that we treat the individual patient rather than the approximate pathological diagnosis or category, the intelligent student can hardly fail to wonder why it is necessary or useful to talk about "diseases" at all.

Speaking from my own experience, I can think of four good reasons why a pathological orientation that applies generically to large groupings of individuals is still relevant to homeopaths of all persuasions. First, I will cite the accumulated experience of untrained laypeople using remedies for first aid and self-care, a technique of proven worth for over a hundred and fifty years. Both to examine the validity of self-care as a concept, and to appraise its scope and limitations in a classical framework, it is necessary to draw on that experience.

Second, within the realm of more serious conditions usually seen by a professional, conventional diagnostic categories like pneumonia, breast cancer, or multiple sclerosis offer our collective experience with their average, approximate, or expected course as points of reference against which the remedies most often effective in these conditions may be compiled and measured. My own experience with *Belladonna, Bryonia,* and *Phytolacca* in acute mastitis, for example, has greatly simplified the process of choosing a remedy in such cases, by providing familiar standards against which the more unusual possibilities are quickly recognized and identified.

Such approximations are particularly valuable in epidemic diseases such as measles, scarlet fever, or cholera, where the main features of any given outbreak impose themselves somewhat uniformly on almost every patient, so that the remedy most closely resembling it can be offered preventively to incipient cases, definite or suspected contacts, and others at high risk. Indeed, with *Belladonna* for scarlet fever, *Pulsatilla* for measles, *Bryonia* for pleurisy, *Sepia* for morning sickness, *Arnica* for blunt injury to soft tissues, *Ignatia* for acute grief, and the like, the pathogenesis of the condition corresponds so closely to the essence of the remedy that each illuminates the other. Under these circumstances, the remedy may appropriately be thought of as "specific" for the condition, and given out in early cases or preventively to those at high risk of developing it or with a history of having benefited from the remedy for it in the past.

Unfortunately, there is no simple rule or formula for the untrained or inexperienced to distinguish these wholly legitimate practices from the shortcuts of those merely impatient with the discipline of the totality of symptoms. Matching common ailments with lists of remedies for treating them and adding a few easy indications for each to differentiate one from the other, texts like those of Jahr, Dewey, or Lilienthal make it possible for a busy or lazy practitioner to forego the labor and discipline of interviewing patients, grading symptoms, or studying remedies at all. Another reason for studying pathology is thus simply to help navigate a path through this minefield.

Third, the central features of many ailments, like the remedies best suited to healing them, are limited in scope to a relatively specialized area of functioning. In otherwise healthy patients bothered by headache, constipation, neuralgia, menstrual cramps, or vaginitis, for example, the narrow focus of the problem may itself provide the first and best clue to the indicated remedy. Clearly recognized and considered at length by Hahnemann himself, these seemingly one-sided or "local" ailments are shown in fact to represent latent chronic diseases of a more generalized character, which are apt to break out in full force if suppressed with conventional drugs. In some cases, with few underlying constitutional symptoms that patients tend to ignore out of familiarity, the picture remains circumscribed even after skillful case-taking, and the indicated remedy must also reflect that pattern. Many remedies both famous and obscure are known primarily for limited applications of this type, though more detailed provings may well reveal their more "constitutional" features in the future.

Fourth, as all these examples illustrate, the practice of homeopathic medicine culminates in the riddle of chronic disease, a problem to which Hahnemann devoted himself throughout the final decades of his life, revealing broad patterns of symptomatology that underlie the myriad of individual differences and are traceable even across the generations. To this pioneering work, still controversial among homeopaths today, we owe the theory of miasms, the major nosodes prepared from actual disease products, and an integrated schema of animal, vegetable, and mineral remedies related to them, both of which have greatly deepened and enriched clinical practice and thus stood the test of time.

For all of these reasons, books like Morrison's that are organized by diseases will continue to serve a valid and useful purpose, as they have always done, however liable to misuse. I regard them as simply another way to classify *Materia medica* information, and as such another possible conduit to the best available remedy, in addition to the strategies of prescribing by keynote, repertory, "essence" information, miasmatic analysis, and various mixtures thereof, no one of which is sufficient, but all of which are helpful at times. These issues are addressed by Roger himself in his brief Introduction:

> The purpose of this book is threefold: It is meant first as an aid to be used at the time of the interview to cue the practitioner toward likely remedies for a particular condition. The second is as a study guide, bringing the main points of the remedies into focus. And [the third is] to give advice about treatment based on the experience of myself and my colleagues at our center.

Another way to think of the book is as the companion piece and logical extension of his earlier *Desktop Guide to Keynotes and Confirmatory Symptoms,* which presents some of the same information organized by *remedies,* a condensed *Materia medica* for the same busy professional I mentioned at the beginning. As he says, both were written "because I wanted [them] for my own practice." Taken together, these two volumes are thus rather like an updated version of Boericke's *Materia Medica and Therapeutics,* intended for the same eminently practical purpose and for much the same audience.

Furthermore, the book is organized in an equally practical and user-friendly way, and incorporates several novel features that are found nowhere else. Thus for every specific ailment a brief introductory discussion concludes with a "Management" section where homeopathic and allopathic perspectives are combined. The next section, entitled "Therapeutic Tips," is likewise divided into homeopathic, naturopathic, and allopathic varieties, and is equally helpful and convenient to use.

Yet another thoughtful innovation, extracted from *MacRepertory* and *Reference Works,* is the listing of useful rubrics in Repertory language, to show the possible connections that have been made so far, and thereby to eliminate the necessity of rediscovering them anew each time, an incredibly useful service to student and practitioner alike. Only then, at the very end, do we come to what is found in all the other books, the remedies he has found most often useful in the condition, with a few simple features for distinguishing them.

Even here, at the point where it most closely resembles the earlier texts of the *genre,* it is clear why books like Morrison's will have to be written and updated continually, because both the definition of pathology and the number of possible diagnoses have expanded in all directions and will very likely do so even more in the decades to come. Indeed, it is in his selection, most especially in the diagnoses he chose to leave out, that the limitations of the present volume are most apparent, presumably reflecting 1) the relatively limited experience with them at his clinic, and 2) the increased medicolegal risk incurred by even the most experienced homeopath in treating them at present.

It is noteworthy, for example, that most of the conditions listed in his table of contents, and even most of the subheadings found in the text, were familiar to Dewey and Boericke and even to Jahr and Lilienthal, while the diseases more recently discovered, like chronic fatigue syndrome, fibromyalgia, and multiple chemical sensitivity or environmental illness, are omitted, as are some infections, like gonorrhea, Lyme disease, mono, and PID, that it might still be unwise to begin treatment for with homeopathy alone. For much the same reasons, serious or potentially life-threatening ailments, like AIDS, serious blood dyscrasias, cancer, etc., are avoided, as are myocardial infarction, which is simply combined with "Angina Pectoris" because the appropriate rubrics for them are more or less indistinguishable, and hypertension, hypercholesterolemia, osteoporosis, and the like, which represent purely technical or laboratory diagnoses, often without symptoms or rubrics at all.

In his Introduction Roger addresses this issue as well, again from the unique standpoint of the practicing physician that underlies all of his works:

> My conviction is that our main duty is to the safety and health of our patients, not to our homeopathic ideals. This sometimes means that we need to resort to allopathic treatment for the short run. Furthermore, the safety of the practitioner is significant. We should never jeopardize our licenses or our reputations in the community. This is especially true in the United States, where homeopathy is still vulnerable to attack. A balanced, conservative approach is our best chance for long-term gains in spreading our beloved therapy.

These bracing and sensible truths should never be far from the thoughts of any practicing homeopath. Yet as the First Edition of a hopefully classic text that will be updated in years to come, I have no doubt that subsequent versions will phase in some of these other more controversial diseases as further experience becomes available, and the integration of homeopathy into the medical profession continues as at present. In any case, the book is splendid and unequalled elsewhere as it stands. It could well become an important achievement for the society at large in the future.

Julian Winston, *The Faces of Homeopathy: An Illustrated History of the First 200 Years**

In all fairness, it is politically incorrect for me to review this book, since I am myself a character in it as well as a friend of the author, and a recipient of an autographed copy for my pains. I decided to risk it, since my rivals for the job would almost surely have been similarly compromised, and I probably could have wangled a free copy in any case. Besides, what could be wrong with simply admitting that I love the book and will do my best to explain why you should do the same? As my mother often says, what's not to like?

In essence, the book is the hard copy and definitive version of the slide shows and videos with which Julian has been educating and regaling audiences around the world these many years. Handsomely bound and printed on glossy paper, with a wealth of magnificent photographs and illustrations, many from the author's own collection or even in his own hand, it covers much the same ground and displays the same inimitable flavor and style that are already well known to his many fans and admirers. Beneath a photo of Carroll Dunham, for example, we find this journal entry, dated February 13, 1996, and imbued with that special, personal touch for which Julian is perhaps best known:

> I had a dream that I found Dunham's phone number. I called, and it rang. Someone picked up and said, *"Dunham here."* I said, *"I've read your works and was wondering if you'd speculate on the future of homeopathy."* There was a long pause. He said something about the new energy of electricity that holds all the secrets -- that homeopathy is just a passing phase, and that electrical therapy will replace it in 50 years. Then I thought, How can I be calling Dunham? They didn't have phones in 1860! And I awoke.

What I found most striking about the book, embodying precisely the odd mix of qualities that our art itself calls for, is its unappeasable appetite

* Book Review: Julian Winston, *The Faces of Homeopathy*, ***Homeopathy Today***, October 1999.

for all things homeopathic, on the one hand, coupled with a gourmet's refined taste for curious facts, colorful anecdotes, ranting opinions, and obsessive calligraphy on the other. As with inveterate collectors of all types, casual browsers who wander in off the street may often feel a bit of a time warp, as if finding themselves in an old attic stuffed with curios and tidbits, many seemingly of dubious value in themselves.

For that matter, even a dyed-in-the-wool aficionado might not need or care to know that Dr. Gram, the first American homeopath, was a Freemason as well as a Swedenborgian, or that Dr. Hempel fathered illegitimate twins who were later found dead in his home under circumstances that suggested *Aconite* poisoning; or that Tullio Verdi came to America with Garibaldi's help, and treated William Seward, Lincoln's Secretary of State, and other Republican politicians and socialites at a time when the G.O.P. stood for the emancipation of blacks and radical social change.

Yet, speaking purely for myself, I treasured these little sidebars, tangents, and footnotes more than almost anything else in the book, because they helped me to relate the lives of real people to the general and social history of their times. Like the video, the book is entitled *The Faces of Homeopathy,* and focuses on *people,* who they were, and what they did, wrote, and said, more than the broad cultural themes that underlie them, or on such elaborate intellectual explanations as an academic historian might seek. This human and personal approach permits Julian to ramble freely over the subject in his own way and at a more leisurely pace than would be suitable in a more formal text.

How else would we ever know that H. N. Guernsey, the homeopathic obstetrician who railed against the practice of routine vaginal examinations in his profession, also wrote for laypeople, in large part to warn parents against exposing their kids to sexual arousal by allowing them to lie prone for a long time, slide down banisters, go too long with a full bladder or rectum, lie in bed awake at night, or do a sleep-over in the same room or bed with their friends?

On the other hand, this informal and highly readable style makes it easy to forget that Julian is also a trained and dedicated scholar, and has contributed an impressive body of documentation for future generations in the form of notes, bibliography, and appendices, compressing a long story and a vast literature into manageable form by a prodigious labor of love that has occupied him for the past fifteen years. In thus seemingly artless fashion, a good many of the larger historical themes do in fact emerge and come to life after all; and the result is a truly magnificent history of the movement that will unquestionably stand the test of time.

This is particularly true of the modern period, where the standard histories of King and Coulter leave off, and about which the dismissive and disdainful attempts of Martin Kaufman in later years have proved sketchy and inaccurate at best. It is a joy to have in hand at last an account of the subject that brings us up to date and does justice to shared and individual experiences alike. More personally, I am especially grateful to him for having taken the time and trouble to give a fair and balanced account of the events leading up to the breakaway of the National Center from the American Foundation in 1981, a momentous turning point in our history, filling in the gaps in the written record by interviewing the players on both sides, and renaming the event "The Great Unpleasantness" with understated relish.

At once a chronological history and an old attic full of dusty memorabilia, *The Faces of Homeopathy* will appeal to two distinct if overlapping audiences, and deserves to be read in two similarly complementary ways. First, as an absorbing story well told, it will reward the serious student or general reader who is prepared to start from the beginning, to proceed in order, and so catch the sweep of the movement as a whole. In addition, as a repository of lore both important and trivial, it will make a perfect gift book for the coffee table of our cured or at least grateful patients, friends, and fellow-travelers who are drawn to or interested in the subject but lack the patience or motivation to wade all the way through its technical details.

Once again, I cannot resist pointing out a few more of the choice bits that caught my eye and gave me food for thought. Early on he speaks of Dr. Pulte's success in treating cholera victims in 1849, a story that has been repeated many times over in connection with other epidemics of other diseases. I have always wondered why historians have yet to document and validate these great victories of the method, which must surely have been recounted in the leading newspapers of the time.

Elsewhere we read of the doctrinal struggle between International Hahnemannian Association "purists" like Lippe, on the one hand, the "mongrels" then dominant in the American Institute of Homeopathy, on the other, and Dunham's heroic efforts to make peace between them, the failure of which evidently hastened the great man's death. Most well-versed students of the method already know or should know that these internecine disputes began with Hahnemann himself and continue unabated today.

There is a wonderful account of a Fincke potency made in 1882, labeled *Belladonna* MM, which found its way to Dave Wember 100 years later in the even more attenuated form of a "dry graft," yet still cured his patient in a single dose. I love to tell stories like these to my patients to elicit their skepticism, and always feel a little uneasy with those who can swallow the Law of Similars and the infinitesimal dose hook, line, and sinker, as if they haven't really felt their bite. Another in the same vein was the seemingly terminal patient of Dr. Stuart Close who revived in a few minutes with a single dose of *Arsenicum* 45M Fincke and lived in good health for 20 years after that. I could go on, of course, but you can read all about it yourself at your leisure.

Nor should anyone miss the superb diatribe by Royal Hayes on the impending demise of homeopathy, which he witnessed all around him but refused to be a party to, or the one by Rudolph Rabe on the unwisdom of currying favor with the orthodox school, a temptation no less prevalent today. There are discussions of the Swedenborgian faith, which Kent, Farrington, and other leading American homeopaths embraced; of radionics, Abrams machines, and the like, which I like to call "experimental homeopathy;" and of the work of other pioneers who were stimulated by homeopathy but later deviated from certain particulars of the discipline, like Edward Bach and Rudolph Steiner. Whatever your taste, there will be plenty here to feast upon. Practitioners especially may relish or be troubled by Vithoulkas' attacks on Sankaran, which sound suspiciously like the "illuminist" criticisms once leveled by the likes of Eizayaga, Künzli, et al., against Vithoulkas himself not so many years ago, as if to remind us that what goes around comes around.

Since it is part of a reviewer's job to detect faults and inadequacies, and I was especially anxious to be scrupulous in this respect, I read the book carefully with blue pencil in hand, but found amazingly little of a substantive nature that the author overlooked, or that would detract from readers' enjoyment. To be sure, partisans of this or that faction or point of view can always object that their position or champion was misrepresented or given short shrift. Except for a good deal on homeopathy in Great Britain, for example, the author freely admits to having little to say about its development outside the English-speaking world, and what he does say is relegated to an appendix. As with any other book of this size and scope, a few typos and misstatements of fact will inevitably be found as well. But Julian never claims or pretends to offer more or less than his own unique, personal selection, his own guided tour through the two hundred years of our history, with its main emphasis on the United States. In any case, I can say without hesitation that he is the most knowledgeable and reliable guide now writing in English, and that every friend of homeopathy will find herein a bounty of unexpected treasures for edification and delight.

A.U. Ramakrishnan and Catherine R. Coulter, *A Homeopathic Approach to Cancer**

I've been eagerly awaiting this newest offering from the pen of Catherine Coulter, not only for its well-chosen words and apt phrases, or its fresh insights and well-seasoned wisdom, all of which we've come to expect, but above all for its subject matter, "the big C," the very archetype of dread and potentially fatal disease, which most classical homeopaths in this country are either wary of treating in the first place, or have had rather limited or disappointing results when they venture to do *so.*

Take me, for instance. After 27 years in practice, I've been able to provide good symptomatic relief to patients on chemotherapy or radiation, had good results with general constitutional support and first-aid remedies for pre- and post-op surgical care, and even had a few cases of dramatic and long-lasting improvement and/or remission. But on the whole, using the single remedy chosen by the totality of symptoms, I've not been able to help patients consistently to shrink their tumors, prevent recurrences, or even get rid of precancerous lesions. Furthermore, both my direct personal experience with Vithoulkas, Sankaran, et al., and extensive familiarity with the writings of Kent, Boger, and the like, confirm my sense that even these great and undoubted masters have not fared all that much better.

Yet on some level I have always known that there has to be a simple and practical way to help cancer patients more reliably using homeopathic remedies and some version of the method we already know to be valid. This book offers and indeed systematically elaborates just such a method, one almost disarmingly easy for an experienced homeopath to use, and indeed so much so as to challenge us all to re-examine what we do and how we do it in a much humbler spirit.

Unlike Catherine's previous books, both the language and intent here are practical and businesslike, rather than artistic and imaginative, her main

* Book Review: Ramakrishnan and Coulter, *A Homeopathic Approach to Cancer*, ***Homeopathy Today,*** November 2001.

roles being those of amanuensis of the scattered case notes and observations of A. U. Ramakrishnan, M.D., a distinguished Indian homeopath whose experience, now augmented by her own, encompasses several thousand cancer cases over the past 25 years. In undertaking this herculean feat of organization, condensation, and synthesis, her primary purpose is simply to identify and formulate his working methodology as clearly and systematically as possible. This task she has certainly accomplished in a clear and readable style, but the finest tribute I can pay to her book, and the fairest measure of its success, is to say nothing further about the literary qualities that have already made her famous, and get down to the often unglamorous details of its content, and how we can use it to improve our results with our patients.

I should perhaps add that the conceptual basis of Ramakrishnan's approach is not nearly as new as it may appear to the average American reader. In fact, it harks back to a style of homeopathic practice that is still widely prevalent in Europe and elsewhere, one that is actually much older than the Kentian method that almost all classical prescribers of my day were taught and still use, including Ramakrishnan himself. Eminent and reputable homeopaths like Hughes and Burnett in the last century, and Clarke and Eizayaga in the present one, have long advocated the use of organ-specific remedies chosen on the basis of more narrowly-defined pathological indications, with less emphasis on elaborate individualization based on personality traits, as favored by some leading teachers today.

Indeed, it would be fair to say that this more medically-oriented style has always been the most popular one with homeopathic physicians the world over, and is so still among members of the LIGA or International Homeopathic Medical League, for example, and especially in Europe, Latin America, and the Indian subcontinent, where the newer schools of Vithoulkas, Sankaran, Scholten, Mangialavori, Sherr, and others are not seldom regarded as "elitist," "illuminist," or speculative interpretations that fail to address the often ugly, unedifying, or inelegant realities of advanced organic disease as commonly seen in clinical practice.

As it happens, Ramakrishnan himself is careful not to take a doctrinaire position on either side of this ongoing and wholly legitimate debate. As National Vice-President of the LIGA for India, and official Physician to the

Prime Minister of India as well, he remains a good classical prescriber who still uses the single remedy in the minimum dose whenever possible, giving the remedy and then waiting for it to act. As he says in his Introduction, he adopted a more proactive and aggressive approach to cancer after the deaths of two close relatives from the disease and his own inability to save them using the best methods available to him at the time.

His thoroughly pragmatic attitude seems to boil down to something like, "This has been my experience with cancer so far, and this is what has worked the best; so give it a try if you want to." What I take from that is just what we already know, that healing pertains to individuals, requires an *ad hoc* decision in every case, and is therefore irreducible to a single protocol, rule, or formula. The apposite quote from Hahnemann would be from *Organon*, ¶1 and footnote, "The physician's high and only mission is to restore the sick to health, not to construct systems [or] hypotheses." Amen to that.

In Chapter 1, "The Homeopathic Approach," the authors justify their modifications of the classical approach on the basis of two considerations that, however plausible or even self-evident they may seem or eventually turn out to be, must still be regarded as hypotheses in need of further proof, namely,

1) that measurable, concrete pathology like cancer calls for a less subtle, less individualized, more pathologically-oriented style of prescribing, featuring the old notion of specific remedies for specific diseases, and others with a particular affinity for certain tissues, organs, or regions of the body, as in the organopathic tradition just alluded to; and
2) that the life-threatening character of the disease generates a real urgency, a "race against time," which requires a more aggressive dosage schedule than simply giving one or a few doses of a single remedy and waiting for them to act.

We may therefore take the present volume as the authors' joint endeavor to make the best possible case for these claims, although it will undoubtedly require the concerted effort of a whole generation of prescribers to persuade the homeopathic community as a whole, let alone the public at large.

As it has evolved thus far, Ramakrishnan's method comprises three main deviations from the classical or "unicist" model, based on the single remedy and the minimum dose:

1) The remedies are given at regular, specified intervals, not on an as needed basis, and repeated over long periods of time, almost always for a number of months.
2) Two remedies are given weekly in alternation, usually an organ-specific or more general "cancer" remedy and a cancer nosode.
3) Remedies are administered either by "plussing," according to the regimen outlined in the text, or by the "split-dose" method in early cases, where each weekly dose is split into four and taken within a single day, from waking till bedtime.

The remainder of the book is largely given over to individual case reports, most of them followed by Catherine's helpful comments on the choice of the remedies and other individualizing features pertaining to that instance.

In Chapter 2, Ramakrishnan's main cancer remedies are listed, subdivided into three groups:

1) cancer nosodes, chiefly *Carcinosin* and *Scirrhinum;*
2) what he calls "wide-spectrum cancer specifics," namely, *Conium, Thuja,* and *Arsenicum album,* each used in cancers of many types; and
3) organ-specific remedies, such as *Aurum muriaticum natronatum* (cervix, uterus, ovaries), *Ceanothus americanus* (spleen, pancreas, liver), *Hekla lava* (bone, bone marrow), *Hydrastis* (stomach), *Lycopodium* (lung), *Phytolacca* (breast, parotid), *Plumbum iod.* (brain), *Sabal serrulata* (prostate), and *Terebinthina* (bladder), to name a few.

In Chapter 3, general rules are formulated for the "Plussing" and "Split-Dose" methods, again with illustrative cases. By far the longest (80 pages), Chapter 4 gives cases of many types of cancer that have responded favorably to remedies given in this fashion, including several sites and cell types where conventional treatment has had the poorest record, such as brain, esophagus, lung, stomach, pancreas, skin (melanoma), and ovary.

The authors' pragmatic, down-to-earth approach is equally evident in the later chapters. Chapter 5, for example, discusses palliative treatment in more advanced cases where metastasis has already occurred, or where the disease has spread too extensively for remedies to offer any realistic hope of cure. Using exactly the same methodology as before, they report unexpectedly good results even in this group, both in length and quality of life. Chapter 6 continues in similar vein with remedies for pain control in advanced and terminal cases, including some not previously discussed, such as *Euphorbium* and *Ornithogalum.* In Chapter 7, constitutional remedies are discussed as a complement or alternative to the usual method when the total symptom-picture clearly indicates them, for example,

1) if the tumors have regressed to the point that plussing is no longer required;

2) if the treatment has stalled or plateau'd and a more closely-fitting remedy is called for to reactivate it;

3) if metastasis occurs in the wake of an apparent cure;

4) from the beginning, if the constitutional remedy has special affinity with the organ or tissue affected; or

5) occasionally without any other remedies or nosodes in very early cases, e.g., carcinoma *in situ,* or slow-growing cancers (thyroid, etc.).

Special problems, such as prescribing for acute ailments that arise in the course of treatment, are also discussed herein.

Chapter 8, on the role of conventional diagnosis and treatment, offers useful techniques by which homeopaths can collaborate with and assist their allopathic colleagues. Remedies are suggested for radiation, chemotherapy, and pre-and post-operative care, along with using remedies between radiation treatments or rounds of chemotherapy. Valuable lessons are embedded in many of these cases, such as the woman with metastatic ovarian cancer in lungs, bladder, and mesenteric nodes, who lived a good-quality life for years with all her lesions, illustrating the often radical discrepancy between the totality of symptoms, the ordinary language of how patients feel and function, and the technical language of abnormalities, the basis of conventional diagnosis and treatment.

In the concluding chapter, the important subject of cancer prevention is addressed at some length, including

1) protocols for treatment of those with strong family histories of cancer;

2) longer courses of the usual cancer treatment to prevent recurrences;

3) optional use of tissue salts for long-term maintenance; and

4) protocols for reversing documented precancerous lesions, for example, leukoplakia of the oral cavity, cervical dysplasia, or elevated PSA with no observable lesions in the prostate,

using the same remedies and dosages already developed. This final chapter I found especially valuable in addressing the common and valid concerns of patients we all see every day. Like any other text of therapeutics, this book will inevitably attract the same sort of contempt and vituperation that so-called "pathological prescribers" have always endured, not least from the pen of Hahnemann himself. But the most important caveat raised by the book, as the authors clearly acknowledge, is that, while seeming deceptively easy for even a novice to find useful remedies to try in a particular case, the method requires experience and skill to obtain consistently good results, and will thus inevitably be misused at times. As usual, the peculiar or individualizing features of case and response will make the difference, for example, by indicating one remedy rather than another, or dictating when the remedy should be changed. To some extent, these often subtle distinctions can be felt and shown, but never wholly taught.

That is part of the reason why it behooves homeopaths and indeed anyone treating patients with cancer or potentially fatal illness to pay even more care and attention than usual to their ongoing relationships with their patients. It is also why this book will ultimately be most useful for experienced homeopathic physicians and other health professionals, and why lay practitioners and patients, if they use it at all, must do so on their own responsibility and at their own peril. In either case, such work should include regular checkups by the oncology team, and should be conducted with their approval whenever possible.

Nevertheless, since the approach outlined in this book is easier to use and promises to be more effective than the one most of us were taught, I'm more than game to try it, and I would encourage other experienced practitioners to do the same. If it works, as I believe it will, it may also open up new directions for the use of homeopathic remedies in treating other serious pathology with organ damage, like multiple sclerosis, cirrhosis, advanced renal disease, chronic obstructive pulmonary disease, and the like, which are equally difficult to help consistently at present. It turns out that these are just the sort of conditions for which homeopaths like Chand and Ramakrishnan in India, Eizayaga in Argentina, and others in Europe and Latin America have long advocated similarly medically-oriented, organopathic strategies, albeit often differing in their details.

Precisely because homeopathic physicians in America have been marginalized for so long, and so effectively, we are veritable babes in the wood at treating folks with this level of sickness, and thus have the unique opportunity, if not, dare I say, the duty to integrate these two often hostile and seemingly irreconcilable strands of our own homeopathic tradition into a new synthesis that can pass the test of time. The book under review gives ample detail for trained, experienced classical prescribers to treat cancer patients more effectively, and I hope and expect that those of good heart and open mind will use it in that spirit.

Julian Winston, *The Heritage of Homeopathic Literature**

Julian Winston is to be thanked and commended yet again for taking such pains to compile this monumental bibliography of our homeopathic literature, spanning its entire history from Hahnemann to the present. You may ask why he does it, or whether it's worth all that effort. After all, who really needs or uses all this stuff, other than a few antiquarians like myself, who like old vests that have long been out of style and get their kicks from browsing through used book stores?

A few weeks ago, when told of some old homeopathic books looking for an owner, a colleague of mine felt only mildly interested in them, since so much of her library was already on computer that she saw little point in collecting old books merely to watch them continue moldering on her shelves. When Julian asked me to write something about his latest labor of love, I thought of her words and how I could answer them for the movement as a whole, since what we do is linked inseparably to the printed word, and also to how readers can gain access to it, from the leather-bound tomes of Hahnemann's day to the advanced software of today.

Indeed, my own enduring fascination with homeopathy was kindled in no small part from its almost religious devotion to text. With our literature consisting essentially of glosses and emendations of Hahnemann, and even our arguments buttressed by essentially scriptural quotations on every side, I realized early on that homeopaths are indeed "People of the Book," like Jews with our Old Testament, Christians with the New, or Muslims with their Qu'ran, all deriving fresh inspiration from a set of quasi-eternal truths revealed to a distinctly human writer at a definite point in historical time.

Our homeopathic literature is thus no mere repository of information, but also the communal efforts of flawed human writers to approach the

* Book Review: Julian Winston, *The Heritage of Homeopathic Literature*, ***Homeopathy Today,*** April/May 2002.

Divine, such that each book, even one that is no longer used, becomes a kind of historical monument to the Word, which if not quite immutable at least doesn't change every year or two, as the concepts and methods of modern "scientific" medicine are explicitly designed to do. It tickles my fancy to imagine a day in the far-distant future when medicine as we know it no longer survives, and an archæologist unearths a huge trove of artifacts—tools of incorruptible stainless steel, instruments for diagnosis and surgery and the like—while the only enduring traces of homeopathy will be the idea of it, expressed in words and preserved for all time in these sacred texts.

On the other hand, a bibliography for today must also and above all be useful, not only to scholars and antiquarians, but also to students and practitioners, who bear the responsibility of applying the words to their Hahnemannian task of curing and healing the sick. That is why it need not and cannot include every last volume or article written on the subject, why it necessarily involves a selection.

It is here in particular that I feel most deeply indebted to Julian, who in addition to his many other talents is a splendid archivist, scholar, and librarian, in that his omnivorous appetite for all things homeopathic extends not only to hunting, gathering, preparing, and serving up all this stuff, but also to tasting, devouring, and digesting it for our benefit, quite possibly even more than his own. While he stops well short of including every last domestic manual, for example, there are more than enough here to satisfy every conceivable taste, and he's earned my thanks for leaving the rest out.

The result is a leisurely guided tour down the main highways and through many forgotten back alleys of our literature, according to the inclinations of his fancy, the mature likes and dislikes of a connoisseur, and his own unashamedly personal opinions about everything and everyone you can think of, as well as quite a few you will discover for the first time. The travelogue is a perfect companion piece to *The Faces of Homeopathy,* his equally idiosyncratic ramble through the people of our history, and it deserves to be savored just as he wrote it, with each section in nearly chronological order, as well as by sampling assorted tidbits, as in a book of reference.

Quite apart from its considerable entertainment value, its practical usefulness was brought home to me while reviewing Ramakrishnan and

Coulter's new book on cancer, which is firmly rooted in the organopathic tradition, sorely maligned by classical fundamentalists from Hahnemann himself on down to many in our own time. From reading Burnett, a great 19th century prescriber, and Clarke, his disciple of a generation later, I already knew that they were successfully treating patients with cancer and other advanced organic pathology many generations ago. Although they give only the most tantalizing clues and hints about how they proceeded, their books at least made me ready and eager to investigate Ramakrishnan's method, even more than I might have been without knowing that history.

Not counting the Preface and Introduction, the bibliography proper is divided into fifteen sections -- the *Organon, Materia Medica*, Repertory, Therapeutics, etc. -- and three appendices, consisting of all the books arranged by date, by author, and Woodbury's "five-foot shelf" of indispensable books, published in 1931. I can't begin to enumerate even a small fraction of the wonderful snippets, tangents, anecdotes, and curmudgeonly rants contained in these pages. But I'll mention a few surprises that caught my eye and made me want to read them, in some cases for the first time.

Several were in the section on Therapeutics, that neglected and despised bastard child of pure homeopathy and pathological diagnosis, which still does useful service in many more cases than most purists would care to admit. The monumental achievement of a long and illustrious career, Jahr's *Therapeutic Guide,* also known as *Forty Years' Practice,* was the digest of his clinical experience, and contains a lot of useful information that is still relevant today. It is the mature and perfected version of his earlier *Clinical Guide*, used by Mary Baker Eddy, the founder of Christian Science, who was also quite a skillful prescriber and had homeopathic physicians visit her, albeit by the back door, when she herself fell ill. I've owned copies of both books for years, and Julian's mini-review has given me the impetus I needed to begin reading them in earnest.

Worthy successor to Hering's *Domestic Physician* (1838), the first of its kind, Laurie's *Domestic Medicine* went through at least 12 editions in less than 50 years, and helped many a pioneer family in their pilgrimage to the west by covered wagon. I own the 4th American edition (1849), and Julian's plug for it has finally gotten me to take it off the shelf.

In the Philosophy section, *A New Synthesis,* by Guy Beckley Stearns and Edgar Evia (1942), was a cutting-edge essay into homeopathic research that prophesied and actually began the development of kinesiology, made original contributions to radionics, and dared to sketch out a philosophy of these still esoteric frontiers of homeopathy at a time when such matters were a lot further beyond the pale of respectable science than they are today. I've already bitten off a lot more than I'll most likely be able to chew, and these are only the beginning.

As perceptive and opinionated as ever, Julian is one of that very small fraternity whose favorites, pet peeves, passions, and prejudices are always worth paying careful attention to, because he has thought them through and can give cogent reasons for what he thinks. Although they may well infuriate some, his broadsides against Sankaran and various other "illuminists," for example, are witty, always thought-provoking, and do make some attempt to give credit where it's due. But don't expect a neutral, detached attitude. He's passionate about homeopathy, he has a point of view, and isn't afraid to play favorites and advocate for what he believes. That is precisely what makes this collection so valuable.

Like any good librarian, he has included virtually everything of importance; like every discerning critic, he displays our subject through the medium of his own sensibility; and in so doing he reveals us to ourselves. I have to admit that the lady friend and colleague I mentioned was right to the extent that the new software does in fact contain the best of the old volumes, and that the originals are best preserved and stored for posterity in some museum where those of us who simply like the look and feel of them can kvell to our hearts' content. The obvious bridge for keeping the old world of bound volumes connected with the new world of computer software is the modem research library, equipped with the most up-to-date technology, and a well-trained professional staff to locate, reprint, and reproduce selected items from the literature for the benefit of scholars and practitioners alike, so the Word may continue to be made flesh, as it was and ever shall be. If we ever get our act together to create such an institution, Julian should logically be in charge of it.

Isaac Golden, *Vaccination & Homeoprophylaxis: A Review of Risks and Alternatives* and *Homeoprophylaxis: A Fifteen-Year Clinical Study**

This self-publishing venture is an excellent treatise on homeoprophylaxis, the long-term use of homeopathic nosodes, or disease-specific remedies like *Drosera* for whooping cough if the nosodes are unavailable, as an alternative to conventional vaccines for prevention of the corresponding diseases. The author, whose engaging photo on the back cover conjures up the likeness and aura of a Talmudic scholar, is a naturopath and homeopath who has studied the subject for a very long time and with exemplary thoroughness, based on his own experience and that of his colleagues in Australia.

I should begin by confessing my own prior lack of enthusiasm for this practice, also of long standing, which made me reluctant at first to undertake this review at all. I have always championed the use and effectiveness of nosodes and specific remedies in treating and preventing acute contagious diseases, as was clearly shown by Hahnemann for scarlet fever and confirmed repeatedly by his successors in epidemics of cholera, typhoid, influenza, and the like, all the way into our own time. But these brilliantly successful if oddly forgotten applications were limited to short-term protection over the months of an actual outbreak.

Employing them for long-term and indeed lifelong protection, as an alternative to our current mandatory vaccination laws and policies, is of much more recent and to my mind more dubious provenance, dating only from the 1940's, when the major industrialized countries, led by the United States, began waging systematic warfare against not only smallpox, but also

* Book Review: Isaac Golden, *Vaccination and Homeoprophylaxis*, ***American Journal of Homeopathic Medicine*** 99:149, Summer 2006.

diphtheria, pertussis, and tetanus, the toxoids of which were added at that time. Since then, we have made, marketed, and mandated more and more vaccines against an ever-growing multitude of acute contagious diseases as our automatic, first-line defense against every such ailment that captures our attention and in the absence of any public-health emergency, simply because it lies within our power to do so, virtually without regulation or oversight, and of course reaping extravagant profits for the industry, with no end in sight.

In the 1940's, when smallpox and DPT were the only vaccines available, prominent homeopaths like Elizabeth Wright-Hubbard used these nosodes as a way of circumventing the already strict enforcement of our mandatory vaccination laws, giving them semi-covertly as simple intercurrents at comparatively rare intervals in the course of their constitutional treatment, signing them off as genuine vaccinations, passable imitations of the real thing, and also conferring a modicum of short-term protection in the process.

As long as the public health authorities remained unaware of or at least turned a blind eye to the subterfuge, it never interfered with the relatively strict yoga of classical homeopathic practice significantly enough to cause leading prescribers like Dr. Hubbard to lose any sleep over it. But at present, when a newborn baby is either required or expected to receive twenty-five different vaccinations before they're two years old, many of them combinations of several different ingredients, like DPT and MMR, plus another 25 by the time they go to college, using nosodes in lieu of vaccines for long-term protection against so many different conditions entails giving a large number of remedies repeatedly throughout life, with very little unmedicated time or space in between for the organism to be capable of responding freely and maximally to constitutional treatment without such interference.

In short, what began as an intercurrent against the background of constitutional treatment began gradually to crowd out and ultimately replace the foreground or basic context of receptivity for homeopathic self-healing to proceed. At any rate, this has always been my concern, as well as my reason for preferring to work on changing the laws to make the vaccines optional, as they are in most other industrialized countries, and for opposing the *goal* of lifelong protection itself as generally unattainable, unnecessary, and even at times undesirable, whichever methods are employed to achieve it.

But I suppose that this old and inveterate prejudice on my part also made me very curious to learn how Dr. Golden would respond to it. I was surprised and delighted to learn that he is quite familiar with this "purist" objection, as he calls it, and that he has answered it in a wonderfully cogent, persuasive, and disarming manner. A Talmudic scholar, after all, is one trained and even devoted to considering every possible aspect of every question, with a systematic thoroughness that includes an amalgam of learned textual exegesis, broad life experience, and a strain of personal reflection that weaves them together. Happily, Dr. Golden's book contains an abundance of all three, because it is about much more than homeoprophylaxis alone.

Its real subject comprises the dangers and adverse consequences of conventional vaccines, which are summarized here as well as anywhere else in the literature. Another major subsection discusses the natural history of the corresponding diseases, about which he likewise provides a wealth of useful information. Purely as a safer, more practical alternative to conventional vaccination, homeopathic prophylaxis does make some sense; and it occupies only about a third of the text. His scriptural commentary encompasses the writings of reputable homeopaths from the whole of our history, including Hahnemann on scarlet fever, Bœnninghausen on cholera, Burnett on smallpox, and Shepherd, Blackie, Eizayaga, and Sankaran the elder in more recent times, when more diseases were involved and a more general strategy seemed to be called for.

His ingenious and eminently practical solution to my scruples about giving too many nosodes and specific remedies too often, thus blanketing the vital force of the patient for many years, is simply

1) to limit his protocol to major diseases that he believes truly warrant long-term protection, namely, tetanus, whooping cough, pneumococcal and HiB disease, polio, and meningococcal meningitis;

2) to give them not throughout life, but only for the years of highest risk, in most cases from birth to age six; and

3) to keep the number of such remedies sufficiently low to remain "intercurrent," in the background of their ongoing constitutional treatment, which he likewise strongly advocates.

While omitting measles, mumps, rubella, influenza, and chicken pox, he does provide *Morbillinum, Hepatitis* B, and *Oscillococcinum* as needed for actual outbreaks of measles, Hep B, or influenza, if they are imminent or threatening.

I would still take issue with his choice of HiB and pneumococcus, mutant strains of organisms in the normal pharyngeal flora, and of meningitis and polio, which are serious but not common enough to warrant routine protection necessarily. But the *principle* of his selection is basically sound, and his practice seems enlightened and sensible, so that my remaining objections are merely pragmatic and involve subtler issues about which serious practitioners will always reasonably differ.

Perhaps the most distinctive part of these works lies in the author's extensive review of his own cases and those of his colleagues who follow his protocol, using modern statistical methods wherever possible. After years of painstaking data collection, he concludes that long-term prophylaxis with nosodes and/or specific remedies is not only considerably safer than conventional vaccination, and comparably effective, as seems entirely plausible to me, but also safer and more effective than no treatment at all, i. e., in those children who are given no nosodes or vaccines and simply left alone, a fascinating conclusion that needs further comment.

To claim that his protocol is just as effective as conventional vaccines in preventing the corresponding diseases, and also much safer, with fewer adverse effects, is already quite a mouthful, since in the category of adverse effects he includes exacerbation of the ordinary diseases of childhood, such as asthma, eczema, otitis media, allergies, and behavioral problems, precisely the same bread-and-butter stuff that I've been blabbing about for decades, and for which any vaccine will do. That is already sticking his neck out, because these global and nonspecific effects have been largely ignored by almost all other writers in this field.

With plenty of data to back him up, he also contends that the children following his protocol are much less prone to these ailments, or at least suffer from them less severely, than those who are not given such prophylaxis at all. In other words, he believes that using these nosodes and specific remedies routinely for everyone, without individualization or classical prescribing, confers a significant and perhaps comparable general health benefit of the same kind.

To test this assertion, it would be necessary and also fascinating to compare the long-term health history of children receiving his protocol alone with two other groups, namely, those receiving constitutional treatment alone, and those receiving both, which he seems to regard as optimal. Would we not be amazed and more than a little chagrined if his protocol-only group turned out to be the healthiest of the three? I know I would be! Would that simple program not be a whole lot cheaper and simpler than the elaborate rigamarole on which we now pride ourselves? Just for the record, I'm still dubious that that would be the result; but the possibility that I might be biased in favor of my own habitual assumptions is the best reason I can think of to carry out this further investigation, and I can think of nobody more admirably qualified to do so than Dr. Isaac Golden, perhaps in his Seventh Edition.

Dana Ullman, *The Homeopathic Revolution: Why Famous People & Cultural Heroes Choose Homeopathy**

This book is not only delightful to read, but well worth the effort. On the most obvious level, it is about celebrities, standouts, and leaders in various walks of life, whose prominence makes them fair game for general interest, entertainment, or simple curiosity. In this sense, it is also a direct expression of its author's own distinctively outgoing and gregarious temperament, with his notable talent for publicity and natural bent for networking.

More importantly, it is also a consummation of the author's life work, to publicize, explain, and celebrate homeopathy, that improbably effective method of healing the sick, together with the uniquely elegant and coherent philosophy that underlies and makes it an ongoing challenge to the reigning medical orthodoxy of our time. Within the homeopathic world, Dana Ullman is himself a genuine hero, having championed both the method and the philosophy, and kept them indefatigably in the public eye for more than 30 years.

Before his debut as a successful lay practitioner in California in the mid-'70's, Dana was a founding member of the Bay Area Study Group, a small but dedicated cadre of physicians, licensed health professionals, and laypeople who met on equal terms for the sheer love of homeopathy. This group included such students as Bill Gray, David Warkentin, Roger Morrison, Nancy Herrick, and Lou Klein, all soon to become leading thinkers and practitioners of a new generation, at a time when homeopathy itself seemed on the verge of extinction in America.

It was Dana's good fortune, and ours, that he was arrested for practicing medicine without a license, which led him to change direction in spite of being acquitted of the charges. Without missing a beat, he found his true

* Book Review: Dana Ullman, *Why Famous People and Cultural Heroes Choose Homeopathy*, ***Journal of Alternative and Complementary Medicine*** 16:517, 2010.

calling as author, teacher, and impresario of this discipline he has loved so faithfully. His mastery of all things homeopathic, his talent for public speaking and public relations in the wider sense, his ease and familiarity with celebrities in many fields, and not least his love of our homeopathic history, have all conspired to make *The Homeopathic Revolution* an authentic culmination of his professional life.

Perhaps impatient with the abiding mystery and esotericism of its basic concepts, and the consequent difficulty of explaining them to an understandably skeptical public, he has long been intrigued by the readiness of celebrities and prominent figures in society, perhaps less subject to the ruling inhibitions and prejudices of their time, to embrace homeopathic medicine for themselves, and even to advocate for its wider acceptance by society at large. His book duly appraises the influence of homeopathic theory and practice upon modern culture, as seen through personal experiences with it and public utterances about it on the part of celebrities and prominent figures in various fields, both past and present, both here and abroad.

As such, it makes thoroughly entertaining and even fascinating reading for anyone, with or without any prior experience of, interest in, or even sympathy for the subject, purely on account of the prominent cultural status of his characters. The allure of celebrity itself is of course a staple truth of the advertising industry, since the opinions of prominent people for or against something are widely used for leading and shaping public opinion in the same direction. But Dana's intention goes well beyond mere name-dropping and big-name advertising, as is made clear in the Introduction, which features a critique of modern scientific medicine, and the first two chapters, which are entitled, "Why Homeopathy Works and Makes Sense," and "Why Homeopathy Is Hated and Vilified," and present a simple exposition of homeopathic philosophy, and a brief history of its persecution by orthodox medicine ever since its creation.

This ulterior purpose is implicit in the book's subtitle, "Why Famous People and Cultural Heroes Choose Homeopathy." Yet for Dana, as for myself and every other practicing homeopath, the great unanswered question is not why illustrious people choose and even prefer it to conventional medicine. To the contrary, it is why the general public and popular culture remain so hesitant to follow their lead, despite its many successes, and why its concepts still seem obscure, opaque, and outdated to most people, as well as an object of ridicule to the profession that stands in direst need of it. To this riddle, alas, the book provides no answer. What it does show, quite beautifully and in extravagant detail, is that celebrities and culture heroes continue to favor homeopathy, and for perfectly good reasons. It is therefore even more mysterious and troubling that homeopathy remains to a large extent unrecognized and unappreciated as a complement to the system now prevailing.

It can hardly fail to excite an open-minded reader who knows nothing of the method that such legendary figures as Goethe, Darwin, Mark Twain, George Bernard Shaw, and Mahatma Gandhi thought so highly of it, and in some cases used it to heal their own illnesses, or that contemporary celebrities like Ravi Shankar, Paul McCartney, Cher, Tina Turner, Tony Blair, Prince Charles, and Queen Elizabeth still do. To that extent, the book does succeed magnificently, if not in solving the mystery, at least in posing it more starkly.

In addition, the author displays painstaking and careful scholarship in tracking down and tracing out the tangled skein of homeopathic history through so many famous and exemplary lives. Dana's enthusiasm for promoting homeopathy as widely as possible sometimes leads to what seem like gross exaggerations until one reads the fine print. Consider, for example, his assertion that Darwin could never have completed *The Origin of Species* had he not successfully healed himself of intense, disabling ailments with the help of homeopathic remedies many years earlier. Sounding at first like utter hyperbole, that conclusion was actually reached by Darwin himself, as a careful reading of his letters makes abundantly clear.

In other cases, Dana's zeal for the odd fact leads him to assert connections that are indeed tenuous and would better have been omitted, such as an unduly long section about the various false rumors that Hitler used homeopathic remedies on a daily basis. If true, this would not only be antithetical to the standards of good homeopathic practice, but also hardly a resounding tribute to the method, in view of its catastrophic results in this particular case.

But these quibbles should in no way detract from the value of the work as a whole. My only more principled reservation follows from homeopathy's precipitous decline in the 20th century, and one reason that Dana himself cites for it, that so many homeopathic physicians were quick to incorporate insulin, antibiotics, blood transfusions, and other technical achievements of orthodox medicine into their practices, and became to that extent less and less scrupulous about adhering to homeopathic principles and methods. This simple and widely acknowledged fact tends to consign all of his legendary tales from an earlier time, however fascinating they were and may still be, to a chapter long past in the history of medicine, whereas his original contention has even more pointed relevance and bite in the present, when both the parlous state of the medical system and his own alternative agenda would seem to demand center stage for the celebrities and culture heroes of today.

That the contemporary examples he provides are neither as numerous nor as prominent as the likes of Goethe, Darwin, Twain, or Gandhi is hardly his fault, merely a sobering fact of life at the moment. But it does indicate an important obstacle in the way of his purpose for the book, that of promoting homeopathy throughout the world by trading on the fame of its adherents, which remains to be overcome in the future.

Massimo Mangialavori, M. D., *PRAXIS: Method of Complexity**

Massimo Mangialavori's latest work is strong and valuable medicine for homeopaths of all persuasions and at all levels of experience. Simply reading it for this occasion has already enriched and sharpened my practice. Beyond that, it is also a pleasure to read. It is written with *intelligence,* which is to say, perceptively, with careful attention to detail, yet never losing sight of the "big picture." Better still, it requires a comparable intelligence on the part of the *reader*, to ponder it, digest it slowly, and take it to heart, rather than taking a fast look and putting it back on the shelf. And perhaps most of all, it engages me as a work of *philosophy,* quite in the spirit of Hahnemann, beginning with the elementary precepts that we all know, and reshaping them according to the needs, problems, and insights of our own time in a way that makes logical and practical sense. To me this is no small achievement, since I've been practicing for so long, and making the same mistakes so consistently, that getting me to change in *any* way is bound to provoke serious resistance.

So I guess the phrase "a pleasure to read" needs further clarification. How pleasant is it to have to re-examine every step of what we do and every rationale for how we think? Or to have our noses rubbed in the flaws and limitations of our early training, not to mention even more bad habits than we knew we had? Fortunately, it's the kind of medicine that I know we all *need*, since it mostly teaches what we already profess to be true, but haven't yet figured out how to accomplish, or have simply become too lazy or complacent to make the effort. Even what is most innovative and controversial about it is firmly rooted in the homeopathic philosophy that we all share, devoutly respectful of that history, and fully conversant with the best that hard science and current philosophy can offer. So once you've

* Book Review: Massimo Mangialavori, *Praxis: Method of Complexity,* ***Spectrum of Homeopathy*** (Germany) 2010, p. 134.

made up your mind to take it, I can at least assure you that the medicine tastes good and won't upset your stomach.

Massimo is of course already well-known and esteemed by homeopaths everywhere for his ongoing courses in Italy, his seminars on *materia medica,* and a growing library of books based on them. The present work is his major theoretical statement, beginning with methodology, followed by an overview of the "Drug" family and its principal themes, and concluding with illustrative cases involving six drug remedies, mostly lesser-known ones.

Its subtitle, "The Search for Coherence in Clinical Phenomena," announces its guiding purpose, which is to discover and teach a deeper, more meaningful similitude between our remedies and patients than any list of unrelated symptoms, like those from which our Repertories, provings, and case reports are compiled. Fortunately, we know when we've found one, because its various symptom-elements fit into and indeed can be derived from a coherent whole, a totality of symptoms that exceeds the sum of its parts and makes intuitive sense to doctor and patient alike. In short, what he is after is the mystical, elusive, and often ridiculed "essence" that master homeopaths like Kent and Vithoulkas have long sought, and that Scholten and Sankaran are now seeking. It is Massimo's way of discovering that unity, and of describing and understanding it once found, that is uniquely his own.

Because of limited time and space, I will simply highlight a few choice nuggets that caught my fancy along the way, to show that it hangs together as a system. Naturally I loved the beginning, a brief essay on the Doctrine of Signatures, in which he agrees with the fundamentalists that trivial resemblances, as between the yellow color of *Chelidonium* and that of the bile, fall short of a real affinity. Often hinted at in the common names of medicinal herbs, the levels of meaning that Massimo is interested in arise from their unique physical, chemical, and mythic properties as systems of adaptation to and within their natural habitat, included their time-honored uses in folklore and medicine.

At times these multi-layered resonances can seem almost spooky. I have always wondered, for example, why, how, and by whom our most important snake was named for *Lachesis,* one of the three Greek goddesses who fix the span of life, given the improbable circumstance that Constantine Hering, who first proved the venom in 1828, died on the fifty-second anniversary of that event, almost to the day. Signatures of this sort are laden with meaning, because they plumb deeply into the history of our culture, and weave what first seem like unrelated details into a tapestry that becomes cogent and persuasive.

Massimo's "Method of Complexity" is so named because it includes such diverse fields of endeavor as anthropology, ethnography, and folk medicine; physiology, biochemistry, and toxicology, on the scientific side; classical homeopathy, with its history and literature; and the art of clinical medicine, which ties them all together by means of the interview, combining the insights of psychology with an easy, understanding, and empathic way of being with sick people, arising from real life and acquaintance with human nature more than any book learning.

Massimo differs from other teachers chiefly in this multi-systems approach, his quest for resonance and corroboration on many levels, and his insistence that no one method or formula of case-taking or remedy study will cover every case, that homeopathy is at bottom an art that cannot simply be taught, must be experienced anew with every case, and is never finished or "complete." All of this talks my language. Yet from start to finish *Praxis* is still a textbook on *method:* warning that the method is difficult is not to say that there is no method at all.

This brings me to his first great heresy, contrary to all we were once taught, that provings are *not* the best source for *materia medica* study, because they yield vast amounts of *information,* in long lists of detailed symptoms, whereas what the student needs to know is how *important* they are for prescribing the remedy, a judgment which must include their *context* in the totality of symptoms of the prover, the same level of similitude that a curative prescription must embody.

Reliable remedy information adequate for prescribing on thus requires some system for organizing and prioritizing the data. Perhaps more than any other leading teacher today, Massimo prefers *cured cases* for this purpose, because they alone can provide the richness of context that allows us to see the whole of the remedy in the whole of the patient, to connect up the various threads that led him to prescribe it, and thus to stimulate the kind of thinking by analogy that could be applied to other patients needing the same remedy, and also to patients requiring different but related remedies. These connections he calls "themes," and from *them*, rather than disembodied symptoms standing alone, he constructs his *materia medica,* based on his own experience, just as we all do.

During my home birth years, I remember racking my brains over *Cimicifuga,* trying to make sense of the disembodied rubric "Fear of insanity," which rarely seemed to fit my cases. Then one of my patients carried to 42 weeks, still had not gone into labor, and the imminent prospect of hospitalization finally prompted her to tell me that her previous miscarriage and D&C had been the most traumatic experience of her life, and that she felt "unhinged" by the very real possibility that the greater intensity of labor would send her over the edge into a state of disintegration from which she might never return. At my office a few days later, and well along in labor, she indeed appeared wild-eyed and out of control, as she had foreseen; her speech was fragmentary, and her gestures disconnected and woeful. In that instant I understood not only the rubric, and why she'd been so reluctant to speak of it, but also many physical symptoms of the remedy in relation to it, so that I too was alarmed for her sanity. Although remaining flagrantly psychotic for the rest of her labor, she made rapid progress on two or three doses of *Cimicifuga* 200, gave birth normally, and made a full recovery, not long after which I began prescribing the remedy to a wide variety of patients with notable success.

Massimo's criteria for a "cured" case are so strict that many of the successes we love to report at conferences would fall far short of satisfying them. For chronic cases, he accepts a remedy as *simillimum* only after a follow-up of at least two years, preferably longer, during which the remedy has continued to act in a curative manner; and only if the remedy is also effective in overcoming seemingly unrelated *acute* conditions developing in the interim, even injuries and other common domestic ailments, in lieu of the usual first-aid remedies.

Remedy themes emerging from cured cases also provide the ideal framework for organizing the mass of symptom-data that provings generate, which can then in turn be used to help confirm, refute, or modify the themes that should and must ultimately connect them. *Materia medica* study thus becomes an ongoing process of integration, rather than a rote memory exercise.

Other priorities are evaluating the relative importance of symptoms, identifying the themes to connect them to, and rewriting and re-organizing the Repertory in light of them, three monumental but fortunately interrelated tasks that will nevertheless require the collaborative efforts of a whole generation of dedicated homeopaths, just as the older Repertories did, and indeed continue to do. I especially love his case of the patient with a passion for toy trains, cured with the help of *Allium sativum,* whom he uses to illustrate how to *clarify* a symptom, to make it relevant to a theme. To render his success in symptom-language, rubrics like "Passion for model making" or "Plays with toy trains before supper" seemed good candidates, since they disappeared after the remedy, as did his other disabling pathologies, his general health improved as well, and they were precisely the kind that we stuff our Repertories full of. Yet they mislead by giving so much detail as to obscure deeper meanings that could provide useful analogies for similar cases, a consideration that led him to add the remedy to the rubric "Childish," upgrade it to a theme, and identify and cure several other patients with equally consuming hobbies.

I also loved his ascending scale of coherence, beginning with "symptoms," the lowest level, whether verbal or non-verbal, subjective or objective, and obtained from provings or cases, which may or may not be associated with a theme. To illustrate, he uses the remedy *Camphora,* some recognized symptoms of which are connected to characteristic themes of the remedy, e.g., "Ailments from loss of fluids," or to fundamental themes of the Drug family in general, like "Sense of isolation" and "Sensitivity to cold," while others are not and thus of little value.

The next higher level of meaning he calls a "coherent symptom group," a *collection* of such symptoms assembled from different parts or functions of the body, exemplified by a group connected to the same *Camphora* theme, "Ailments from loss of fluids:"

Mind:	*Anxiety, during stool;*
	Delirium, with thirst;
Stomach:	*Thirst, burning, vehement;*
Rectum:	*Cholera;*
	Diarrhea, in hot weather;
Stool:	*Profuse;*
Female:	*Metrorrhagia, with coldness of body;*
Extremities:	*Coldness, with diarrhea;*
Perspiration:	*Cold, with vomtiting.*

It is obvious that these Repertory extractions are facilitated and inspired by various kinds of computer software, such as MacRepertory and Reference Works, both of which Massimo makes frequent and extensive use of, and without which such projects would not be technically possible.

A still higher level of coherence is provided by themes that he calls "characteristic," or distinctive of the remedy and often present, but not always, because they are limited either to certain phases in the evolution of the remedy, such as the *Belladonna* tendency to acute inflammation, which occurs mainly in childhood; or to either side of a polarity if the patient is compensated, or its opposite, if decompensated. Many such themes are to be found in well-known keynotes of polychrests, and *overidentified* with them as a result, like the classic creativity of *Cannabis indica,* which can quickly vanish when the patient is at his worst.

In contrast, the highest level of coherence are "fundamental" themes of the remedy, that is, "an essential, structural component of the remedy and its adaptive strategy," and "nearly always present in a case," although not necessarily *voiced* in so many words and thus having at times to be inferred by the homeopath. These "permeate" the remedy, "describe [its] deepest level," its "core and structure," and provide the ultimate basis of its similitude. He chooses the theme of "Isolation" in *Camphora,* which provides a matrix for connecting many symptoms of the remedy, although many of them would not *look* connected until the theme is recognized, and which turns out to be fundamental not only to *Camphora* itself, but also to the entire homeopathic "Drug" family.

In contrast, "Sensitivity to cold," the famous keynote of *Camphora,* is a *characteristic* theme of only its most decompensated cases, while a more usual, compensated patient might actually *defy* the cold. This is the kind of nitty-gritty scholarship which I found especially characteristic about the book, and it's everywhere, as well as elegant and sublimely beautiful at times. His elucidation of themes is masterful and easy to grasp, although as the fruit of a long experience their actual *discovery* probably looks a lot easier than it will prove to be in practice for someone encountering the idea for the first time.

It all culminates in his concept of the Homeopathic Family, precisely the point where his method comes closest to that of Sankaran and Scholten, and also where he diverges from them, and charts a path most uniquely his own. The attempt to classify homeopathic remedies into "families" has a very old pedigree, and consists of two possible strategies, based on *taxonomy,* the place of the remedy within Nature, like the Periodic Table for the mineral remedies, or on the homeopathic characteristics of the remedies themselves.

Much easier to understand and accept, the taxonomic approach was envisioned by Farrington, and in our own time has been elaborated most convincingly by Sankaran and Scholten. Massimo prefers the second or homeopathic approach, which is purer and more difficult; but in practice he incorporates elements from both strategies. Frequently his first suspicion of a family arises from a treatment failure involving the best-known representative of a natural biological or chemical grouping, and usually a polychrest, like *Lachesis* for the snakes. Next it will include a few others taxonomically related to it, such as *Crotalus, Naja,* and *Bothrops,* but insisting on a purely homeopathic definition, based on the fundamental themes they have in common. Eventually, having identified these themes makes it possible to recognize and add other remedies with the same themes that are taxonomically unrelated, often "small" or at least unfamiliar and under-represented in the literature.

The same idea has fruitful applications for the situation where one remedy has acted curatively for a period of years, but then stops working, and therefore needs to be changed. In my earlier training, based on Kent and his successors, this was a clear signal for retaking the case and prescribing a new remedy, perhaps but not necessarily complementary to it. But if the major themes are still at work in the patient, as one would expect them to be from the length and strength of the curative reaction, Massimo's family concept argues strongly for choosing a different remedy from the same family, a strategy he has evidently employed with great success.

Reading his case reports in Volume II, I marvel at how he gets his patients to confide in him as they do, to spit out their deep inner truths, in the absence of which we are apt to substitute a Review of Systems, for no better reason than that's all we can think of to fill up the time. This is the abiding mystery of case-taking, which is really the "sleeper" factor that distinguishes great homeopaths from merely competent ones, and ultimately it can't really be taught in a linear or discursive fashion, because it also involves and engages the subjective experience of the homeopath as a human being, not only a doctor, scientist, or healer.

The objective of the Method of Complexity is to identify the patient's basic adaptive strategies *at work,* which are exhibited in physical symptoms no less than mental, just as the characteristic and fundamental themes of the remedies and their family groupings are represented in many if not all sections of the Repertory. In other words, the distinction between "Physical" and "Mental" symptoms is itself artificial, and meaningless in many cases. This is the kind of iconoclasm that makes this book so valuable, and that Sankaran and other leading teachers of today have independently discovered and advocated in their own fashion.

As always, the emphasis is on facilitating a free-flowing narrative, and allowing the patient to experience what emerges spontaneously, rather than trying to force the conversation in a certain direction, becoming frustrated if the effort is unsuccessful, and asking questions that require logical explanation. The hardest part is learning to tolerate those long, pregnant silences, and to trust the innate wisdom of the patient to reveal or hide itself, without feeling the need to amass more information in as many areas as possible. This involves focusing on the relevant detail, and finding the whole story there, recognizing the theme or signature pattern in every part as it is offered.

The cases in Volume II are beautifully presented, and a pleasure to read. Each remedy is introduced with a brief but scholarly essay on its natural history, its uses in folk medicine, and its pharmacological, toxicological, and homeopathic characteristics, such that the cases seem to arise and emerge from this background, each with its own unique individuality, yet with clear and vivid analogies to the others. Rather reminiscent of the remedy introductions in Clarke's *Dictionary,* but much richer, more detailed, and beautifully written, these little gems were for me highlights of *materia medica* writing that surpass or at least equal the very best that we possess; and the cases that follow are always sensitively taken, and full of deep confidences from real people that embody and bring to life the method that he has outlined and elaborated for us.

Many of the actual case reports are followed by commentaries by Dr. Giovanni Marotta, Massimo's long-time mentor, collaborator, and friend, almost an *alter ego,* whose more reflective style is nevertheless so perfectly attuned to the method which was created and developed by both men in tandem that it adds a further richness to the work and in no way detracts or distracts from its mission.

Unfortunately the same is not always true for the small army of other people who were involved in the project of rendering the original Italian edition into English, or for the sometimes unclear division of labor between them. A sizeable portion of Volume One, Chapter 1, for example, was a learned but at times barely intelligible essay written by Professor Alberto Panza, an academic colleague who tried to identify themes in modern European philosophy, science, and culture that were congruent with the teachings of homeopathy, a supremely worthy project that could have taken the work to a whole other level of meaning. Unfortunately, the writing, the translation, and perhaps some of the sources cited revolved around technical terms that will be unfamiliar to most of his readers, difficult to translate, and too abstruse for most people to understand, even those who have met them before. So this splendid idea was for me at least a dismal failure.

Another example was the last chapter of Volume 1, the longest in the book, which was a summary of the main teachings of modern psychology with special interest and relevance for homeopaths. For the Italian edition, this project was undertaken by Dr. Marotta, while for its English-speaking audience it fell to John Sobraske, the General Editor, whose coverage of the subject was certainly thorough and well-researched. But coming after Massimo's more engaged, incisive, and goal-oriented style, this section seemed dry and boring to an extent that I found almost jarring. Sobraske's Introduction to Volume 2, on the other hand, which is essentially a brief summary of Volume I, is excellent, thoroughly competent and readable throughout. My only quibble is that I see no reason for doing it, except as a "pony" or shortcut for those choosing to omit Volume 1, which contains some of the finest writing on homeopathy that I have ever read and would be a huge mistake to miss.

In addition, there were a sizeable number of translators and editors, including such dedicated homeopaths as Betty Wood, Krista Heron, Bill Gray, and Maria Kingdon in North America, and several others in the UK and Europe, and their work certainly deserves hearty commendation. But their task was made almost superfluous by Massimo's own excellent command of English, and almost impossibly difficult by Prof. Panza's much greater need and unfamiliar subject matter. In the end, I was left with the suspicion that there were too many good cooks, and no master chef to keep them in line.

But these are minor quibbles. I have no doubt that this work is among the very best our method has produced in its long history, not only for its considerable literary merit, but above all for the cogency of its ideas, which I predict will change how homeopathy is taught and practiced, now and in future.

Catherine Coulter, *The Power of Vision: Life of Samuel Hahnemann**

Catherine Coulter's *Life of Samuel Hahnemann*, her latest book, was written primarily for adolescents and young adults, and for the most part in simple language that even pre-teens can understand. Although the chapters expounding his principles and methods will naturally be a bit dicey even for most eleventh- and twelfth-graders, some such shift in voice and tone is probably unavoidable, since her target audience encompasses the long formative period that extends all the way from late childhood into puberty, adolescence, and young adulthood, from chapter books to history texts. Any book that would span that distance must have something for youngest, oldest, and everyone in between: a tall order.

Hence it seems entirely fitting that her account begins as a tale of high adventure, worthy of Harry Potter or the Hardy Boys, yet finds its ultimate fulfillment in a discussion of ideas appropriate for a college lecture course. For Hahnemann's exemplary life does in fact embody both perspectives. What's more, quite unlike any previous biography, this one centers on his own childhood, adolescence, and young adulthood as a unique vantage point, from which his maturity and old age actually make a new kind of sense.

What I found most refreshing about this emphasis on his early life is its invitation to the reader to regard Hahnemann first and foremost as a man, rather than merely an icon or object of worship, and indeed most emblematically as a youth and a young man, long before he became famous, a time when his greatness was nevertheless clearly foreshadowed by predilections, habits, and inclinations already pre-eminent in the boy. We are thus reminded that his outstanding intellectual abilities were assiduously cultivated by his father, a semi-educated, impoverished painter of porcelain, who often took it upon himself to lock the studious ten-year-old

* Book Review: Catherine Coulter, *The Power of Vision: Life of Samuel Hahnemann*, ***Homeopathy Today,*** Spring 2012.

in his room, set him an intellectual problem, and keep him there until he had solved it. This well-known vignette thus itself becomes iconic, like the ill-fated cherry tree that the young George Washington could not lie about.

Ms. Coulter's emphasis on his early, formative years also helps us appreciate how much inner work was required before Hahnemann's ideas suddenly burst forth fully formed from his brain like the goddess Athene from the head of Zeus, and astonished the world. We who know him mainly from his published work and the standard biographies of Bradford and Haehl are apt to overlook those long years of grinding poverty, which dogged him from earliest childhood, throughout his schooling and licensure, his marriage and family life, and his career as a young physician. For decades he eked out a meager living as tutor to his fellow-students, and later as a translator of medical works, while moving his growing family from town to town to seek a better living and to stay ahead of the doctors and pharmacists who were harassing and hounding him.

We similarly tend to forget that he was in his forties before writing his first article on the subject that would commandeer the rest of his life, and that *The Organon* did not see the light of day until well into middle age. Reframing his long and immensely productive life as an epic of struggle and high adventure thus gets it exactly right in a way that his previous biographers, for all their erudition and attention to detail, tended to lose sight of.

As always with Ms. Coulter's work, these virtues are wonderfully enhanced by the beauty and elegance of her writing, doubly so in this case by the purity and simplicity of her language, almost like that of a fable suitable for reading to young children. Here too, these literary qualities are highlighted by her emphasis on Hahnemann's childhood and early life, which are so thinly documented in the literature that she is free to invent several important characters from whole cloth, with at most a few clues, hints, and offhand remarks to go on.

Two notable examples are Ernst, his inseparable boyhood friend, and Frau Martha, the wise and kindly herbalist who takes him under her wing, teaches him the lore of plant remedies, and thus initiates the boy, hitherto steeped only in book learning, into the study and experience of the natural world, a whole new cornucopia of inexhaustible beauty and healing power. Whether or not these persons actually existed, they might well have; and in any case they help to illustrate and explain those signal qualities and admirable traits in the man that were so highly developed in and indeed central to his work.

I was equally charmed by her way of elaborating on other salient features of Hahnemann's life and character that are much better-known, such as his extraordinary gift for languages and indeed for all academic work, which he pursued with a dedication to excellence that even the severely straitened circumstances of his parents could not discourage. I loved her anecdote of the 12-year-old Hahnemann, who after his father had sent him away to learn a trade in a distant town, simply defected, came back home, and hid in his parents' attic, first with the help of his sister, then with the connivance of his mother, and at last winning his father's pained but truly chastened acceptance. Once again, Ms. Coulter makes a plausible conjecture thoroughly convincing, solely through the power of her language.

The same theme of intellectual prowess developed by persistent application is then retold at various stages of his life, until it becomes a recurrent *leitmotiv* that provides meaning and context for everything that follows, like the old American legend of Horatio Alger, that rags-to-riches saga of industry and perseverance that was routinely preached to schoolchildren in days gone by. Thus, after the débâcle of his apprenticeship, we learn that Hahnemann was taken in by the town schoolmaster, Herr Muller, awarded free tuition, the only way he could possibly have attended, in exchange for tutoring and otherwise assisting his fellow students, and was graced with special kindness, affection, and esteem by teachers and students alike. Throughout his medical training, he was likewise singled out for favored consideration by a succession of teachers, mentors, and benefactors.

I also took particular delight in Ms. Coulter's imaginative rendering of some members of Hahnemann's family who are little more than footnotes in the biographical information that is generally available. Two of his children come particularly to mind, namely, Friedrich, who though often surly and difficult, was also extraordinarily gifted, sensitive, and unselfish, and eventually became an accomplished homeopath in his own right, but died young and unhappy; and Amalie, her father's favorite, who was closest to him emotionally and spiritually, and assisted him in his work after her mother died, yet graciously stepped aside in favor of Melanie when she came to Cöthen to marry him and whisk him away to Paris for the remainder of his life. They appear both as children and adults at various points in the narrative; and both come vividly and almost palpably to life in a way that helps us to understand their father more authentically than any recital of his ideas and accomplishments possibly could.

My only reservation about the book is the question of its audience. I enjoyed it thoroughly, on many levels; but I am a homeopath, already steeped in the lore and mystique of the man and his creation, with my youth far behind me. This biography is intended for young people, to persuade them to become homeopaths themselves, or at least to pique their interest in and enrich their understanding of the man whose teachings their parents have had reason and occasion to value. When I raised this question with Ms. Coulter, she expressed the hope that such parents would want not only to give but also in some cases to read it to their children, which I think would work quite well for the narrative, but less so for the didactic parts. By the time these children would be capable of tackling the Law of Similars, they would no longer need or want to be read to, and would long since have graduated from chapter books and the Hardy Boys to *Dungeons and Dragons,* video games, and the like, so that reading the expository sections would not be a top priority either. In short, I'm not at all sure that the book will succeed for a large part of the audience she has in mind, which is a pity. But I have no doubt that it will delight and enlighten their parents and grandparents, and might then spill over into the culture at large, as I very much hope that it will.

Prafull and Ambrish Vijayakar, M. D., *Predictive Homeopathy**

AIH Seminar, New Orleans, 2014

Exactly one year after Karl Robinson's inspired last-minute walk-on for them in Chicago, the Vijayakars, father and son, finally arrived in the flesh; and I'm happy to say, it was well worth the wait. Although spring was slow in coming, Irene Sebastian, a Louisiana native, picked another winner for our hotel, which was tastefully appointed, well-staffed, and strategically located in the heart of the French Quarter.

The added excitement generated by what we were about to receive was evident in the impressive cohort of old-timers who showed up, many of them experienced teachers in their own right, to glimpse and draw inspiration from something radically new and different, even at this late date in their careers.

To be sure, a lot of what drew us all to New Orleans were the dramatic cures the Vijayakars presented, and the well-earned fame they enjoy as a result of them, as in one video case, when somebody opened the door to their waiting room, and for a brief moment we caught sight of the throngs outside in their dozens, these legions of the grievously sick and disabled, waiting their turn and hoping for a miracle.

What gave particular meaning and emphasis to these vignettes were two very different social and political realities, almost polar opposites of each other. The first was the high level of esteem that our colleagues enjoy in India, where homeopathic medicine is taught in dozens if not hundreds of full-time training colleges throughout the country, and is officially recognized, promoted, and licensed by the government, such that homeopathic doctors are treated as equals and given numerous inpatient and outpatient referrals by their allopathic brethren, even and especially

* Seminar Review: Prafull and Ambrish Vijayakar, *Predictive Homeopathy*, ***American Journal of Homeopathic Medicine*** 107:77, Summer 2014.

for the treatment of grave, incurable, and terminal conditions. It would be difficult for their American counterparts not to feel envious of this achievement, which is without parallel in the world, and far above the mere toleration that we may at last be close to achieving in this country.

On the flip side was the sobering fact that our own level of training and expertise, while admirably suited to maintaining a general practice of ambulatory medicine, is largely inadequate to do justice to the extreme patient loads and advanced pathologies that the Vijayakars are seeing and helping on a routine basis. These spectacular cures were accordingly intended mainly to illustrate their new way of understanding and ultimately predicting them, just as their title had promised. I daresay no one present could have failed to be thrilled at being taught how to succeed with precisely the kinds of patients we tend to hit the wall with in our own practices, those with acute, life-threatening emergencies, or cancer and other advanced diseases, that apart from some rare, lucky hits, we more often try but fail to help very much, not to mention congenital anomalies that have always seemed beyond the reach of remedies entirely, even in the most skillful hands.

Although we were not told how they arrived at the remedy, few among us will ever forget the video of the young girl born without corneas, pupils or lenses, whose eyes appeared totally white and opaque. Three months after a single dose of *Merc. sol.* 200, corneas were clearly evident in both eyes, and she could grasp objects with her hands; after 12 months she could follow objects with her eyes; after 18 months she could see and grasp whatever interested her; and after 2 years she could get herself a drink without assistance.

Witnessing such a miracle also helped me to appreciate the fact that Prafull himself, a son and grandson of allopaths, had undergone an evolution quite similar to our own, beginning as a "mongrel" using both methods, i. e., precisely the kind of "half-homeopath" for whom Hahnemann reserved his most savage criticism, then later deciding to follow the *Organon* and Law of Similars exclusively and achieving some cures, but mainly of acute diseases and those that were self-limiting to begin with. Virtually everyone present could recognize and identify with this history, which was the same predicament that led Hahnemann to study the chronic diseases and ultimately write the *magnum opus* of his later years on that subject.

These parallel biographies thus helped me grasp the reality that not only Hahnemann and Vijayakar, but indeed all homeopaths before and since, were and are in much the same boat, helping our patients recover from their acute ailments and episodes by finding the most similar remedy for that situation, only to watch their underlying and often invisible chronic diseases continue to progress and worsen over the years, erupting repeatedly and needing further treatment each time, without ever being truly and permanently cured.

This universal difficulty helped explain Prafull's insistence that Hahnemann's greatest discovery was not the Law of Similars, the defining principle of homeopathy, as we'd always been taught, but rather his theory of miasms, which has always remained so controversial that many pre-eminent homeopaths both then and now have abstained from following him into this forbidding terrain at all. An appealing corollary of Prafull's iconoclasm lay in his determination to integrate the theory and practice of homeopathic medicine into the vast corpus of contemporary science, and thus make effective use of the full range of knowledge so painfully won over the past two hundred years since the *Organon* was published. For the Vijayakars, embryology has provided a valuable scientific explanation of Hering's Laws of Cure, as well as further corroboration of their importance in clinical cases, in the light of which the thorough and permanent cure of chronic diseases has been shown not only to be possible, but also to proceed in a direction that is largely predictable, if often at variance with what we have been taught and what our common sense has generally supposed.

As an illustration, Prafull's son Ambrish cited a case of psoriasis developing soon after the disappearance of asthma under homeopathic treatment. Rather than a cure, according to Hering's Second and Third Laws, from inside outwards, and from more vital to less vital organ, as we would ordinarily assume, both their embryological studies and their clinical work suggest quite the opposite, that it represents a suppression into more advanced pathology, because the characteristic lesions of psoriasis, while manifesting on the skin, actually originate in the dermis, which according to their schema arises from a deeper layer than the bronchiolar lining.

Although I'm still trying to understand exactly what "deeper" means in this context, I was powerfully drawn to this line of thinking as a reaffirmation of what on some level we already know, or should know, that since homeopathy does embody an authentic truth, it must therefore be compatible with and indeed ultimately confirmed by the best and most advanced scientific knowledge available.

In the same vein, albeit less explicitly stated, was their rehabilitation of pathology and the various basic and clinical sciences allied with it, mainly anatomy, physiology, biochemistry, and genetics. As both Prafull and Ambrish repeatedly insisted, homeopaths must "treat the *man* with the disease," and not "the *disease* in man," as our allopathic brethren just as proudly aspire to; on this point at least, all classical prescribers, fundamentalists and innovators alike, can unanimously agree. But Hahnemann's theory of the chronic miasms, backed up by the Vijayakars' huge volume of cured cases, reinstates the concept of pathological entities that do in fact "exist" on some level and in some fashion independently of the individual patient who happens to exhibit them. Although all patients react uniquely and must therefore be treated as individuals, acknowledging the miasms as real allows and indeed obliges us to study and track their diagnosable diseases by the same laboratory abnormalities that are detectable even before the patient is aware of them, just as we learned in medical school. Predictive homeopathy thus reminds even the purist classical prescriber that pathology does indeed matter, for the same reason that Künzli once savaged "essence prescribing," that the hypertensive patient who feels better emotionally after the remedy is still not better in the way he needs and wants to be if his blood pressure remains unchanged.

That is why the main body of the seminar began not with the usual "hot" topics, such as *materia medica* or choosing the remedy, but more prosaically, with the nuts and bolts of the follow-up visit, and especially how to decide whether or not the disappearance of symptoms is proceeding in accordance with Hering's Laws. In a direct assault upon our more laid-back approach, both father and son repeatedly insisted that a genuine and permanent cure of chronic disease *must* by definition follow this kind of sequence, and that only acute diseases can disappear without necessarily passing through accumulated layers of suppression from the past.

The first day was therefore largely devoted to Prafull's seven-part "hierarchy of suppression," based on the three main tissue layers of embryonic development and their further subdivisions, which are quite complicated to explain and deserve more detailed scrutiny than this limited space allows. A fuller version appears in a chart at the end of his first book,

Predictive Homeopathy, Part I: the Theory of Suppression; but I will reproduce a bare-bones outline of it here:

1) *The ectoderm,* comprising the skin and appendages, i.e., *the outermost layer* of the body. Its ailments include boils, rashes, conjunctivitis, etc.

2) *The endoderm,* consisting of *the cells lining the upper respiratory, GI, and GU tracts.* Its ailments include colds, coughs, heartburn, UTI's, etc.

3) *The mesenchymal* or outer *layer of mesoderm,* comprising the *connective tissues* (bones, joints, muscles, etc.), dermis, teeth, blood, and lymph. Its ailments include alopecia, psoriasis, arthritis, anemia, etc.

4) *The mesothelial* or inner *layer of mesoderm,* which forms the heart, blood vessels, and the parenchyma of lungs and kidneys. Its ailments include hypertension, atherosclerosis, renal and pulmonary diseases, etc.

5) *The endocrine system,* i.e., *pituitary, thyroid, adrenals, pancreatic islets, ovaries, and testes.* Its ailments include thyroiditis, diabetes, etc.

6) *The neuroectoderm,* comprising *brain, CNS, autonomic, and peripheral nervous system.* Its ailments include neuritis, epilepsy, MS, etc.

7) The *genetic code,* i. e., basic cellular structure and function; and *mind.* Ailments include psychoses, auto-immune disease, cancer, gangrene, etc.

Generalizing from the insights of Hahnemann and Hering, their hypothesis is that effective suppression of any disease, whether from allopathic drugs or an incorrect remedy, will *necessarily* lead to a disease at the next higher or "deeper" level, while a curative response, at least for the chronic diseases, must proceed in the opposite direction, i. e., back through a sequence of ailments at successively lower levels.

Ambrish then showed how closely Hering's Laws parallel what we now know as the earliest stages in intrauterine development, and thus uncannily foreshadowed the birth of the science of embryology that was still many decades away:

1) Hering's First Law, *from above downwards,* corresponds to the *apical dominance* which develops very early in embryonic life, with the differentiation of cephalic and caudal poles (the head and tail end, respectively) from the central axis, with the former becoming dominant as the structure from which the brain and CNS develop.

2) Hering's Second Law, *from inside outwards,* from center to periphery, corresponds to the formation of *the proximo-distal gradient,* followed by the endocrine glands, the parenchyma of visceral organs (heart, lungs, kidneys), the musculoskeletal system and connective tissues, and the skin and appendages, i. e., in the reverse order of the stages of suppression.

3) Hering's Third Law, *from more vital to less vital organ,* follows the same sequence.

4) Hering's Fourth Law, *that symptoms reappear and disappear in the reverse order of their appearance in the life history of the patient,* traces out the same sequence through time, the deeper and more recent symptoms disappearing before the more superficial symptoms from longer ago.

I will leave aside for further study the same doubts and qualifications that should properly greet every scientific hypothesis, namely,

1) *Is* there such a hierarchy?

2) If so, is theirs *the right one?*

3) In either case, yes or no, *what does it all mean?*

It is far from intuitively obvious, for example, that the endocrine organs should qualify as "more vital" organs than either the heart or the lungs, or that their diseases should therefore outrank in importance such notorious killers as atherosclerotic coronary disease, COPD, and end-stage renal disease, or that arthritis sits higher on the totem pole than bronchitis or asthma, as Ambrish was at such pains to point out. Nor is it entirely clear in what sense the mesoderm, comprising the musculoskeletal system and connective tissues, is a "deeper" layer than the endoderm, or easy to accept that the inner lining cells of a cavity, e. g., the endocardium, endothelium, and *endoderm*, aren't more "important" or "vital" than their supporting structures, connective tissues, or membranous coverings (pleura, pericardium, mesothelium, etc.).

Because the Vijayakars undoubtedly discovered and in any case have amply confirmed the truth of their seven-part hierarchy on the empirical evidence of their cases, it is more than reasonable to use it as a practical schema for conducting the follow-up visit, without expecting them to provide such "explanations" for it; nor can it be their fault if "deeper" and "more vital" in Hering's terminology don't always translate perfectly into modern embryological language. In short, the persistence of these riddles simply provides an added incentive to continue our studies with the Vijayakars in a more comprehensive way at a later date.

In any case, at least part of their resolution undoubtedly lies buried deep in the heart of their other main topic, the three miasms of Hahnemann, psora, sycosis, and syphilis, which were discussed more systematically on Saturday, and featured a detailed analysis of their respective pathological styles, how to identify them clinically, and how to use them in choosing the remedy and evaluating the cure at each follow-up.

Their studies in this area brought to mind the late Proceso Ortega of Mexico, whose seminal work, *Apuntes sobre los Miasmas,* identified psora with physical and/or mental *deficiency,* sycosis with *excessive growth* or mental elaboration (OCD, hysteria, anxiety, etc.), and syphilis with *perversion, ulceration, and destruction* in body or mind, and correlated them with an exhaustive, scholarly exegesis of rubrics in Kent's *Repertory.* Stressing the importance of mastering the physical, mental, and general symptom-characteristics of each, the Vijayakars again ingeniously updated them with cross-references to familiar pathological processes:

1) *Psora,* the most basic defense mechanism, i.e., *inflammation, a process occurring solely on the biochemical and physiological plane, without permanent organic or tissue changes.*

Corresponding to acute, self-limiting diseases, when the mechanism is sufficient to control and ultimately cure the condition, psora is also the most important of the three, in that the other two both develop from it when it fails, and entail some form and degree of morphological or structural change. Acute ailments of the psoric type may also provide useful "entry points" for the prescriber, by virtue of the sheer number and variety of their symptom-complaints, many indicating some form of physical, mental, or emotional hypersensitivity.

When the psoric mechanism fails to contain the problem, it tends to progress to

2) *Sycosis,* characterized by phenomena of *accumulation* (congestion, effusion, swelling, or deposition of fats, as in obesity, atherosclerosis); *induration,*

involving synthesis of fibrin or elastin (scarring, fibrosis, and contractures, or prolapse, varices, and hemorrhoids); and finally, *proliferation* (hyperplasia, endometriosis, warts, moles, cysts, tumors, polyps, etc.).

These may be accompanied by mental and emotional expressions of excess, such as OCD or phobias; but sycotic symptoms seldom furnish useful entry-points, because they represent the individual's lived mythology, typically buttressed with self-regard, and are therefore apt to be deceptive, misleading, or at least incomplete. When these in turn prove insufficient or break down, they may progress to

3) *Syphilis,* involving *destructive or self-destructive processes and/or behavior,* in which a part may have to be sacrificed in order to save the whole, or the symptom-picture goes *out of control* and assumes *extreme forms:* bleeding, ulceration, gangrene, and auto-immune or degenerative diseases; or hallucinations, delusions, hysteria, perversions, and suicidal or murderous behavior.

In chronic cases, the Vijayakars stress leaving aside the psoric and sycotic elements and going straight for the syphilitic as their entry-point for choosing the remedy, because they are the most extreme, dangerous, life-threatening, often the "strange, rare, and peculiar" symptoms that we've always been taught to look for, and because, as the deepest pathology, they must be cured first in any case, before the process can complete itself by regressing "backward" through the other two miasms. These ideas I found among the most stimulating and rewarding of the whole seminar, once again by reinstating the central importance of anatomic, physiological, and biochemical pathologies in our clinical work.

Although Prafull recognizes only Hahnemann's original triad of psora, sycosis, and syphilis in his written work, and explicitly rejects Sankaran's addition of "intermediate" miasms -- ringworm, typhoid, malaria, cancer, tuberculosis, and leprosy -- in the seminar he described his own cases as "psoro-sycotic" or "syco-syphilitic" often enough to cut what had sounded like a real difference down to the size of a semantic distinction. What I liked about it was the consistency of his emphasis on the three main disease-making styles and their correlation with well-known pathological processes.

In conclusion, since nearly all of us in attendance were clinicians primarily, no review of the event would be complete without at least a sampling of cases. For limitations of space, it is impossible to reproduce the details of how they were analyzed, how remedies were chosen for them, how well they worked, or by what paths the cures evolved; so I've settled for simply listing them with their remedies, followed by some "pearls" that we were blessed to receive along the way.

Cases:

Young girl, sclerocornea	*Mercurius sol.*	200
Boy, 4, too weak to stand	*Pulsatilla*	200
Boy, 18 months, asthma	*Mercurius sol.*	200
Man, 45, psoriasis	*Natrum mur.*	200
Man, severe 3° burns, in ICU	*Magnesia sulph.*	200
Man, severe cellulitis of face	*Sulphur*	200
Man, chest pain, anxiety, in ER	*Stramonium*	200 by olfaction
Man, high BP, diabetic gangrene	*Pulsatilla*	200 by olfaction
Boy, 4, seizures, cysticercosis	*Stramonium*	1M
Girl, 9, asthma, fungal septicemia	*Arsenicum alb.*	200
Man, 85, paralyzed, in coma	*Arnica*	
Man, 90, afraid to die	*Baryta carb.*	
Woman, schizophrenic	*Sulphur*	
Woman, endometriosis, liver, brain	*Acetic. acid.*	
Boy, 8, "like vegetable," can't walk	*Opium*	
Boy, 7, his brother, also can't walk	*Hyoscyamus*	
Girl, medulloblastoma	*Platina*	
Boy, 5, blind, can't stand, walk, talk	*Pulsatilla*	
Child, sclerocornea from birth	*Sulphur*	

"Pearls:"

The ability to predict outcomes means that the science has been perfected. Homeopathy is the most advanced medical science; only our knowledge falls short.
The human body is perfect, mathematical, just like the natural world as a whole.

Modern medicine accepts nothing but the body, and what is provable to the senses; it treats only half the man, gets only half-results.

The disappearance of symptoms is not cure: if the Laws of Cure are violated, the direction is wrong, and the remedy must be changed. The disease that is manifest at any particular time is only the tip of the iceberg; if the remedy is right, the reversal is more transient and less intense than before.

For acutes, when changes are purely physiological, give the phenotypic simillimum; once structural changes are present, acute remedies are no longer sufficient.

In emergencies, give remedies by olfaction or rubbing into the skin.

The first pillar of Predictive Homeopathy is the follow-up visit; the goal of treatment is not simply to relieve suffering, but to eradicate the disease.

In adults, the history is dominated by sycosis, the facade we project for others to see; the real miasm is easier to see in children. Go "below" the history to uncover it.

Every remedy can exhibit symptoms of all three miasms.
Miasms aren't "good" or "bad," just different kinds of reaction to morbific stimuli.

The syphilitic patient no longer loves life nor fears death.
Sycosis is the selfish love of life, of gratification of the need for money, sex, or power.

I don't know what else to say, except that, like almost everyone else, I was blown away by the Vijayakars: by their results, and by the system of homeopathic, embryological, and pathological ideas that they developed to explain and endeavor to perfect them. The best part is now, in taking it all back to my own practice, imbued with a feeling of renewed excitement in being with my patients, and enlisting their help, as always, in finding the best way to help them.

Karl Robinson, M. D.,
*Small Doses, Big Results**

Homeopathic books come in many varieties, from textbooks to testimonials, from introductions for the curious with no previous experience to detailed treatises for the serious student. This one is like a smorgasbord, with tasty tidbits of all the above, and more. It includes snippets of personal narrative, didactic explanation of basic principles, nuts and bolts of case-taking and analysis, repertorizations, *Materia medica,* and an oversized main course of cured cases, some of them quite spectacular. But what gives life to it all and sets it apart from the rest is the distinctive *voice* of its author, which anyone who knows Karl will instantly recognize as unmistakably his own, a real achievement for any writer.

To begin with, he is an accomplished raconteur. Perhaps dating from his earlier career as a journalist, which one would like to hear more about, he writes much as he speaks, in a pithy, earthy, style that eschews fancy language, revels in the idioms and cadences of everyday speech, and is easily accessible for the average person to read and understand. Here's a random sample from page 39, describing a classic *Colocynthis* case of lower back pain:

> "What gives me the greatest relief is for me to lie on my stomach and my wife to stand on my buttocks and hamstrings. She's around 230 lbs., and the pleasure of that release is so great, I fall asleep right away." Can you begin to make sense of his problem? He had muscle pain in the buttocks and hamstrings which was better from hard pressure. *Very hard pressure.* Not the usual pain that yields to a good massage. No. This pain only yielded to EXTREME pressure, to a 230-pound woman standing on his buttocks (!).

The book is full of vivid mini-stories like this, such that the reader doesn't want them to end. That too is high praise.

---

* Book Review: Karl Robinson, *Small Doses, Big Results,* ***American Journal of Homeopathic Medicine*** 107:145, Fall 2014.

But there's more besides. Although you might not have noticed it, Karl is also an evangelist. While recuperating from an infected wound in the hospital founded by the late Albert Schweitzer in West Africa, he came under the spell of the older man's exemplary life, and had a sudden epiphany that his true vocation lay in medicine, a field that he'd shown no interest or aptitude in before and was totally unprepared for, taking the great missionary's words to heart as a kind of personal mantra:

> Ethics is nothing else than reverence for life.
> The purpose of human life is to serve [with] compassion and the will to help others.
> Do something wonderful, [that] people may imitate it.
> I don't know your destiny, but the only ones among you who will be really happy are those who have sought and found how to serve.

After completing his prerequisites and entering medical school, he soon recognized the numberless ways in which his chosen profession fell short of the ideals for the sake of which he had entered it, and thus naturally gravitated to homeopathy, which for him has always meant not only practicing it, but also promoting its radically different point of view by teaching it to others. Facing mainly indifference and hostility from his allopathic colleagues, Karl like almost every other physician practicing homeopathy in America today would have felt obliged to preach that gospel in any case; but for him it was an inseparable part of the spiritual revelation that led him to become a physician in the first place.

When I first met him in the '70's in New Mexico, he had already attracted a small following of students, both licensed and otherwise; and more than a few have stayed with or near him ever since. More recently, with years of teaching and practicing under his belt, the missionary aspect of his work has blossomed into the Homeopathy School of the Americas, a peripatetic enterprise centered in Guatemala, Honduras, and El Salvador, which began as a project of Homeopaths Without Borders, but is now largely subsidized out of Karl's own pocket, with some of his best students even supplying cases for this book.

A similarly admirable zeal is evident in his eagerness to learn from as many world-class homeopaths as possible, and his willingness to go literally to the ends of the earth to find them. A frequent visitor to India in particular, he has studied with Dhawale, Sankaran, Vijayakar, his latest teacher, for whom he has an especially high regard, and quite a few more, I believe, whose names have long since escaped me. Since earning an MFHom. from the Royal London Hospital School in the '70's, he has studied with Vithoulkas in Greece, and many, many others, including Nuala Eising in Ireland, justly famed for her psychospiritual and mystical faculties, and the subject of a wonderful chapter in the book. It is impossible not to admire and be grateful to him for his dedication and perseverance in tracking such people down, wherever they may be, and in bringing back, sharing, and redistributing the riches he has amassed from them; he is truly the Marco Polo of our art. Few of us will ever forget his willingness to step in at the last minute for the Vijayakars last year in Chicago, when they defaulted on account of Prafull's illness, let alone the virtuoso performance that he improvised for the occasion.

These, at any rate, are some of the qualities of the man that made something like this book inevitable and provide its unique character and style. As to how well it succeeds in what I take to be its mission, to disseminate the homeopathic point of view as widely as possible in his native land, one good reason for optimism lies in its genial, user-friendly ambiance and refreshing lack of pretense to being the last word on the subject. Its thrust is mainly to tell stories from life, and to evoke the infinite diversity of complaints and situations for which homeopathic treatment is not only appropriate, but in many cases more effective than the prevailing form of medicine, and even life-saving at times. It will, I'm sure, be comforting to many to learn how a fine, experienced homeopath thinks about his patients, and how varied are the complaints, problems, ailments, and yes, *diseases,* for which homeopathy can work miracles in skilled hands.

Even a cursory glance at its 45 short chapters will suffice to give a rough idea of their range: back pain, dementia, meningitis, colic, herpetic keratitis, depression, warts, PTSD, psychosis, dyslexia, Rocky Mountain spotted fever, Lyme disease, concussion, a teen-age "zombie," eczema, drug abuse, deep-vein thrombosis, a premonition of death, a paranoid *pistolero,* asthma, epilepsy, sciatica, pneumonia, chronic diarrhea, exhaustion, emaciation, vertigo, osteoarthritis, pyelonephritis, ADHD, fracture not healing, brown recluse spider bite, altitude sickness, euthanasia, and radiation sickness. In short, it encompasses virtually the whole spectrum of general and family medicine, yet another feature that bodes well for its success.

A quick look at the remedies presented -- *Alumina, Belladonna, Sulphur, Mercurius, Ignatia, Causticum, Arnica, Arsenicum alb., Baryta iod., Sepia, Opium, Elaps, Calcarea carb., Thuja, Mercurius sulph., Antimonium tart., Tellurium, Phosphorus, Croton tig., Gelsemium, Natrum mur., Cocculus, Tarentula, Bryonia, Lachesis, Coca, Granite, Marble* -- likewise reveals a pretty fair sampling of the entire *materia medica,* including all three kingdoms, several polychrests, some unusual remedies, snakes, spiders, and even a few of the seemingly non-medicinal substances, like salt, chalk, and sand, that the homeopathic process has transformed into powerful remedies in their own right.

I'll single out a few, to demonstrate both his genius for cut-to-the-chase prescribing and the direct, down-to-earth style of his teaching. In his chapter on isopathy, for example, he tells the story of a septuagenarian patient whom he and other well-known homeopaths had been treating for decades without success, until he learned at a conference that black tea contains a lot of aluminum, and then from his own study that its absorption was greatly enhanced by adding lemon. The black tea connection immediately rang a bell, because his patient had stopped drinking coffee at his request, substituted black tea and lemon for it, and thus, he surmised, had very probably been ingesting what for her were toxic levels of aluminum over a period of thirty years. That conjecture was amply borne out when she conquered her asthma with the help of low potencies of *Alumina* daily and successfully weaned herself from her meds. Of the aluminum in black tea and its enhanced absorption from adding lemon, I knew nothing until Karl presented them at his walk-on seminar in Chicago last year.

Here's another one, in his own words, which I chose primarily for the uncommon remedy he came up with:

> Marta had been suffering from right-sided sciatic pain, [which] traveled from the low back down the back of the thigh to the ankle. She could only fall asleep on her left side, and if she turned on to the right, the pain woke her. [It] was worse [from] sneezing, lifting a suitcase, and straining at stool. Her symptoms corresponded to the element *Tellurium,* which in homeopathic form is known

> to relieve sciatica which is worse from coughing and straining. Curiously, it is known to act on right-sided sciatica.
>
> Many homeopathic medicines predominantly affect either the right or left side. Skillful homeopaths play close attention to laterality. When most of the symptoms point to a medicine but the laterality doesn't correspond, it probably should be discarded.
>
> She was given a dose of *Tellurium* 200 and improved dramatically within days. Seven months later, she relapsed. As before, the pain was worse from coughing, sneezing, and straining at stool. She also mentioned that she liked apples. It so happens that in the proving of *Tellurium* some provers experienced a desire to eat apples. So once again her symptoms fit. Two days after another dose, she was able to sleep flat and rise from bed without pain. At one month, she was 75% better. She went on to a full recovery. [Fifteen years later] she had a recurrence, and again *Tellurium* 200 put her right in days.
>
> When she came to me for allergies and loss of voice, I thought I'd give *Tellurium* a try because it had acted so swiftly, even though it is not well-known in that area. The allergies ceased in a few days. The conclusion I draw is that *Tellurium* was probably her constitutional medicine, because it acted curatively in two separate conditions. Homeopaths believe that all illnesses, all complaints, are connected.

OK, I can't resist: just one more. "In the following example," he says, "a woman improved significantly with homeopathic treatment when there was no plausible physiological explanation:"

> She had no ileum. It had been surgically removed over 4 years before. As a result, she was having frequent diarrhea and had to be extremely careful about everything she put into her mouth. She was 70 and had trigger-quick diarrhea immediately after eating or drinking. Anything more [than] small quantities set off diarrhea within minutes.
>
> Could homeopathy help in spite of the fact that she was missing a long segment of her intestine? I took the following symptoms from the Repertory:
>
> *"Diarrhea immediately after eating"*
> *"Diarrhea immediately after drinking"*
> *"Diarrhea, sudden"*

> These symptoms suggested *Croton tiglium,* made from croton oil, [which can] cure sudden, gushing diarrhea. She took a single dose, and *the diarrhea ceased.* She was able to eat and drink normally. This kind of result cannot be explained physiologically. After removal of the ileum, the remaining gut [may] partially take over [in] about 2 years, [but] even then most people will still have diarrhea. The annals of homeopathy contain innumerable unlikely cures.
>
> But my patient may not have needed to have her ileum removed. [Years earlier] she was diagnosed with endometrial cancer. The uterus and ovaries were surgically removed. She then underwent chemo and radiation. It was the radiation that nearly did her in. *"I was sure the treatments were harming me. I begged my doctors not to do any more." She was part of a research protocol; {so they refused}." Then they did a CT scan which showed the ileum was non-functioning. {So} they removed {it}."*
>
> The doctors were wedded to their protocol and refused to alter it. Yet she knew the radiation was harming her. Why is it difficult for doctors to listen to patients? Had she not had the radiation, would the cancer have returned? No one will ever know. The surgeon cleaned up the mess caused by too much radiation, and *Croton tiglium* was able to undo some of the havoc caused by the loss of her ileum.

That's the best part of all: what we get is not simply the technical aspect, the nuts and bolts of finding the remedy, but the real-life context in which the need for it came about. This is what I like to call "plain doctoring," at its best.

He could have spent a little more time, energy, and money prettying up the cover and interior design; but I'm sure he was motivated to keep the price down so more folks would buy it, and at $12.95 it certainly is a bargain. In short, I wish for this book a great success. Whether you're a newcomer, a beginner, or an expert, I guarantee that you'll have fun reading it, and that you'll learn things you didn't know before. If you're new to homeopathy, you'll see what the fuss is all about, and why you might like to try it; and if you've been doing it for years, you already know why you can't resist coming back for more. As the great Yogi Berra once said, it's *déjà vu* all over again.

V. Obituaries.

"Elinore Peebles (1897-1992)"

"Maesimund Panos, M. D.
(1912-1999)"

"Julian Winston (1941-2005)"

"Christine Luthra, M. D. (1951-2006)"

"Harris Coulter, Ph. D. (1952-2009)"

"David Warkentin (1951-2010)"

"Catherine Coulter (1934-2014)"

*Elinore Peebles (1897-1992)**

Following a long life of service, this lively, intelligent, and altogether remarkable woman died in a nursing home on July 13, soon after her 95th birthday. Having had the privilege of knowing her as a friend, I would like to leave behind this short remembrance of her to the homeopathic community, on whose behalf she gave so much of herself, and with whose history her life was inseparably connected for nearly a century.

Elinore was born in 1897, the year that her father, Charles Cutting, M.D., graduated from the Hahnemann Medical College. The family settled in Newtonville, near Boston, where Dr. Cutting set up his medical practice, and Elinore learned homeopathy directly from him, helping out in his office during clinic hours, accompanying him on home and hospital visits, eavesdropping on case conferences with his colleagues, and, of course, savoring the mysterious globules when she fell ill.

From the age of seven, her sole ambition and fondest wish was to go to college and become a homeopathic physician. But when Elinore was 16, financial reverses abruptly put an end to both her dream and her childhood. This great and incalculable disappointment remained engraved forever in her heart, left its mark on her character, and also cheated the people of Massachusetts of the truly fine and dedicated physician that she would undoubtedly have become.

Never one to indulge in self-pity or brooding about the past, Elinore soon married Waldo Peebles, an old friend of her childhood, and devoted herself to raising a daughter, two sons, and a flock of grandchildren, as women have always been expected to do. Like her mother, she also became active in the Swedenborgian Church, a notable influence on other eminent homeopaths from Hering and Kent to Pierre Schmidt and Elizabeth Wright-Hubbard in her own time. In later years, Elinore loved to go to the supermarket wearing her favorite T-shirt, with "Here comes a Homeopath" imprinted on the front, and "There goes a Swedenborgian" on the back, bearing witness to the close spiritual kinship between the two.

* "Elinore Peebles (1897-1992)," ***Homeopathy Today,*** October 1992.

One son and one grandson became fine and reputable physicians, graduating from Harvard Medical School, where her son still teaches and practices, never using homeopathy for himself, yet ever protective of it for her sake and eager for her remedies when he himself fell ill. The bittersweet irony of watching her loved ones reach for and attain the pinnacle of her own chosen profession by turning away from her beloved homeopathy must have brought her such commingled joy and pain as would have been difficult to distinguish throughout the later years of her life.

In the 1940's and '50's, with homeopathy clearly on the decline and the Boston homeopaths beginning to die off without anyone to replace them, Elinore devoted herself to homeopathic education and self-help with a zeal and ability that were an inspiration to all who knew her. She became active in the Boston Homeopathic Laymen's League and the Ladies' Auxiliary of Hahnemann Hospital in Brighton, a small homeopathic community hospital that she helped found in the 1940's but was soon dominated by the more lucrative allopathic style of practice. During the 1950's, with the help of James Stephenson, MD, and Dorothy Cornish, she organized the Homeopathic Information Service and published a number of excellent and wonderfully concise pamphlets about homeopathy for the general public that bear comparison with the finest available today; several of these she wrote herself.

During this period she was also invited to speak to Harvard medical students, and helped organize a series of lectures at the medical college of Boston University, which had actually been founded as a homeopathic school in 1875. For all these labors she was awarded an honorary life membership in the American Institute of Homeopathy, whose professional meetings she regularly attended. Her brainchild, the Homeopathic Information Service, remained active until the 1970's.

But no recital of accomplishments can do justice to her sparkling intelligence, lively wit, and dedication to her core values of family, Church, and homeopathy that she lived and breathed throughout her long life. I first met her in 1982, within a few days of my arrival in Boston, on sabbatical and incognito as I thought, with no desire to start up a practice right away. I remember feeling a little taken aback by this frail octogenarian quizzing me on Hahnemann and Kent in my own living room. But when, in a voice that brooked no contradiction, she told me that there hadn't been a homeopath in Boston for 25 years and that I'd better get busy, there was suddenly nowhere to hide.

Despite her many infirmities and illnesses, each one threatening to be her last, she somehow managed to pull out of them, although more by her indomitable will and sheer life force, it seemed to me, than from any particular skill or remedy of mine. Once she came down with pneumonia, and with typical stubbornness asked for antibiotics only at the end to speed her recovery, long after her son had pleaded with her to take them to no avail. At times she could be downright cantankerous, most predictably when anyone suggested that she give up her old house in Auburndale for more suitable lodging.

Elinore was a delightful companion and friend, a keen and astute observer of the latest doings in homeopathy, and of every aspect of its past, present, and likely future. Although a strict Kentian by experience and inclination, she envisioned a non-sectarian integration of all healing paths, advocated that homeopathic physicians first be trained in allopathic medicine of the highest calibre, and had little use for the idea of separate homeopathic schools. I shall never forget the 1986 NCH meeting in Boston, in which she and three other old-timers held us all spell-bound with tales of homeopathy in the "good old days" and its problems so much like our own.

She leaves behind three children, many grandchildren and great-grandchildren, and innumerable friends and admirers, among whom I shall always be proud to count myself. Good-bye, Elinore! Wherever you are, you may take comfort and pride in a life both long and rich, with an uncommon share of heartache and fulfillment alike. We who love homeopathy shall not forget you, nor soon see your like again.

*Maesimund Panos, M. D. (1912-1999): Stateswoman, Friend, and Mother of Us All**

Like Bill Gray, Dave Wember, Sandra Chase, Karl Robinson, Nick Nossaman, and others who learned homeopathy in the '70's, I knew Maisie first as a teacher and mentor, beginning with her classes on Kent's *Repertory* at the NCH Summer School, which in those days was almost the only show in town. In that rôle, she was not at all charismatic in the idiosyncratic and histrionic style of a Vithoulkas or Sankaran, but rather more dry and methodical, in the no-nonsense, businesslike manner of an old-fashioned schoolmarm in a little country town, perhaps a trifle impatient with the limited minds and attitudes of her pupils in that backward time and place.

Although her father, grandfather, and first husband had all been homeopathic physicians before her, even when following in their footsteps she remained true first of all to her own experience as wife and mother, and taught with the same practical, down-to-earth flavor that came from years of first-aid and acute prescribing for her family, and made her so beloved of her patients as well. In my very first class at Millersville, for example, I remember asking her what potency to use, and receiving the following answer, so typical of her blunt, plain-spoken, and economical style: "Just use whatever you have!"

As often as I heard her repeat them over the years, these little pearls and maxims of hers have seldom failed me; but she was too far away to serve me well as preceptor or supervisor, which of course was my loss. In those days, it was not uncommon for young GP's like myself, trained in the "see one, do one, teach one" fashion of the time, to go into practice after a one-year rotating internship. In much the same spirit, with nothing but the two-week NCH Professional Course to cut our teeth on, we were turned loose on our patients to learn homeopathy more or less by the seat of our pants,

* "Maesimund Panos, M. D. (1912-1999): Stateswoman, Friend, Mother of Us All," ***Homeopathy Today,*** October 1999.

just as our teachers had, because that was as much formal instruction as was available back then.

Sometimes I'd call her in desperation to ask for advice or guidance in treating patients with advanced organic pathology, like one I remember with metastatic cancer, only to receive her sympathetic and motherly assurance that I was doing just fine and should keep up the good work! Eventually I realized that what I was really hoping for was for her to take charge, to relieve me of the burden of caring for very sick people, which made me feel totally out of my depth, and that simply helping me to accept that weighty responsibility was all that was necessary or possible under the circumstances.

In these very practical ways she was indeed a mentor to me, as I'm sure she was to many of my contemporaries. But it is above all as stateswoman and guardian of the homeopathic movement that I will always honor Maisie and cherish her memory, for without her steadfast and dedicated leadership the National Center and I daresay the whole history of American homeopathy in the last 40 years would have been very different, and indeed might not have been at all.

When we first met at the NCH Summer School in 1974, Maisie had already served as President of the American Foundation for Homeopathy for about 15 years, keeping the movement alive in spite of declining attendance and public interest in homeopathy generally, until signs of a modest revival finally became apparent. When the NCH was created as a public, non-profit "umbrella" organization for promoting homeopathy and spending the funds that the AFH gave it, Maisie naturally became its first President.

By the time I was elected to the Board in 1980, she already had a strong and clear vision of the future of classical homeopathy in America and of the NCH's mission to train physicians and allied health professionals in the highest standards of practice available in the world. Almost single-handed, she sponsored George Vithoulkas to teach in this country and had created a scholarship fund to assist young doctors like Bill Gray, George Guess, and Roger Morrison to study with him in Greece.

This was also the time of what Julian Winston with classic understatement has called "The Great Unpleasantness," the painful maturation process of the NCH as it grew apart and eventually broke away from the AFH, its parent but increasingly niggardly sponsor. Once again, Maisie not only foresaw this development, but also helped to engineer it in a typical behind-the-scenes maneuver. In 1980, after the AFH Board had used several proxy votes to elect compliant new Directors to the slots that had fallen vacant, Maisie paid them back in their own coin by creating several new slots and filling them with her own supporters, including myself, like a latter-day Franklin Roosevelt trying to "pack" the Supreme Court with his political allies, with the significant difference that she succeeded.

Now openly seeking to transform the NCH into a national membership organization, the new majority of the Board began to investigate our financial and legal relationship with the AFH; and when the latter group warned us to desist or face expulsion, for the next six months the NCH had to operate on a shoestring out of Dave Wember's basement; but we were free at last. All Maisie really did was to expand the Board with young blood who shared her vision and were eager to do her bidding. While of course she flattered us with the illusion that we were the activists who made it happen, in reality she had done most of the heavy lifting before we ever got there.

But it was at the NCH Board meetings in Washington that I first got to know Maisie as a friend and colleague, as well as a leader to admire and emulate. Both before and after the formal events of the day, a group of her protegés would gather in her daughter Annie's house, where some of the out-of-towners like myself had also been invited to stay. At such times the whole company were amply supplied with good food and drink, as well as regaled and kept in high spirits, while current gossip was exchanged, much important and useful business was discussed, rehearsed, and all but transacted behind the scenes, and visions of the future were sketched out, poems recited, and songs sung, often into the wee hours of the morning.

To a degree that few today can appreciate, the history of American homeopathy over the last forty years revolved around the steady, relentless life force of this extraordinary woman, who almost single-handedly created an interlocking directorate of personal friendships, movement loyalties, and multi-institutional officeholders that endured for as long as she was willing to do the often tedious work of presiding over it and holding it together, almost always with her persuasive, coaxing, usually indirect, but occasionally bullying management style.

For all the years that I served on the Board, I never knew her to shirk or shrink from doing whatever needed to be done; yet behind all the feasting and camaraderie, it was often difficult and in fact unnecessary to see the powerful intelligence, will, and vision that had masterminded and co-ordinated it all, seemingly without effort, and less by what she actually *did* than by what she facilitated and allowed us all to do, as if it were our own idea. Rather like a Washington hostess, she accomplished a great deal by simply bringing people together in an atmosphere of fellowship and good cheer; but she also provided a special ethos of her own, which valued enthusiasm and hard work and never hesitated to encourage, promote, and model them. This was the basis of her moral force and the incalculable influence that she exercised over all of us, as in effect the mother of a whole generation of homeopaths.

I feel truly blessed and honored to have been given the opportunity to contribute to her vision, even by disagreeing with her when it seemed necessary. Although she was a passionate democrat and card-carrying member of the ACLU, it was mainly when she refused to go along with the general consensus that the stubborn, feisty, cantankerous, tough old bird in her would sometimes emerge, often with relatively little prompting from the outside. I still remember the steely looks and gruff mutterings she sent my way when the Board was evenly split over dropping the old English diphthong "œ" from our name, and it fell to me as President to break the deadlock.

In 1985, when Sandra Chase stepped down as NCH President and I was nominated to take her place, Maisie invited me to Ohio to discuss our growing differences over the future of the National Center and the lay movement in particular. "Invited" is perhaps too polite a term for what Maisie had in mind, which was actually a detailed and prolonged interrogation that I knew I had to pass in order to qualify for the job; but I never questioned her right to decide my fate and the National Center's in this high-handedly autocratic manner, which her unstinting dedication had earned many times over.

At the time, she was rightly exercised about my declared sympathy for the concept of lay practice, an issue that still divides our membership to this day. The thrust of my argument was that lay practice was already a *fait accompli,* with many of our greatest masters untrained, unlicensed, self-taught, like Boenninghausen, Vithoulkas, Coulter, et al., and knowing vastly more homeopathy than most doctors, so that the primary task of the National Center as a large membership organization had to be to teach and disseminate information to anyone willing and able to understand and use it.

Maisie adhered no less firmly to the opposite persuasion, that our mission had always been limited to training doctors and licensed health professionals, and that trying to do the same for lay people was not only bad homeopathy and bad medicine, but also illegal and thus dangerous to the future of the movement.

We went around and around on the issue all weekend, unwilling to change our own minds and unable to convince each other, both equally certain that our views were carefully thought out and worthy of serious consideration. Although she disagreed with me strongly on almost every point, I never had reason to fear that she would disqualify me for that reason alone, or hold it against me in our friendship. That shows the caliber of human being that she was.

While she continued to send me Christmas cards and was always friendly whenever we spoke by telephone, after I retired from the Board in 1987 we rarely saw each other again until the NCH's 25th Anniversary shindig last April in Fort Lauderdale, when I had dinner with her for what proved to be the last time. On that occasion she seemed to me rather withdrawn and uncommunicative, not at all from incapacity, or something personal that had come between us, but simply from what I interpreted as indifference, as if, with her life's work completed and her personal goals fulfilled, there was little in the public or social arena that could still grab or hold her interest for very long. For that reason I was not at all shocked or surprised to hear the news that she had died, and that her exit was peaceful and free of pain or struggle.

What seeing her again did revive was my old sense of an inscrutable mystery at the core of her that I've had to work around in these pages, by restricting myself to what she believed about a certain issue or what she did on a particular occasion. Basically I found her to be a complex and rather inaccessible person, whom I knew best by the causes she stood for and the people she inspired, rather than through the intimate play of her imagination, which has always eluded me and remains an impenetrable enigma to this day. Inevitably I am drawn to the paradox that the well-known image of her that we all loved and admired was also richly imbued with everything human and personal, which is also what her life and work were really about. Upon just such ironies do great lives revolve, and hers was surely one of the greatest in our midst. We shall not soon see her like again.

*Julian Winston (1941-2005): In Loving Memory**

I first met Julian in 1980, when he was helping with registrations at the NCH Summer School. As always, his main contribution was *himself,* by which I mean not only the plant walks to identify the remedies that grew nearby, or the down-home musical evenings with pedal-steel guitar, or the incredibly knowledgeable and fact-filled slide shows on homeopathic history, but most of all the stunning array of talents, interests, and eccentricities that they represented, that miraculously coexisted in his person. I sensed in him a kindred spirit, and so we became friends.

Some years earlier, Dr. Raymond Seidel, a veteran prescriber in Philadelphia, had cured him of a persistent bladder infection with a few doses of *Merc. iod. flav.* 3X, 6X, or some such thing. From sitting in with Dr. Seidel, but most of all through his own study, Julian was already so knowledgeable by the time he appeared on the scene that his meteoric rise to a succession of leadership posts in the NCH seemed entirely natural, if not heaven-sent. Within a year he was named Registrar of the Summer School, and later its Dean (1987), as well as NCH Librarian, Board member (1982), and Editor-in-Chief of *Homeopathy Today* (1984), his most influential position, which earned him a worldwide reputation, and in which he served an unbroken tenure of more than two decades. Yet while homeopathy had already become a ruling passion and a labor of love for him, he continued to earn his living as Professor of Design at the University of the Arts in Philadelphia. In this prodigious outpouring of life energy in so many fields at once, he was truly the Benjamin Franklin of homeopathy.

The early 1980's were exciting times for homeopathy in America, full of rapid growth and interest on the one hand and deep philosophical divisions on the other, in part generational, and embodying radically different conceptions of the role of the lay movement and the legitimacy of

* "Julian Winston (1941-2005): In Loving Memory," ***Homeopathy Today,*** July/August 2005.

lay practice. Under Dr. Panos' dedicated leadership, the NCH Board was transforming itself from a self-appointed, privately funded charity into a large national membership organization that could represent the American homeopathic movement as a whole.

Although Julian was not a physician and never aspired to practice, he tackled these issues in his typical hands-on fashion. In the summer and fall of 1981, he traveled around the country at his own expense, meeting and talking with homeopaths of all shades of opinion and every style of practice, including physicians, naturopaths, and other health professionals, as well as a number of committed laypeople, many of whom were not only treating their own families and friends, but also teaching the principles of homeopathic first-aid and self-care to study groups in their own communities. His monograph, "Some Notes & Observations on the State of Homeopathy in America," a concise but detailed summary of his travels, described the growing infrastructure that already existed then, and still makes fascinating reading today. His lively scholarship and the improbable revival that it uncovered provided a cogent and persuasive rationale for the Affiliated Study Group concept that the NCH Board initiated in 1985, both to expand its membership and support these grassroots efforts.

Buying and renovating an old firehouse in Philadelphia, he filled it to bursting with old books, journals, medicines, and paraphernalia of every description, the sheer quantity and variety of which, while doubtless beautifully organized, threatened to crowd out the possibility of sharing his life with anyone else. This veritable museum of homeopathy also housed his ever-expanding computer and on-line capability, which likewise kept him far ahead of the curve.

One of the most interesting and attractive aspects of his nature was his remarkable facility for squaring the circle of seemingly irreconcilable traits. Alongside a devoted scholar's penchant for all things antiquarian, he was blessed with an artist's eye for design and a geeky flair for information technology and all of its latest applications. His ability to orchestrate and harmonize all of these talents yielded a rich harvest of learned yet immensely accessible works for which we and our descendants will be forever in his debt.

Unquestionably the greatest of these is his book and video, *The Faces of Homeopathy,* originating from his ever-popular slide shows, celebrating the pageant and sweep of homeopathic history as a multi-media entertainment, and featuring the people who lived it and the influences that shaped them. Lavishly produced and illustrated by his own hand, often with memorabilia from his own collection, this classic reference text blends rare archival sources, photographs, and portraits with intelligent commentary, much of it based on personal acquaintance or gleaned from careful study. His seemingly artless style make it deceptively easy for readers to miss the rigorous scholarship that always backed it up.

Its companion volume, *The Heritage of Homeopathic Literature,* offers a guided tour through the entire bibliography, of which his knowledge was encyclopedic and his selection always intelligent and worth looking at, especially when his opinions were controversial, as they often were. The inestimable value of his many contributions to homeopathy includes his rare courage in holding to his opinions and gut feelings even when they were eccentric or unpopular, because they typically illuminated hidden aspects of the field that most of us had never considered before.

As his fame and reputation grew, he was much in demand as a lecturer on the international circuit. In 1992, while teaching at the Wellington College of Homeopathy in New Zealand, the old bachelor, collector, and pack rat finally met the love of his life, Gwyneth Evans, who just happened to be the Principal of the school. In 1995, he married her, moved to New Zealand, and settled into a marital bliss that he had never known and indeed stoutly resisted until then, and that he continued to enjoy for the remainder of his life. How and to what extent Gwyneth managed to find room for all the priceless treasures that he brought over with him is a tale that is hers alone to tell or leave out.

While of course I was happy for him, his flight to the far side of the world left a gaping hole in my life that neither his ongoing editorials nor my own halting online replies could ever replenish. He may well have taken umbrage at my suggestion that he resign as Editor, and he continued to take the measure of homeopathy in America from across the sea, insisting that the Internet had abolished any difficulties of time and space.

As the years passed, more narrowly ideological differences inevitably arose between us. Julian was always a champion of classical homeopathy and the Hahnemannian tradition in particular, as am I, and had long been of two minds about the authenticity of Vithoulkas' "essences," though I, like most practicing American homeopaths of my generation, had been inspired by George's example. From the mid-1990s, the new teachings of Sankaran, Scholten, and others likewise became increasingly popular with a growing number of students in Europe and America, including me, while Julian sensed in many of them a threat to the integrity and survival of the movement itself. With a bloodhound's nose for the real and the phony, in both his editorials and the overall content of *Homeopathy Today* he sparked a major backlash against these innovations, based on the fear that they were speculative in nature and thus not strictly homeopathic at all.

What really bothered me, I have to confess, was not his philosophy *per se,* as much as the chilly reappraisal of my own writings that followed from it. Two years after soliciting my review of Nancy Herrick's new book of animal provings, for example, he felt the need to supplant it with a much more damning one of his own, even though I'd already voiced many of the same reservations in a more friendly tone. That hit me where it hurt. I signed Roger Morrison's letter in Nancy's defense, knowing full well that my public endorsement of it would hurt him plenty. Apart from the justice or injustice of what was said, I feel sure that it was mainly wounded pride that made me strike out in that way.

Needless to say, things went downhill from there. In the ensuing months Julian ran a large series of letters in support of his position, as well as Andre Saine's learned diatribe, "Homeopathy vs. Speculative Medicine," as a lead article, but refused to publish my rebuttal of it. For me that was the last straw. I told him that as a partisan in the dispute he should resign as Editor, that I would no longer write for *Homeopathy Today* until he did so, and instead proposed that he contribute a regular column in which he could rant and rave to his heart's content. Needless to say, he never accepted my offer. When I relented some months later, he accepted my apology, and we resumed our e-mailing back and forth as before; but things would never be quite the same between us.

Like the entire homeopathic world, I always esteemed and admired him for his stubborn insistence on being himself, no matter what it cost, even when I had to take my lumps for it. Yet no matter how well we knew and loved him, that was the part of him that always remained elusive and beyond our grasp. For all of these reasons, his untimely passing leaves us with a grief that will be hard to assuage and a void that will never be filled.

But I would also pay homage to the occasionally brutal honesty with which he followed his path, and express my deep gratitude for all he gave that will enrich all of our lives for years to come. So farewell, old friend, and rest assured that we will not forget you.

*Christine Luthra, M. D. (1951-2006): Dedicated Homeopath, Dear Friend, Inspiration to Many**

I am writing to commemorate the life of a dedicated homeopath and a splendid human being whose name and accomplishments are not as widely known as they deserve to be. Christine Luthra's recent, untimely death left a serious void in the hearts of a great many practitioners in America and Europe who knew her, and in the lives of thousands of individuals and families throughout New England who felt blessed and honored to have been in her care.

I first met Christine around 1982, not long after we both moved to Boston, she fresh from her family practice residency, with two small children in tow. Born in Belgium to French-speaking parents, she was educated in philosophy and medicine at the University of Louvain, a venerable Catholic institution dating back to medieval times, and she remained a serious intellectual all her life, with far-ranging interests in philosophy, literature, fine art, music, and poetry, not to mention more esoteric fields, such as anthroposophy, psychospiritual healing, Jungian psychology, astrology, and indeed homeopathy itself.

Back in Belgium after an extended spiritual pilgrimage to India, she met Dev Luthra, her future husband, emigrated with him to the U.S., and there gave birth to her two children, a son, Yannig, and a daughter, Lakshmi. Her marriage was short-lived, but the yoga of running a busy practice as well as raising two children on her own gave her life a concrete, practical focus that engaged and sustained her and brought her deep joy and fulfillment throughout her life. Christine's practice quickly grew and flourished, and as her friend and neighbor I found her distinctive blend of homeopathy and philosophy both congenial and complementary to my own.

---

* "Christine Luthra, M. D. (1951-2006): Dedicated Homeopath, Dear Friend, Inspiration to Many," ***Homeopathy Today,*** November/December 2006.

I treasure the memory of our lunch meetings and walks in the Arboretum, where we let our fancy take us, conversing about everything under the sun with a warmth of heart and a freedom of imagination that sometimes left us both nearly breathless with pleasure, and made me deeply grateful for the existence of a soul-companion such as one meets but seldom in the course of a life. Yet at the same time I knew that this was just one side of her multi-faceted nature, and that other friends were having very different kinds of experiences with her that were just as treasured and memorable.

I knew and valued her first as a skilled physician and homeopath, faithful to the essence of the old teachings, yet ever seeking to expand her horizons and deepen her knowledge. Also learned and practiced in the use of anthroposophical remedies, Christine often used them as intercurrents or more generic prescriptions for basic, energetic support when the exact *sìmillimum* appeared elusive, or when she was reluctant to repeat it just yet. At the same time, she was receptive and indeed dedicated to many of the newer teachings, especially the pioneering work of Jan Scholten, and the charismatic style of Lou Klein, whose highly personal synthesis she followed diligently for many years. I think it must have been in Lou's classes that she first became acquainted with many of the best students and practitioners of her own generation, and soon began teaching some of the younger students as well.

Our methods and styles of practice were similar enough that we often referred patients to each other when we had given them so many remedies that we realized we were part of the problem rather than the solution; and I know for a fact that many of my referrals to her benefited greatly from the exchange. With Betty Wood, M. D., another long-time friend and colleague, Christine was a founding member of the New England Homeopathic Academy (NEHA), which sponsors seminars by leading homeopaths from throughout the world.

Yet Christine herself remained a bit shy in her adopted country, and published very little in English, despite her remarkable fluency in it. She was a dedicated physician, who always put the interest of her patients well ahead of the purity of any doctrine. A gifted and intuitive diagnostician, she used laboratory tests both for screening and confirmation, prescribed antibiotics and other conventional drugs when indicated, and interfaced freely and effectively with specialists and hospitals when needed. But above all, Christine was a friend and a *soul*—a warm, lively, and attractive human being who related easily to others, and whose own spirituality was well-grounded, fully engaged in and by no means disdainful of ordinary life on this far from untroubled planet.

Indeed, I would have to say that both her unique gift and an exquisite vulnerability lay in this sphere, for her empathy with others in pain and indeed with the state of the world at times became more intense than her sensitive nature could easily tolerate. This quality first became apparent to me and took me by surprise in the aftermath of the terrorist attacks of September 11 and the U.S.-led invasion of Afghanistan that followed soon after. Early in 2002 she was hospitalized with severe, acute abdominal pain secondary to an intermittent intestinal obstruction that laid her low for weeks.

Always interested in and knowledgeable about world affairs, she had become quite alarmed by the latest turns to the right in American politics, from the disputed election of 2000 to the invasion of Afghanistan. By the time I visited her in the hospital, we both knew that the Iraqi invasion had already been decided upon. For me this was largely a political matter, a violation of international law, to be opposed with marches and demonstrations of public outrage. But talking with her in her hospital bed, I realized that Christine felt this war literally, intensely, and in every cell and fiber of her body, as though the mechanism by which most people manage to compartmentalize and defuse such unpleasantness was simply not available or acceptable to her.

Eventually she overcame her illness, but about a year later she discovered a lump in her breast that proved to be cancer of an exceptionally aggressive type. Immediately after surgery, she began a punishing course of chemotherapy in spite of her serious misgivings about using the drugs, not only because of their side-effects, which were intense and worrisome in themselves, but also because their cell-destroying purpose went against every instinct that she lived by and every philosophy that her practice was based on. Although she was a wise, experienced physician and by no means a fanatic for homeopathy or unalterably opposed to conventional medicines when indicated, it must have pained and saddened her beyond measure when she herself felt the need to resort to methods of brute force that on some level she always detested.

Nevertheless she did what she knew she had to do, supplementing the drugs with the best alternative treatments available, naturally including homeopathic medicines. For two years she went into remission and did quite well, although greatly weakened and unable to resume her active practice. Not long afterward, she sold her house in Boston and moved herself and her practice to Maine at the invitation of a new man in her life, with high hopes of beginning a new and less hectic mode of life.

But neither the plan nor her new romance survived the recurrence of her cancer this past February, with metastases in several places. Once again, in spite of the same highly aggressive pathology, she rallied repeatedly and heroically in one of the most remarkable displays of physical and emotional fortitude that I have ever witnessed. Although severely emaciated and weakened by the chemotherapy, and even on the brink of death several times, she almost always brightened up when friends dropped by. When I visited her this past May, we talked animatedly for hours on sundry topics, just as we had in days gone by. That was the last time I saw her alive. By then Yannig and Lakshmi, who were now fully grown, had put their lives on hold to be with her and care for her in the final months, as well as sending out regular e-mail communiqués to her many friends and well-wishers, while her mother, sister, and brothers visited from Europe as often as they could.

Christine's last days were peaceful and serene, without pain or torment. She died in late August at the age of 55. The funeral service at her church in Portland, Maine, was quiet, deeply affecting, and memorable, not only for the love and warmth that were felt and expressed by the many friends and family members who spoke of her, but also for the depth and variety of her friendships and interests, as personified in the diversity of her mourners, who included colleagues and patients, poets and painters, fellow-parishioners and atheists, with each of whom she had shared experiences that were unique, yet always seemed to go further, toward that spiritual realm wherein all souls are one.

She was a dear friend and an inspiration to many, not only as a homeopath and a physician, both roles which she practiced with skill, grace, and distinction, but above all as a fellow human being, a loving parent, a beloved daughter and sister, and a wounded soul, like all of us, on the path to enlightenment and capable of great beauty that touched the sublime. Although she had her share of foibles and frailties like everyone else, she always kept her gaze fixed on the divine, on what was best and truest about each one of us, and so reminded us to look for and even helped us to see this in ourselves and in others as well. She will be missed.

*Harris Coulter, Ph. D. (1932-2009): Devoted Scholar, Keen Intellect, Soldier for the Cause**

Harry was my very first personal contact with homeopathy, one which began in 1970, four years before we actually met. A doctor who knew of my interest in home birth and my already jaded perspective on the medical system mentioned his name as a medical historian who had written sympathetically about homeopathy. But at the time this was a subject I was wholly unfamiliar with, and would undoubtedly have looked askance at it if someone had tried to explain it to me. It took me four more years of doing home births and dabbling in whatever herbs were growing near where I lived in the Colorado mountains to realize that in fact there were other methods and philosophies of healing out there that deserved a closer look. In 1974 I finally enrolled in the NCH Summer School at Millersville, Pennsylvania, in the heart of Amish country.

Harry's words were among the first I heard in that course, and were a big part of what hooked me once and for all. More than anyone else, he showed me that homeopathy was no mere New Age cult, but a philosophy and method that were deeply rooted in the history of medicine and had already endured for two hundred years, a longevity which seemed almost miraculous when compared with the dizzying pace of change that modern medicine quite rightly prides itself upon. In short, he was no hippie, but a serious scholar and intellectual who had devoted years of his life to studying the subject, and who taught it in a way that made rational sense, not as dogma to be learned by rote, but as an important subject that merited careful and dispassionate investigation.

In those days, American homeopathy had become a very small fraternity, a shadow of its former self; but Harry was always right in the thick of it, and never one to hold back from an argument or keep his opinions to himself,

---

* "Harris Coulter, Ph. D. (!932-2009): Devoted Scholar, Keen Intellect, Soldier for the Cause," *American Journal of Homeopathic Medicine* 103:7, Spring 2010.

even when controversial, as they often were. At meetings and conferences he was personally acquainted with and esteemed by prominent homeopaths from all over the world, and much sought after as a speaker and lecturer, with a lucid style of presentation that made arcane, learned, and difficult concepts readily understandable to others without such background. In short, he was a brilliant teacher, and an authority on all things homeopathic, whose views I always sought and took seriously, even when I disagreed with them, of which more later.

Also gifted with a clear, direct, and persuasive literary style, he was known perhaps best of all as a writer. His *magnum opus,* the four-volume *Divided Legacy: A History of the Schism in Medical Thought,* arose out of his doctoral thesis at Columbia, on the conflict between homeopathy and orthodox or allopathic medicine in 19th-Century America. In a prodigious *tour de force* requiring decades of concentrated scholarship, he eventually located and identified similar tensions between what he called "empirical" and "rationalist" strains that helped shape and define the entire history of Western medical thought and practice, from its Hippocratic origins to the rise of scientific medicine and extending into our own time.

Published in 1973 as *Science and Ethics in American Medicine, 1800-1914,* his dissertation became Volume III of the final work; Volume I, on Ancient and Medieval Medicine, and Volume II, on the early modern period, followed in 1975 and 1977; and Volume IV, *Twentieth-Century Medicine: the Bacteriological Era,* appeared in 1994. Characteristically, he insisted on publishing it himself, rather than submitting it to editorial scrutiny by a large commercial publisher, who would probably have rejected it in any case, because of its limited marketability and polemical style, since he never hesitated to take sides or stake out a clear rhetorical position of its own. Always true to himself, Harry believed passionately in the superior cogency and power of the homeopathic philosophy, and unapologetically upheld it as a mirror to what he perceived as the scientific excesses and moral deficiencies of organized medicine.

Among his other written works, two others were especially influential on me, and also deserved a much wider audience. Published in 1991, *The Controlled Clinical Trial* looked long and hard at the theory and practice of the double-blind or Random Controlled Trial (RCT), the "gold standard" of modern clinical research, exposing numerous flaws and limitations in both design and execution that are seldom examined or taken seriously. Here again, like a *samurai* of the spirit, he ventured even into the lions' den to get at the truth of what he believed and felt.

Perhaps his most famous piece was *DPT: A Shot in the Dark,* published in 1985, and written with Barbara Loe Fisher, whose child was severely brain-damaged following a DPT shot. Compiling the stories of dozens of similar cases, it was so explosive and aroused such a furor among the medical community that the publisher took it off the market, and it had to be re-issued under another imprint at a later date. It was one of the first books in the Postwar period to challenge the theory and practice of routine mandatory vaccination of young infants, and helped Ms. Fisher found Dissatisfied Parents Together (DPT), an advocacy group which grew into the National Vaccine Information Center (NVIC), sponsors yearly conferences, and maintains local and regional chapters of concerned parents and their friends and supporters throughout the country. This was Harry putting his intellect to work in the service of patients and indeed *victims* of that same establishment, an activist rôle that he certainly relished. As I look back on the trajectory of his work, I am struck by the extent to which I myself have been following many of the same paths that he pioneered, and I regret that I never adequately recognized or thanked him for this kind of modeling while he was alive.

That may in part have been due to the circumstances of our falling out, which took place rather abruptly in 1980-81, shortly after I joined the NCH Board, and began a long estrangement that lingered on for many years after the issues that led to it were no longer relevant. I was one of a new crop of younger physicians that included George Guess, Sandra Chase, and Dave Wember, who were brought onto the Board at the instigation of Dr. Panos. At that time, Harry was an officer and long-time member of the American Foundation for Homeopathy, which exercised total control over our extremely meager budget and tiny, aging membership. When we began to look more carefully into the fine print of this overly intimate and seemingly redundant relationship, the AFH leadership threatened to cut off our funding unless we desisted, and Harry as their spokesperson lost no opportunity in denouncing our impertinence in their newsletter. Matters came to a head when he tried to crash one of our Board meetings, and it fell to me to show him out, the upshot of which was that the NCH became independent, and Harry and I weren't on speaking terms for months, although I never stopped reading, valuing, and indeed praising his writings.

In 1985, I became NCH President, and helped to organize its annual meeting, which was held at Emmanuel College in Boston. A highlight of that occasion was the visit and lecture of Dr. Tatanya Popova, a Ukrainian homeopath who operated the clinic that her father had founded in Kiev. Inviting her with the help of a Russian physician at Harvard Medical School who had studied with her, I asked Harry if he would give a simultaneous translation of her lecture, knowing that among his other talents he had once moonlighted as a Russian translator and interpreter at the UN. Needless to say, he did so willingly and with his usual flair and facility.

But after that I saw very little of him until his massive stroke in the late 1990's and his surprise appearance in a wheelchair at the rededication of the Hahnemann Monument in Washington in 2000. By then severely crippled but still sharp mentally and as always very much himself, he greeted me warmly, and all of our past unpleasantness was suddenly washed away as if it had never been. To this day I'm still ashamed that we both let it go so long for no good reason.

In the years since then, he often phoned me to while away the hours of helpless tedium and loneliness in the nursing home where he lived. Ever capable of lively conversation, he was also solicitous about his estranged wife Catherine, the superb homeopath and author who had moved to the Boston area after their divorce, was renting my office to train licensed physicians, and had become a close friend. Although I often had my hands full trying to avoid being drawn into these remains of their drama, I finally grew to love and grieve for him as a friend and colleague, someone whose wit and acumen I still treasured and admired, and whose ever-growing incapacity I could do nothing to allay. Much as I mourn his passing, and will miss his companionship, I take comfort in the assurance that his passionate commitment and important contributions to homeopathy will long endure.

*David Warkentin (1951-2010): An Appreciation**

David's recent illness and untimely death were profoundly shocking on every level, because he was not only a great friend and benefactor to all homeopaths, and an epitome of the best that we have to offer, but also the very embodiment of robust health and the ideal of a balanced life, combining enlightened work, physical fitness, and love of wilderness and the outdoors in a socially-conscious way. To almost everyone who knew him or knew of his work -- and there are very few among us who didn't -- his passing has an impact that will long endure.

I knew very little about his personal life, except that he loved to lead whitewater river trips, attracted lovely and accomplished women to his side, and had innumerable friends in every corner of the world. Yet I suspect that at bottom he was rather a private person.

I first met him in 1977, at the California State society meeting in San Diego. Then 27, he was already an experienced Physician Assistant, a skilled and devoted prescriber, and an active member of the famous Berkeley study group, which later morphed into the storied Hering Clinic. In short, he sat on the cutting edge of the improbable revival of classical homeopathy in America. Among the attendees were such future notables as Dana Ullman, Bill Gray, Bob Schore, Corey Weinstein, Lou Klein, Murray Feldman, Peggy Chipkin, Randy Neustaedter, and John Melnychuk, to name the few that are still accessible to my aging memory.

Of course, there were no computers in those days, and our cases had to be solved in longhand, by laboriously writing out the remedies under the rubrics we chose, as of old, and tallying up the number of rubrics and the grades of the remedies in each. But already, even in that talented company, long before his remarkable inventions, David stood out for his keen intelligence, lively wit, attractive personality, and an affable, engaging

* "David Warkentin (1951-2010): An Appreciation," ***American Journal of Homeopathic Medicine*** 103:179, Winter 2010.

manner that seemed open to everything and everyone, without being in the least showy about his own personal contribution.

Largely because of distance, I didn't see a lot of him for more than a decade after that, until various brands of software appeared, claiming to streamline the repertorization process; and soon MacRepertory towered above them all, universally acclaimed as the best, most thorough, and most user-friendly program available. I freely confess that I myself, a traditionalist by nature, and a confirmed technophobe who entered the computer age only reluctantly and under duress, was thoroughly skeptical of the whole project at first, counting it a virtue to continue taking as much time as possible in doing my cases. Against that sort of headwind, to have converted the likes of me to the use and even the celebration of MacRep and Reference Works must surely rank among his most difficult and least important achievements. In recent years, when the newer versions I bought had become incompatible with my old machine, I tried mightily to resist this planned obsolescence, reverting to longhand for some months, but gave in when forced to admit how pleasant and easy they had made my chosen work, and how little reward my purist scruples and inveterate habits had earned me for my trouble.

Today his software is used, loved, and appreciated by grateful homeopaths of every stripe, in every country where remedies are prescribed. Throughout his career, he always acted and thought of himself as our benefactor, a claim amply borne out by his consistent presence at our seminars and conferences, both here and abroad, and his unfailing patience in instructing and guiding us, no matter how long it took or how dense or recalcitrant we proved to be. In that sense, he was *everybody's* friend.

He was a true American genius in the best sense: an inventor, a tinkerer, with a rare gift for improvisation, and an equally rare capacity for systematic thought and detailed scholarship at the same time. Yet these flowerings cannot be understood apart from his roots as a fine and dedicated homeopath, who understood from the inside what successful practitioners need, and who applied the new information technology to the heroic task of computerizing the vast body of homeopathic literature into a single database, far exceeding the memory capacity of any living individual, and making it instantly accessible to us at the moments when we need it.

As built into MacRepertory, Reference Works, and their various competitors, these technical innovations have also prefigured and indeed made possible the important conceptual innovations of Sankaran, Scholten, Mangialavori, et al., in their attempts to systematize our *materia medica,* and to develop practical applications of our most difficult notions, such as "miasm" and "family," a monumental task which pioneers like Farrington envisioned long ago but lacked the technical capacity to carry out. This great, transformative project is of course a labor of many generations, and far from being completed, if indeed it ever can be; but David's vision and inventiveness have played such an indispensable part in its history, and ours, that his own too-brief sojourn on earth can be fitly summarized by the epitaph which Hahnemann wrote for himself, *non inutilis vixi,* "I have not lived in vain."

*Catherine Coulter (1934-2014): A Remembrance**

Although she was eighty years old, with a full, rich life already behind her, Catherine's unexpected death a few weeks ago came as a shock to me, and even more so to Marian and Elizabeth, her daughters, who had lived with her for decades and were well acquainted with her remarkable talent for recovering from a variety of illnesses in the past. For that reason, even at the risk of speaking out about matters ordinarily left unsaid, I feel impelled to begin this celebration of her life with a few words about the manner of her leaving it, because it seems so emblematic of her nature.

First of all, she never breathed a word about any indisposition, either to me or my wife Linda, with whom she was also very friendly; I had actually telephoned her a few weeks earlier to arrange a date for us to visit in the spring, without her giving even a hint of any illness or health problem. When the girls called with the news of her death, Marian told me that she had been seriously anemic for several months, that her breathing had become labored and wet-sounding recently, and that she finally went to the hospital seeking a transfusion. Diagnosing congestive heart failure, the doctors insisted that her cardiac condition be stabilized first and gave her several allopathic drugs for that purpose; but neither these nor even the blood gave her much relief. When further testing was proposed to detect any deeper pathology, she adamantly refused, left the hospital soon after, and died at home a few days later, in a manner reminiscent of another great homeopath, E. A. Farrington, who similarly refused allopathic treatment on his deathbed, saying "I would rather die a Christian!" Such were her principles, and such her determination to live by them.

She was equally passionate about many other things in addition to homeopathy, such as animal rights, her concern for the poor and less fortunate, and above all her love of literature, which fed and sustained her throughout her life. Indeed she was well-stocked with strong and

* "Catherine Coulter (1934-2014): A Remembrance," ***Homeopathy Today,*** Summer 2014.

well-developed opinions on many subjects, which were sometimes controversial but always worth listening to; she thought about things very carefully, and often persuaded me that there was another side to the matter that I needed to take account of.

Her parents were both Russian, and left the old country in 1917, in the wake of the Revolution; Catherine was born in London in 1934, but the family moved to America soon after and settled first in Long Island and eventually in New York City, where she lived until her marriage. As a child she attended an elite private school, and always ranked among the top of her class, as well as excelling in athletics, although allergies, migraine headaches, and other complaints sidelined her from serious competition in her teens. Interestingly, in view of what was to follow, her mother had no faith in doctors, and encouraged her to work through her ailments without drugs, relying on ocean air, healthy food, and plenty of rest, and stoic, uncomplaining acceptance of whatever ailments defied such measures. In Marian's estimation, the result was that

> she grew up a very self-reliant person, unconventional in her ideas, and a strong critical thinker. Unlike most people, she never let even her intense family attachments interfere with her sense of true and false or right and wrong.

Earning her B.A. in literature at Barnard College, she completed an M.A. in Russian Studies from Columbia, where she met Harris Coulter, her future husband, and also taught literature; soon after marriage, they relocated to Washington, D. C., where she continued teaching at George Washington University. In 1960, on a trip to Paris, she first became acquainted with homeopathy when a friend recommended it for her allergies. Just how these pluralist treatments *à la français* actually turned out, I cannot say; but once back in the States she obtained a copy of Boericke's *Materia Medica,* read it from cover to cover, and was hooked, like so many others before and since.

In her practice, she was largely self-taught, at a time when there were very few lay prescribers, and even fewer doctors willing to train or supervise them. Although both she and Harris traveled widely in homeopathic circles and knew Wright-Hubbard, Whitmont, and many of the best-known homeopaths of the day, her own instruction as a prescriber came almost entirely from reading, especially Boericke, and Boger's *Synoptic Key*, the texts she consulted regularly, with Hering's *Guiding Symptoms* as a backup or last Court of Appeal. Like all successful prescribers, she learned most of what she knew from her patients, and above all from her own cured cases.

In the 1970's, when American homeopathy as a profession had nearly died out, she began teaching some younger doctors who at last were showing interest in the method, acting as their preceptor and supervisor, and sharing some portion of the fees they collected. Over the years she trained a sizeable number of excellent homeopathic physicians in this fashion, almost all of whom are still practicing today, as well as at least one Professor of Integrative Medicine I know of who wanted to be acquainted with the method without necessarily practicing it himself. In later years, at least partly in recognition of her policy of training M. D.'s and D. O.'s exclusively, she was named an Honorary Member of the American Institute of Homeopathy, which at that time was open only to licensed physicians and strongly opposed to teaching or encouraging the practice of unlicensed persons, an irony I imagine she must have relished.

Once established in Washington, D.C., she became active in the American homeopathic movement, and remained a faithful supporter of the National Center for Homeopathy throughout her life. In 1980, when the NCH finally cut loose from the American Foundation, its sole financial support, and began raising its own funds as an independent membership-based organization, she never wavered in her loyalty, even though its physical presence at the time amounted to little more than a few boxes in a corner of Dave Wember's basement. Her unshakable allegiance to the National Center may even have contributed to her divorce, since as an officer of the Foundation Harris was just as strenuously opposed to what he considered a reckless and destructive move.

By the time I met her, she was already in the process of writing *Portraits of Homeopathic Medicines,* the classic series of in-depth remedy pictures for which she is best known; these eventually ran to three volumes and continue to be widely read and put to use today, not least for their felicitous prose and piquant references to famous cultural figures and beloved characters from literature. These remedy portraits occupy a unique place in the homeopathic literature for the beauty and elegance of her writing, which add immeasurably to their practical value in bringing the remedies to life for the prescriber. When I was given the privilege of reviewing the second volume of the series, what struck me most of all was the rich and fertile interplay of these two very different, equally distinctive, yet somehow closely-related perspectives, her love of language and literature, on the one hand, and her devotion to pure classical homeopathy on the other, both of which had become and would always remain the guiding passions of her life.

But even these two limitless worlds of study could not fully encompass the extraordinary range and diversity of her interests. Prominent among them were the esoteric realms of consciousness, including not only homeopathy itself, with its unique position astride both the material and immaterial worlds, but also astrology, in which she was particularly learned, as well as psychic phenomena and all forms of spirituality, which in her case spilled over into a deep concern for animal rights, passionate opposition to vivisection, and a living sense of the cosmic unity of all creation.

In the early '90's, when we taught together at the NCH Summer School, I recall her asking Julian Winston, who was then our Dean, to assign her a sleeping room that faced a certain way, the exact details of which have long since escaped me. What I can say with some assurance is that, at a time when few in the West had even heard of it, let alone credited it with any meaning or value, this little bit of *Feng shui* was no mere affectation on her part, but simply a practical expedient for mitigating the various pains and discomforts she had long been subject to, as well a more sensitive way of experiencing reality that most people, including myself, are largely unaware if not incapable of.

Eventually she moved to Arlington in the Boston area with her two daughters, and continued her training program for aspiring homeopathic doctors, for which purpose she rented my office in Watertown part-time, while also discreetly maintaining her own private practice in her home. This arrangement required some delicate negotiations to protect us both from the risk of prying, harassment, and possible disciplinary action at the hands of the Massachusetts Medical Society and/or the State Board of Registration in Medicine; but it worked perfectly well for many years, until Catherine bought a larger home and transferred her entire operation over there.

During this last phase of her life, she met A. U. Ramakrishnan, the esteemed Indian homeopath, and became his valued co-worker and amanuensis, eventually compiling and summarizing his extensive experience and detailed methodology for treating the various forms of cancer into the ground-breaking book, *A Homeopathic Approach to Cancer,* a significant departure from the strict classical tradition that she had always practiced and taught. In her willingness to adapt the principles she had previously lived by and insisted upon to new situations and unanticipated needs, she demonstrated a resiliency and flexibility of mind that may well have aroused the ire of fundamentalists of every stripe, but earned her the gratitude of a whole new clientele of patients, many with little else to hope for. Here again, she displayed that same moral courage and independence of mind which her daughters were rightly so proud of: she followed the dictates of both intellect and conscience, wherever they might lead, and whatever the opposition, trusting her own intuition and needing no further assurance of what the outcome would be.

By this time, we had become good friends, and enjoyed seeing each other socially, along with my wife, Linda, and sometimes other mutual friends as well. When it came to world affairs, culture, art, literature, and politics, she was a delightful companion, probably one of the most outspoken people I have ever known on a wide variety of topics, with strong opinions that were almost always well thought out and worth paying attention to, no matter how improbable they might at first appear. Even a casual phone conversation was likely to continue for much longer than either of us had planned, just for the sake of hearing each other's words and forming our own in reply. I have known very few people in my life with whom I could talk so freely about so many things, and who spoke so well about them that the art of conversation itself became the main purpose of our connection and the chief pleasure that we both derived from it. A friend to cherish, and a colleague to be proud of, whose contributions we will all be forever grateful for, she lived a life to which we all might well aspire, a life of heart, intellect, and imagination in the service of others in need.

I will conclude with something that Marian told me about her last days that could almost serve as a fitting epitaph for the rest:

She was deeply dedicated to her work; she was working until the week before she died, talking to clients on the phone and preparing remedies for them. Although we could see how weak she was, and how weak her voice was when she talked to us, on the phone her voice became strong again and she sounded just like her old self. Her love of homeopathy was what carried her through.

VI. Letters.

To Harold Morowitz, Ph. D.

To Gerald Weissman, M. D.

To Jennifer Jacobs, M. D., and the Homeopathic Research Network

*Moskowitz vs. Morowitz, or Harvard vs. Yale**

[Editor's Note: *The July issue of* Hospital Practice *contained an article on homeopathy entitled "Much Ado About Nothing," by Dr. Harold J. Morowitz, Professor of Molecular Biophysics and Biochemistry at Yale; it is reprinted here with the permission of* Hospital Practice. *He is answered by Richard Moskowitz, M. D., a Phi Beta Kappa graduate of Harvard and Director of Publications for the National Center for Homeopathy.*]

Dr. Morowitz:

On a number of occasions lately I have observed otherwise rational, intelligent individuals extolling the virtues of homeopathy. Not wishing to be more narrow-minded than is absolutely necessary, I decided to investigate the claims of the followers of Samuel Hahnemann (1755-1843). His doctrine turns out to be an unusual olio of sophisticated advanced concepts and sheer nonsense, defying the most firmly established laws of physics. Curiously enough, in spite of the strange mixture, there were periods during the nineteenth century when homeopathy was probably the best treatment available to most sick individuals.

Hahnemann's original theory can be divided into three postulates:

1) disease is a whole-organism property, an aberration from the state of health;
2) like is healed by like, which means that substances causing symptoms at high doses will cure those same disorders at low doses; and
3) the effect of a remedy is inversely proportional to its concentration.

The first tenet of homeopathy -- the integrated view -- occurs as an accepted idea within current system-theory studies of health and disease. Earlier concepts of simple one-to-one correlations between causes and effects have proved of limited value in a large number of pathological

* "Moskowitz vs. Morowitz, or Harvard vs. Yale," ***Homeopathy Today,*** October 1982.

conditions. From Virchow to Dubos, medical scientists have spoken of multiple etiologies. The organismic approaches can be completely reductionist, as in the various mathematical models of physiological systems; or they can have a much larger psychological component, as is seen in contemporary holistic medicine. Indeed, it is on the fringes of holistic medicine that one finds many present-day homeopaths. They have adopted the perceptive and far-seeing part of Hahnemann's natural philosophy without critically evaluating the scientifically untenable portions of his doctrine.

The second postulate of homeopathy, that like is healed by like, is often referred to by the Latin *similia similibus curantur.* The principle is presumably a generalization from experience, but little is offered by way of the exhaustive data that must support such a synthesis. Moreover, the test of falsifiability, a foundation-stone of scientific epistemology, is never invoked to deal with those cases in which *similia similibus non curantur.* Homeopathy is acutely aware of the experimental, and there are constant references to "provings," whereby healthy individuals are dosed with a drug to find out the symptoms that it will supposedly cure. Once the substances are so "proved," there is the assumption that the dilute chemical will work as predicted. Homeopaths don't require an empirical test of the general principle; that is for them a given, a dogma of the discipline. There is thus the pseudo-science of invoking experiments at one level and ignoring the necessity of extensive data at the deeper and more important level of the validity of the general postulate.

The third aspect of the theory, that dilution increases efficacy, involves starting with a drug and successively diluting it by factors of 10. The number of dilutions is designated by a factor called the potency. Thus, potency 3 is one part in a thousand, potency 6 is one part in a million, etc., out to potency 30, which is one part in a thousand billion billion billion, or considerably less than one molecule per dose. This postulate comes into conflict with an underlying principle of thermodynamics, so fundamental that no special name has been assigned to it. This basic assumption asserts that an isolated system will come to a state of equilibrium dependent on its physical parameters, such as temperature, pressure, volume, and composition, and independent of its history, that is, independent of how it was prepared.

Let us take an example. Start out with two samples: the first, a 1% solution of sodium chloride and the second, an extract of ground-up honeybees. Sequential dilutions are made in pure water until they have reached a potency of 30. At this dilution each final sample is just water, regardless of the starting material: the odds are less than one in a million that a cubic centimeter of the final samples will contain a molecule of the starting material. At that point no physical measurement can distinguish the two final dilutions. According to the laws of physics, the two samples are in every way the same. According to the laws of homeopathy, they will have different effects when administered to a patient.

If homeopathy is correct, either living organisms must operate independently of the laws of physics or one of the most basic assumptions of physics must be wrong. Either way, homeopathic medicine is in direct confrontation with some of the most firmly established branches of human knowledge. Given the paucity of any positive evidence, these violations of natural law place the third postulate of homeopathy in the category of scientific nonsense.

In spite of our dim assessment of homeopathic theory, it must be conceded that it enjoyed considerable success in the 1800's and early 1900's and was widely sought after. I believe we would now admit that during the early and mid-1800's, before scientific medicine began to take hold, most sick individuals would have been better off under homeopathic treatment than under the care of a standard physician. The reason is that the pharmacopoeia employed by orthodox medical professionals listed a large number of highly toxic materials, while those of the homeopath were harmless, since they contained little or no active substance. Using just water or sugar tablets as their medical armamentarium, the homeopaths were unlikely to do any harm. In addition, the allopaths -- physicians other than homeopaths -- practiced bleeding and similarly dangerous rites. Patients of both types of practitioners were able to enjoy placebo effects and psychosomatic gains and to benefit from the fact that most illnesses resolve spontaneously. Clients of homeopaths were spared additional risks of treatments, which were often harsh and dangerous.

Given the state of knowledge through much of the 1800's, it was often better to do nothing than to do something; and that is what the homeopaths were doing: nothing. Our story is not without a moral. It is easy to look back at a past age and suggest the values of doing nothing. It is difficult in the extreme to examine our own behavior and conclude that there are times when no action is the optimal course of action.

This is true in every field of human endeavor but particularly so in medicine, where one is presented with complaining and suffering human beings. One advantage that accrues to the homeopath is never having to admit that he is doing nothing. He always presents his patient with what appears to be an active, vigorous course of medication. The fact that the medicine is as vacuous as the theory is unknown to both the healer and the healee, thus allowing the full range of psychodynamics. Lacking these advantages, the practitioner of normal scientific medicine must nevertheless be prepared, on occasion, to make the decision that doing nothing is the best course of treatment.

Why has there been a return to homeopathy in the current age of science? The answer is a familiar one. In the face of difficult questions or problems that lack answers or solutions, individuals turn to doctrines that are without a rational basis but have a ring of conviction about them. The history of human folly is, after all, rich in examples of such ideologies. The movements arising from such doctrines offer solace to the sick and the confused. In the case of homeopathy, nothing has gone and continues to go a very long way when that nothing is accompanied by hope and faith.

Dr. Moskowitz:

I am writing in reply to Dr. Morowitz' recent column on homeopathy. Having practiced classical homeopathy for the past eight years, I may possibly qualify as one of those "otherwise rational, intelligent individuals" he is talking about. With all due respect for Dr. Morowitz, his understanding of homeopathy is very limited, and, to use his own words, considerably "more narrow-minded than is absolutely necessary." He is certainly correct that in homeopathy the patient is not always cured, but that is true of any method of treatment. He is also correct that the principle of treatment by "similars" is a fixed postulate of the method, rather than a hypothesis as yet capable of easy proof or disproof. But that is hardly a reproach either. It is rather a property that homeopathy shares with all other formal systems of thought, namely, that some principles are undemonstrable within that system, because they are presupposed in it. This is merely Gödel's famous Theorem. It means that the truth or validity of such a principle cannot be judged apart from the coherence, predictive force, and other formal attributes of the system as a whole.

Precisely the same is true of physics itself, for that matter. Dr. Morowitz cannot prove his "underlying principles of thermodynamics" either: it is, in his own words, "so fundamental that no special name has been assigned to it;" it is, precisely, an assumption. Perhaps *his* basic assumption is more obvious or self-evident to him than *similia similibus curentur.* But to dismiss homoeopathy as "unscientific" merely because it is not equally obvious to him is mere name-calling, and does him little credit.

Secondly, homeopathy does not contend that dilution *per se* increases efficacy. It is true that Hahnemann used and many homeopaths today use microdoses, medicinal substances diluted beyond the level of Avogadro's number. But Dr. Morowitz does not understand that remedies so diluted must also be mechanically agitated or "successed" in a certain way to be medicinally active, and that recent nuclear magnetic resonance studies do in fact demonstrate considerable differences in the physical behavior of successed microdoses in solution as compared with that of the solvent alone. Furthermore, microdoses have been shown to have precisely measurable effects upon biological systems, such as bacterial populations, germinating plants, fruit flies, etc.

Ultradilute remedies are in no way required by the homeopathic "law." They are used simply because they produce fewer harmful side effects; and they act for a longer period and on a deeper plane than the same substances given in their grosser "chemical" form, which are subject to catabolic degradation. Such action therefore cannot be understood on the chemical plane: it obliges us to look deeper, at the purely dynamic or energetic plane, analogous to the *ch'i* of acupuncture or the "subtle body" of Hindu philosophy. We homeopaths freely admit that we do not understand any more than this how our remedies actually work. But, once again, it is pathetic to see a grown man of Dr. Morowitz' stature feel compelled to dismiss summarily what he cannot understand. Exploration of the mysterious is, after all, a lot of what science is supposed to be about.

As a matter of fact, the action of very dilute substances is not so far from our common understanding in everyday life. When we walk down the street and smell the lilacs in bloom, we are moved quite profoundly by lilac molecules in immeasurably small concentrations. Our response is therefore a function of the deep qualitative affinity or resonance between what we might call the "essence" of lilac and the human beings who are so moved by them, while we would surely be overwhelmed by more concentrated odors in the vicinity, such as exhaust fumes or, for that matter, a huge vat of purified lilac extract. If we are near a lilac bush and wish to savor its fragrance, we sniff the air very lightly, because there is some very minute concentration that optimally enhances the sensitivity of our olfactory receptors. That is precisely the sort of affinity that homeopaths seek and sometimes are blessed to find between our remedies and our patients.

If the so-called "laws" of physics cannot accommodate subtle phenomena of this kind, doesn't that fact cast some doubt upon the universal applicability of those laws as currently understood? Newton's laws of motion are still valid, but they fail Einstein's test at very high velocities, just as Einstein's laws will themselves be superseded one day, or rather included as special cases within some still broader and deeper understanding. To that end, we are all students on the path, and nobody has a monopoly on the truth, or even on the definition of what is true.

In conclusion, if Dr. Morowitz would like to witness for himself the action of dilute homeopathic remedies on my patients, I will gladly provide a demonstration, which he may then report back to the readers of this Journal. If homeopathy passes this test, we may continue to argue at our leisure about what it means. For the test by which the medical art has always been judged is simply and precisely, how well does it work, how well does it help people to heal themselves? Homeopathy wishes for itself no other, and I very much doubt that even Dr. Morowitz could devise a better one.

Truly yours,
Richard Moskowitz, M. D.

*Reply to Gerald Weissman, M. D.**

[Editor's Note:] *Richard Moskowitz, M. D., sent us a copy of the November 1992 issue of* MD Magazine, *which contained an editorial by Gerald Weissman, MD, entitled, "Dancing with Fairies, Sucking with Vampires." In it Dr. Weissman recalls the superstitions governing the Salem witch trials and continues as follows:*

Dr. Weissman:

Puritan stock is very much alive in the 20th Century and has run into the rapids of unreason. In these nebulous '90s, we seem determined to limit the nation's medical bill while we dribble away funds to a murky throng of homeopaths, herbalists, holists, hallucinators, channellers, clairvoyants, and New Age Mohegans in search of 'unconventional medical practices.'

Now all of this would be fun and games were it not for the more sinister implications of New Age healing. The Senate Appropriations Committee has mandated that the NIH set up an office of Unconventional Medical Practices (UMPs) with an initial funding of $2 million per annum. The NIH failed to object and summoned "experts" in the fields of Ayurvedic, naturopathic, Chinese herbal, and homeopathic medicine, and designed large-scale controlled trials of UMP's. They held plenary and breakout sessions in which they agreed that UMP's have associated belief systems. Well, of course they do: one calls them 'religions.' Before scientific medicine interfered with traditional practices, few folks lived to be old, and the sorry public health statistics of our inner cities are not due to inadequate access to folk remedies.

To paraphrase Lincoln Steffens, we already know the future of UMP's: They don't work! Meanwhile research grants remain unfunded, because an alliance of homeopaths and New Age toe-ticklers have gotten hold of a dotty senator or two. In 1842, Oliver Wendell Holmes' book, *Homeopathy*

* Reply to Gerald Weissman, M. D., ***Homeopathy Today,*** March 1993.

and Its Kindred Delusions, took up his pen against the persistent cult of delusional fantasy that keeps banging its belief against Avogadro's number.

Dr. Moskowitz:

Dear Dr. Weissman:

I was both saddened and amused by your memo, "Dancing with Fairies, Sucking with Vampires," which begins by heaping scorn on the fanaticism of Jonathan Edwards and the Salem Witch hunters and ends with a diatribe against "New Age" thinking as uninformed and intolerant as any of them.

Two strategic omissions left a very one-sided impression: first, you neglected to say that Nathaniel Hawthorne and other learned members of the famous Saturday Club continued to study and practice homeopathy in spite of Oliver Wendell Holmes' best attempts to discredit it; and second, that the illustrious Dr. Holmes also said that if the entire *materia medica* of his time were dumped overboard, "it would be so much the better for mankind and so much worse for the fishes!" The devastation of marine life following recent medical waste dumping off the Atlantic coast shows his words to be even truer if anything for the pharmacopoeia of today.

I agree that the poor health of our inner cities cannot be ascribed to a lack of folk remedies. But neither can it be attributed to a lack of funding of more of the same old research studies that have done little but add to the problem. You and I both know that the root causes are poverty and neglect secondary to racial discrimination and second-class citizenship.

I've been practicing family medicine for 25 years and investigating and using homeopathic remedies since 1974. In short, I presumably qualify for membership in that "murky throng of homeopaths, herbalists, holists, hallucinators, channellers, clairvoyants and New Age Mohegans" against whom you rail so much and about whom you obviously know so little.

I don't know how homeopathy works. It isn't intuitively clear to me or anyone else how medicinal substances that produce certain symptom-pictures in healthy people can thereby elicit curative responses in patients with similar characteristics. Still less has anyone ever satisfactorily explained how medicines diluted past the point of Avogadro's number could possibly do anything, let alone help seriously ill people recover.

Yet, I can assure you that they do. I see patients of all ages, with ailments of every type, both acute and chronic. While by no means all my patients are benefitted from taking homeopathic remedies, enough of them are that I have as many patients as I can handle without having to write prescriptions, not to mention the satisfaction of having helped many of them heal themselves without drugs or surgery.

I can well understand that you, like most of my colleagues, believe that the dilute remedies are essentially placebos. But this argument cuts both ways. If that is true, if my shamanic powers, the self-healing capacity of my patients, and even what you would probably call their extreme and pathetic gullibility are sufficient for them to achieve genuine, long-lasting results without chronic drug dependence or surgical mutilation, who in their right mind would not prefer the gentler, less expensive, and more effective way whenever possible? Indeed, if "placebos" work as well as or better than the "real" stuff, then which one is the placebo, yours or mine?

Personally, I don't think that the remedies are merely placebos, and my patients don't either. I've seen them work quickly and effectively in resuscitation of the newborn, and in animals, comatose people, and even in patients openly scornful of the method. But even if that's all they are, they would still be vastly preferable to the high-tech, high-cost, high-risk treatments that have helped put medicine in its presently critical condition.

The popularity of New Age practitioners, both competent and otherwise, has a lot less to do with gullibility than with authentic deficiencies in the theory and practice of medicine. I assume we can both agree that the detailed knowledge of the structure and function of the human body and the development of medical and surgical technology that have followed from it are among the greatest cultural achievements of human history. But narrowly mechanistic theories of how patients fall ill and recover and similarly one-dimensional priorities for the biomedical enterprise as a whole have alienated huge segments of the population from the medical system in its present form.

In any case, I cannot allow you to negate my entire professional life and evolution as a healer, or the lives and work of thousands like me, simply because we both still lack current scientific categories capable of accommodating them. To be sure, homeopathy, acupuncture, and other holistic approaches are belief systems, philosophies, and even religions, if you prefer. They are integrated theories, attitudes, and methodologies of healing, derived from principles and built upon experience, even though not yet capable of the same rigorous cause-and-effect linkage as insisted upon by orthodox medicine or what passes for science these days.

But orthodox medicine and all other sciences are likewise belief systems, philosophies, and indeed religions in precisely the same sense. Indeed, the stricter its laws may be, the more rigid its methodologies for generating "truth," and the harsher the penalties it would exact from those who choose to depart from them. Yet new ideas and belief systems are still required for all scientific progress. I am interested in homeopathy and other holistic approaches precisely insofar as they presuppose the existence of a more inclusive bioenergetic science that is still in its infancy.

Conversely, for all of its achievements, allopathic medicine has not yet outgrown the reductionist philosophies of Virchow and Claude Bernard, which are still splendid and useful in many ways, but no longer the last word on how living systems work and break down. You refuse to venture beyond the frontier of Avogadro's number, as if the concepts of the atom and the molecule have delimited religion from science for all time. You sit as if in judgment of heresy, as smug in the knowledge of absolute truth as the judge who condemned the simple townspeople of Salem for healing ordinary folk with herbs and calling it witchcraft.

Truly yours,
Richard Moskowitz, M. D.

*Letter to Jennifer Jacobs, M. D., and the Homeopathic Research Network**

Dear Jennifer:

Once again, thank you on behalf of the entire homeopathic community for the publication of your research in *Pediatrics,* a landmark achievement for us all. This time, I am writing to discuss the problem of animal testing, which was raised by Catherine Coulter in *JAIH,* Autumn 1994, and to invite you and your colleagues in the Homeopathic Research Network to use future issues of the *AIH Journal* as a public forum on this most pressing albeit unpopular subject.

My own interest in animal testing began after my Junior year at Harvard as a summer trainee in biochemistry at the Jackson Laboratory in Maine, a facility devoted to the breeding of genetically pure strains of mice and other mammalian species (dogs, cats, rats, rabbits, guinea pigs, hamsters, monkeys, etc.) for export to medical research centers throughout the world. From a rough calculation of the numbers involved, I understood that medical research is based on the systematic mutilation and killing of unconsenting animals on a global scale. It was and is impossible for me to imagine how valid scientific or ethical standards could ever be built on such a foundation.[1]

When I first began to study homeopathy, I was relieved to discover that the Law of Similars, the totality of the symptoms, and the classical method of proving remedies on healthy human volunteers obviates the need for experimental pathology or animal testing on a large scale. Even in Europe, where most of them have been published, animal studies have been used mainly to show that dilute remedies act in *some* demonstrable way, i. e., to convince the allopathic world that they are not placebos. As Ms. Coulter has pointed out, *in vitro* models using cells in tissue culture and cell-free enzyme systems are now available for the same purpose.[2]

---

* Letter to Jennifer Jacobs, M. D., and the Homeopathic Research Network, ***Journal of the AIH*** 88:9, Winter 1995.

In addition to this ethical argument, there is another equally powerful reason not to follow blindly the prevailing fashions of what passes for science these days. I leave aside the obvious one, which Prof. Benveniste has already taught us, that no matter how many hoops we agree to jump through to appease our opponents, still others of even greater difficulty will be found to take their place. It is rather that animal studies, double-blind trials, and the whole works are required because of an outdated theory of causality whereby we seek to develop biotechnologies like drugs or surgical procedures of sufficient power to override variations in individual susceptibility, in effect to force the organism to do something it has no natural inclination to do.[3] To the extent that causal influences of this degree require deadly force to accomplish them, we naturally prefer to sacrifice animals first before inflicting them on humans later.

A similar realization was no small part of why you and I and many of our colleagues were first drawn to study and practice a more wholesome philosophy and method, preferring the kinds of causality that are content to persuade, allow, or assist the organism to finish what it is already trying to accomplish. To demonstrate subtler influences of this type, animal studies and double-blind trials are actually more likely to obscure the actual effect, because the self-healing capacity of the organism is represented on the placebo or control side of the equation as the baseline which the experimental drug or surgery is designed to surpass.[4] To exhibit the truth that every clinician and every patient already knows, we need to develop new methods of clinical and experimental investigation that are much closer to the ordinary lived experience of how patients actually feel and function than allopathic models need or can ever be.[5]

In that spirit, I invite you and others in the Homeopathic Research Network to use the pages of our AIH Journal to discuss the issues of animal testing and double-blind trials in homeopathy and to seek better and more wholesome ways to exhibit our truth for the benefit of the profession and the public.

Best regards,
Dick Moskowitz

NOTES.

1 Moskowitz, R., "Why I Became a Homeopath," *Homeopathy Today,* December 1982.
2 Coulter, C., "Homeopathic Medical Research," *JAIH* **87**: Autumn 1994.
3 Moskowitz, "Who Needs the AIH? A Brief Pep Talk, *JAIH* **87**:193, Winter 1994.
4 Ibid.
5 Coulter, H., *The Controlled Clinical Trial: an Analysis,* Center for Empirical Medicine, Washington, D.C., 1991.

VII. Interviews.

With Peggy O'Mara, *Mothering* Magazine

With Jane Ryan, C.N.M., *New England Journal of Homeopathy*

*An Interview with Peggy O'Mara, Mothering Magazine**

[Editor's Note:] ***Richard Moskowitz, MD,*** *received his undergraduate degree from Harvard and his medical degree from New York University. He studied homeopathy with George Vithoulkas in Athens, Greece, and recently served as President of the National Center for Homeopathy. After medical school, Dick studied philosophy at the University of Colorado in Boulder, where he became involved in draft resistance and the antiwar movement. In 1967, he finished his internship, and began practicing what he calls "minimalist medicine." In 1969, he attended a home birth for the first time, and the experience changed his life. In 1974, he moved to Santa Fe, New Mexico. Dick and his family moved to Boston in 1982, after 13 years of home-birth experience. He currently practices classical homeopathy at the Turning Point Family Wellness Center in Watertown, Massachusetts. Several of his articles on immunizations have appeared in past issues of* Mothering *and are reprinted in our "Immunization Booklet." Two of his booklets, 'The Case against Immunizations" and "Homeopathic Reasoning," are available from the National Center for Homeopathy, 1500 Massachusetts Avenue, Washington, DC 20005.*

O'Mara: Is there a resurgence of interest in homeopathy today?

Moskowitz: Yes, very much so. Homeopathy has caught on as a primary care vehicle for many people because the idea of self-care that underlies homeopathy has become more important and timely than ever before. As with home birth, people are trying to reclaim decision-making power over their health. Home birth transforms our relationship with our healthcare providers, in that the midwife is a *guest* in the home, and does not automatically presume to tell us how to give birth or how to live our lives. Homeopathy takes this one step further, by showing us a way of thinking about our health that is self-aware. The study of the remedies is

* Interview with Peggy O'Mara, ***Mothering*** Magazine, Spring 1988.

a way of sharpening our awareness of ourselves, of looking at aspects of our health that we do not ordinarily look at.

O'Mara: Does prescribing a remedy for yourself then require you to assess yourself and your condition in a broad sense?

Moskowitz: That's right. "Homeopathy" is really a *thought process* that leads to something very practical. You can experiment with homeopathic remedies under guidelines that are very, very safe if you are willing to take the trouble to study them. In the process of learning homeopathy, people begin to remember their own healing, just as after a home birth they remember that the birth is theirs, that it belongs *to them.* The healing of illness, like birth, is inherent in human beings, all animals, and indeed in all life. Homeopathy is not the only way to heal illness, not even necessarily the best way for some people: but it does work, and can easily be studied by everyone on their own time and in their own way.

O'Mara: When did you first become interested in homeopathy?

Moskowitz: In 1974. I started out as a home-birth doctor, a "barefoot doctor," you might say; that was in 1969. Through my experience with home births, I began to understand that real healing is *possible.* First I began studying herbs, and then acupuncture. Although I'd heard of homeopathy, I couldn't make heads or tails of it; I tried to read a book on it that I found in a used bookshop, but I couldn't fathom what it was trying to say. Once I saw a patient who was very allergic to bee stings, and wrote a letter to an old homeopath in Vermont, asking him if he thought that bee venom would be an appropriate homeopathic prescription for her. He encouraged me to take the professional Course of the National Center for Homeopathy; and as soon as I took it, I knew that homeopathy was what I was going to do. Here was a *method,* a coherent and systematic approach that made sense to me philosophically.

O'Mara: Can you venture a definition of homeopathy?

Moskowitz: The "Law of Similars" is really the basis of homeopathy. It was a discovery that started out, like many discoveries, as an "accident" that happened to a person who was prepared to understand its true significance. Samuel Hahnemann was a well-known German physician and chemist of the late 18th century who discovered that he was unable to cure his own children, using the methods of his time, when they fell ill with various epidemic diseases. He became so discouraged that he dropped out of medicine and began to earn his living by translating medical works from English and other languages into German. In the process, he came across a passage that really struck him.

Quinine bark, which was just being introduced into European medicine at the time, was considered a specific for intermittent fever, which the author he was translating attributed to its bitter taste. The scholastic analogy between its bitter taste and the supposed astringency of its action on the organism seemed totally speculative to Hahnemann; so he decided to take a dose of the bark himself and discovered, to his great amazement, that it produced in him a paroxysm of fever and chills very much like the illness that quinine was treating so successfully. He was so astonished that he let the dose wear off and tried it again, with exactly the same result. He understood immediately that something very important had happened, that the ability of a medicine to heal a sickness is in direct relation to its ability to *produce* a similar sickness in a healthy person.

Still a bit dubious, he began to test his discovery. As an expert pharmacologist, a person thoroughly familiar with the remedies of his time, he started administering them to healthy people on an experimental basis. In a very systematic way, he administered other medicines to whomever he could find for these investigations: himself, his family, his friends, colleagues, and students. In every case, he found that the therapeutic range of a substance did in fact correspond to its power to *produce* a similar sickness in healthy individuals.

O'Mara: How does homeopathy work? Does it stimulate the immune system so that the condition moves on to a new phase?

Moskowitz: First of alL let me just say that nobody can answer that question right now in a thoroughly convincing way. My answer is necessarily somewhat metaphorical: Homeopathy heralds the creation of a science that is not yet born. We are still in the realm of art and philosophy. I like and appreciate the artfulness of homeopathy, because I am able to use it simply as a resource, as a vehicle to train my own unique awareness of a person, here and now. Homeopathy provides a structure, a form, but it doesn't tell me what to do. There is still an element about it that is not quite cut-and-dried.

O'Mara: What happens when a homeopathic remedy is given?

Moskowitz: The illness that we see in a person is already a restorative self-healing *attempt,* rather than simply a "bummer" that we are trying to correct, or an event that we can reduce to a definite abnormality and oppose, control, or manipulate in a certain direction. Illness is a concerted expression of the whole organism, attempting to overcome whatever it needs to overcome, doing whatever it can to heal itself. When people have an illness, they are often *stuck* in it, and some sicknesses are inherently more difficult to heal than others. If we give a remedy which when given to a healthy person will elicit a similar totality of symptoms or responses, then somehow the healing effort of the body is focused in that same direction.

O'Mara: How do you know when you give a remedy that it is the right one?

Moskowitz: Does it help, or doesn't it? That's all you really need to know. But you also have to ask what it means to "help." By our current medical definition, helping means killing the tumor or knocking down the blood pressure. I am proposing a different definition: namely, that the patient feels better, functions better, lives better—and that is *self-validating.*

O'Mara: What do you think about homeopathic dosages and amounts for self-care? Should one be cautious?

Moskowitz: Yes, I think it is very possible to abuse remedies. Although it is widely understood that homeopathic products on the market are very safe, and that anyone can buy and use them, there is some confusion about levels and amounts. The proper guidelines for homeopathic self-care are basically the same as for taking aspirin or any other over-the-counter medicine. If you have to keep using a remedy day after day, week after week, then common sense should tell you that you're barking up the wrong tree. At the very least, you ought to be doing something else as well. By relying on a remedy that is not working, you may be missing a lot. If all you're getting after days of use is a slight palliative effect, then what you're doing is no different from taking aspirin or any other over-the-counter drug in an unwise manner. You're simply masking something that needs further attention.

O'Mara: What's the difference between 6X, 12X, and 30C, the dilution factor?

Moskowitz: In one sense, there's really not much difference. What does matter is that as you go higher on the scale of dilution, you repeat the remedy less and less frequently. Professionals use the higher dilutions because they don't see the patient very often. The lower dilutions are the ones most suitable for repetition, and repetition benefits the acute ailments that you would be involved with in self-care applications: colds, flus, sore throats, and the like.

O'Mara: Is there a rule of thumb for repeating doses of remedies?

Moskowitz: Yes, although, like most of the principles of homeopathy, it's quite easy to state and somewhat harder to interpret. The rule is: Give the remedy until a reaction occurs, then stop for as long as the reaction lasts—that is, let it go on its own for as long as it can. The number of repetitions depends on how quickly the illness develops, and how quickly you need to see improvements. For example, say your baby goes out in a cold wind and comes back two hours later with a fever of 103°. If you give the remedy immediately, you may have to give it only once or twice before the fever comes right down again.

O'Mara: What if nothing happens?

Moskowitz: If nothing happens after a few doses, then you'll need to try something else. Remember, the purpose of giving a remedy is not to slug the person into submission, but rather to stimulate a reaction that's already trying to happen. In an acute ailment, you may have to repeat the remedy several times. People sometimes make the mistake of quitting too early. A flu, for example, has a certain rhythm to it. If it has taken three days to come on, it would be unreasonable to expect it to vanish in two hours. The illness has a certain rhythm, and although the correct remedy will shorten it a little, it will still be recognizable as that illness. So you must be prepared to give the remedy a number of times, maybe even four or five times a day.

O'Mara: How does one know whether to change remedies or continue with the same one, particularly with coughs or more vague or changeable conditions?

Moskowitz: That's the big question, and that's where the self-care concept gets a bit tricky! In the first place, you have to realize that, with an acute ailment, all you really need to do is *help.* If the remedy is pretty close, it's probably going to help somewhat. People sometimes imagine that the remedy is a magic carpet to take a person immediately from total sickness to total health. Although it's amazing how often something like this actually happens, it would be very unwise to count on it. The fact is that many different remedies are likely to be suitable for any given ailment. On the other hand, certain criteria can be used to determine when a particular remedy is not working. In some cases, it will be obvious that nothing is happening. In others, a special intuitive attentiveness will be required. This is the same common-sense awareness that mothers develop from being with their babies and learning to distinguish serious complaints from minor ones.

O'Mara: Is there some way to know when homeopathy is advisable, or some other medical philosophy is necessary? How can a parent know what or whom to seek help from, especially during a panic situation with one's kld in the middle of the night?

Moskowitz: Some *patients* will make the selection. For example, there are people who are not willing to be treated homeopathically, although I'd be willing, because they very properly make the judgment that only they can make: "I have a strep throat, and I want penicillin." Since that is what they believe in, that is what they should do. I'm more concerned about parents who are so turned off by the medical system that they expect to manage their children's health all by themselves. This is a very unfortunate development.

Two questions are involved here, and they're interconnected. One is, When do I ask for help? The other is, What kind of help do I really want? We need to learn how to tell the practitioner—the physician, nurse, or physician assistant— what we would like from him or her, and what we would not like. I can easily imagine a parent saying to an allopathically trained doctor, *"We really need a pediatrician. I would like you to know us. We use self-care, homeopathic remedies, and herbs, and we go to an acupuncturist from time to time. But there are times when this is not adequate, when something that's happening is so disturbing that we really want an expert medical opinion. So we would like to be able to come to you at those times, to help us decide what is really going on with our child. Please understand that this does not necessarily mean we are going to want to hospitalize our child or accept the recommended treatment. But we really appreciate your expertise, and would like an explanation and some advice or recommendation from you. And there are probably going to be times when we will want some very specialized treatment from you, and from some of your colleagues as well. We would like to be able to come to you at such times, and to work out such a relationship."*

How can anyone say no to that? Most pediatricians would love to hear this message. It acknowledges a well-defined area of expertise, and decreases your chances of being dismissed as someone unwilling to make any concessions to the medical system. Addressing a health practitioner in this way defines exactly how the medical system can and should be helpful to you. And it is a definition that everybody desperately needs— especially pediatricians, because they, too, are struggling with this.

O'Mara: Are there any vaccinations that you like? Do you feel differently about the polio, tetanus, or pertussis vaccines?

Moskowitz: I have mostly questions. My basic feeling about vaccinations revolves around questions more than answers, questions so insistent and so troubling to me that I feel they must be answered. Until they are, I cannot subscribe to the practice of compulsory vaccinations. My experience has taught me that routine "immunization" across the board, regardless of the individual's need or sensitivity, is producing high amounts of chronic disease in our population. My sense is that vaccinating transforms the propensity to get acute diseases into the propensity to get chronic diseases. In most cases, I'd much rather take my chances with the acute diseases. With chronic diseases, suffering is amortized over time; you pay for it with interest over the course of your life.

We have to ask how vaccines affect the total health of individuals over a period of 15 or 20 years. However, we don't yet have the conceptual tools to do this, because we don't agree on what the total health of an individual is, and most of the time we don't even think to ask. Infectious diseases come and go; they are part of the biosphere. To think that we can simply eliminate them through some kind of technical engineering is incredibly reckless. I think we are stepping into the genetic engineering department here, and that is a very dangerous thing to do. Vaccines are engineering changes in the genetic material that we really do not understand. I would prefer to accept the reality of sickness—to accept the fact that we do fall ill and that healing is possible.

O'Mara: Are unvaccinated people traveling in other countries more susceptible to illness?

Moskowitz: I'd hate to come down with yellow fever, which is very nasty. But on the other hand, at this point in my life, I'd be much more inclined to trust my own healing power, and whatever healers I would hope to find, than to believe that the vaccine will protect me against yellow fever. I just don't trust it anymore; I've come too far. As much as I'd like to be able to trust it, I see the potential risk, and in some cases I've seen the actual cost. So I'm having to re-examine even vaccinations like tetanus toxoid. I just have these questions, and they won't go away.

O'Mara: Would you comment on fever in children?

Moskowitz: With some exceptions, fever is usually a sign that the child is relatively OK. I like to see a certain amount of fever in a child, because it reassures me that this child has the immunological mechanisms to deal with an acute illness.

O'Mara: Would you feel it necessary to suppress the fever?

Moskowitz: Usually not. But naturally I feel concerned when a child develops a fever of 105° for days. I wouldn't want to see the child have febrile seizures, even though they're usually benign. I would prefer to see the child get it over with. A fever response is an acute response, meaning that it should be and usually is over quickly. Fever indicates movement and vigor; this is the situation where the acute remedies excel.

O'Mara: Why is it suggested that homeopathic remedies be given 15 minutes before or after eating, and that strong smells or strong tastes be avoided?

Moskowitz: The remedies are subtle. They act as energies or "vibrations," rather than as *molecules.* Since they work at the vibrational level, if another strong vibration is present—say, a flavor in the mouth or a strong perfume—then the remedy will have to compete with it. The remedy needs a clear field in which to operate. In this sense the remedies are quite delicate and easily interfered with.

O'Mara: That is part of the thought process that you mentioned, the philosophy of the method?

Moskowitz: I would call it giving respect. You have to give a certain amount of respect to the remedies. You have to give a certain amount of respect to any medicine—to appreciate what it will do, what it won't do, how to take it, and how often to take it. One of the reasons why I dislike drugs is that we don't respect them when we have to take them every day; after a while, we don't even notice them. The way the American

Indians smoke tobacco and eat peyote shows that they have respect for these medicines of the earth. They know what they will do, and they know how to purify themselves to prepare for that. It is a special use for a special occasion. This is the way I see medicines. Homeopathy is very much a part of this tradition. A person has to respect what the remedy will do, what it won't do, and how to take it.

*An Interview with Jane Ryan, C. N. M., New England Journal of Homeopathy**

Ryan: Dick, perhaps we should start with the obvious question: How did you get into homeopathy?

Moskowitz: That's a long story! I was disillusioned with medicine and couldn't yet say exactly why. At first I think it was mainly an aesthetic thing. It all seemed so ugly, gross, and brutal, like the indignity of people dying with tubes coming in and out of them. I'll never forget such a patient from my training at Bellevue Hospital, a middle-aged guy who was hooked up to just about every conceivable device, and I thought, to have to die this way was completely beyond the pale of anything I could subscribe to as a physician. I remember running out of the room, not wanting to be a party to it. Mostly I just played the game, but at such times I would occasionally absent myself.

Another routine chore was having to inoculate mice with pneumococci from our lobar pneumonia patients, a purely academic exercise, since we also did stained smears of their sputum. So there was an unethical and immoral aspect to it as well, but in the beginning I think it was primarily an aesthetic revulsion, which made me disappear or refuse to participate. After my second year, my parents rewarded me with a trip to Europe, where I met a guy from Finland who invited me to visit his country, and I knew if I did I wouldn't make it back in time for the fall term. It was very tempting, but I chickened out because I had no idea about what else to do with my life.

In fact, I came very close to not making it to medical school in the first place. In the summer after my junior year in college I worked at a

* Interview with Jane Ryan, C. N. M., *New England Journal of Homeopathy,* Summer 2000.

cancer research lab doing biochemical research, which involved cutting up a small number of mice every day. Simply by adding these numbers to the much larger total of other experiments being conducted there, I suddenly had a vision of what medicine was really like, and it was abhorrent to me; that lab was a veritable Auschwitz for mice. In addition, they sent vast numbers of genetically pure strains of mice and other experimental animals to scientific institutions all over the world. I was horrified by the enormous scale of this slaughter, upon which the whole edifice of so-called scientific medicine was built. For the better part of the summer, I would hide out in a dark alcove of the library reading Freud, which was about as far away from "hard" science as I could get there.

It was a miserable experience. As you can well imagine, my senior year was a crisis of indecision and self-doubt. I considered law school, grad school, even taking time off. I guess I'm really an academic at heart. By the time I decided to go to medical school, it was late spring, and the classes were all full. The fact is, I really had no business being in that class, but my grades were good, my father knew somebody with connections at New York University Medical School, and they made an extra place for me. Posterity will have to judge how serious a mistake that was, for them and for me! [Laughter.]

The first two years were mostly book learning in the basic sciences. I wasn't thrilled, but certainly interested at times, engaged with my classes, and I could tolerate the small clerkships that met on the hospital wards. It was the clinical years that almost finished me, as I've described in "Why I Became a Homeopath." Somehow I got through school, but when my classmates were applying and matching for internships and residencies, I decided that medicine wasn't for me and doubted I'd ever see a patient again. I took a graduate fellowship in philosophy at the University of Colorado, and flourished in that environment, as I began asking myself what it meant to be a doctor and what the medical enterprise was really about. At the same time my personal life was falling apart. My wife and I divorced, and I had to go to work to support my infant son, which meant doing my internship and getting my license, and certainly didn't excite me very much.

But much to my surprise, and in spite of all my reservations, I actually enjoyed my internship. I discovered that I rather liked playing doctor and felt pretty comfortable in that role. I realized that I did have something to offer patients beyond medicines and procedures, namely, myself, my own energy, if only to help guide them through the medical maze so they wouldn't get hurt too badly. 1 spent a lot of time talking them out of surgery and gave drugs as little as possible. I tried to develop other strategies, really not so far from what I do now. The work was honest but quite difficult, because my only technique or procedure was to make a diagnosis and then put it on the shelf for a while, to try to find a healing path that would fit each patient individually.

But if anyone had suggested homeopathy or herbs or acupuncture or some such thing, I'm sure I'd have thought they were nuts. I was totally closed to such a possibility. For all its faults, medicine was all that I could see with any theoretical rigor or legitimacy. The choice seemed very stark to me: everything was either yes or no, black or white. As time went on, there was less and less that I was willing to do as a physician, and by 1969 I really hit rock bottom, with almost nothing in medicine that I could still wholeheartedly subscribe to.

That was the setting for my first home birth. I was living in Boulder, Colorado at the time, where I'd been active in the antiwar movement and had done some draft resistance work. The bulk of my practice consisted of university students and the young and underage hippies who were suddenly moving into town in large numbers. It was a fun time in many ways.

Ryan: What kind of practice did you have exactly?

Moskowitz: It was mostly students and street people: lots of birth control pills, STD's, gonorrhea, bad drug trips, hepatitis, pneumonia, young teenagers and runaways living in crash pads, many of them half-crazed on pot or acid, with boa constrictors wrapped around their arms. It was a great and wild scene. Then this woman calls me out of the blue. She was due to give birth in four weeks, and no OB would have anything to do with her; but she was determined to have her baby at home with or without help. I thought it was a pretty crazy idea, and naturally I was scared, with no nurses to hand me things, set me up, and make me look good, and no docs or hospital to back me up if things went sour. But I also sensed she was giving me a present, a way to practice medicine without having to lay a trip on anyone; as a guest in her home, I realized it would no longer be my place to tell her what to do or how to live.

When I arrived at her house, I remember wanting to do a vaginal exam right away, to see how labor was progressing, as I'd been trained. But the candlelight, the Bach playing softly, and everyone watching intently made it clear that the exam was my need, not hers. It felt intrusive under the circumstances, without any sign of trouble. I kept asking myself how I'd know if something went wrong, and finally decided my best bet was to sit down and pay attention like everyone else. She taught me the whole course that way, without saying a word. I kept wondering how she knew how to do it, since her other child had been delivered under general anesthesia nine years earlier. There was no book learning.

It was a beautiful and almost religious experience for all of us, but for me it turned around my whole notion of what medicine and healing were all about. It was just before dawn on a clear April morning, and we all just sat there staring at mother and baby as people have always done since the beginning of time. I could swear I saw a faint gray halo of light all around them, like a Madonna of Raphael or Fra Filippo Lippi. It was a revelation I will treasure always. But the birth seemed like an original idea that this woman had thought up out of the depths of her experience. It never occurred to me that anyone else would choose to do such a crazy thing, much less that it would become the mainstay of my practice. It wasn't until a year or so later that a lot of people began calling me, I was delivering babies hand over fist, and before I knew it I was actively involved in what had clearly become a historic movement.

Home birth also opened my eyes to other modes of healing. It helped me realize that Western medicine was based on its power to control human physiology, to force the blood pressure to stay within the limits we impose on it, to manipulate thyroid hormone levels up or down, and so forth. Home birth was my initiation into another realm, a dimension of life energy that prefigured the split into mind and body, into a unified way of studying the human organism as a whole. I began investigating herbal medicine, nutrition, psychotherapy, acupuncture, and anything else I could find out there.

In 1974 I moved to New Mexico to study Oriental medicine with a Japanese teacher whom I came to love and admire. With its holistic and spiritual attitude, his teaching seemed very close to what I had in mind. It was during these years that I began hearing about homeopathy as well. In 1972 or so I found an old British *Materia Medica* by Neatby and Stoneham in a used book store in Denver, which made no sense to me at all and wound up on a shelf gathering dust with dozens of others. An old lady I knew in Boulder was doing some amazing things in the back room of her health food store, including dowsing for homeopathic remedies with a pendulum. At the time I had a patient who was deathly allergic to bee stings, and from what little I knew of homeopathy at the time it occurred to me to give her *Apis.* Fortunately I got the name of an old homeopath in Vermont and asked him if that would be an appropriate thing to do, to which he replied, "Well, sonny boy, I think you'd better come to our summer school!"

I did. That was in 1974. As soon as I got there, I knew it was just what I was looking for, and that I would happily devote the rest of my life to studying and practicing it. For homeopathic medicine offered me nothing more nor less than a philosophy and a method for doing in a more skillful and intelligent way what I was already doing instinctively by the seat of my pants. Even before I'd seen it work for a patient, I was elated because it was also Western, was part of my culture, unlike acupuncture, which fascinated me but seemed fundamentally alien; I feared I'd have to learn Japanese and take on outlandish habits and manners that were foreign to how I wanted to live.

Here at last was something originating from my own history and background that I could be at home with. There was also the added bonus of more rummaging through used book stores, which I love to do anyway. I've been doing it ever since.

Ryan: Were you practicing homeopathy in Boulder?

Moskowitz: No. I didn't open an office or have a formal practice until I moved to Santa Fe in 1974. At first it was mainly acute remedies, *Aconite, Belladonna, Chamomilla,* and *Gelsemium,* first aid for fevers and such, just the remedies I could see. It was all I could realistically know at that level, after that two-week NCH course. But that was also the nature of my medical training: see one, do one, teach one, learning as you go, and by the seat of your pants, making lots of mistakes, sometimes learning from them, and sometimes learning the wrong things, as is still the case.

When I was over my head, I'd call Dr. Panos. I had an old woman with a big tumor that she herself suspected was cancer and didn't really want to do any tests to find out. I gave her remedies for about a year with questionable results, until I felt really scared and overwhelmed by the responsibility of taking care of seriously ill people. At such times Maisie would invariably say, "Sounds like you're doing the right thing," or "Keep up the good work!" As it turned out, the woman did have cancer, and eventually died of it, but only after three years of good quality life, and at home, as I hope to do when my time comes. It was only in the last month that she developed metastases and had to be coaxed in for X-rays. She died in her bed with the help of her neighbors, and was buried in her back yard at her request, which was still legal in New Mexico back then.

Little by little, my homeopathic practice grew. Often at a birth I'd be searching through my Yingling to come up with something, but in the clutch all the remedies sounded pretty much the same. When my own learned prescriptions failed, as they often did, a woman whom I took to births with me would sometimes dowse for remedies and crank them out on the spot using her Rae machine.

Ryan: A Rae machine?

Moskowitz: It's a radionic device that purports to be a large magnet, with a card for each remedy, a distinctive configuration of concentric circles and radial interference lines drawn through them at various angles, supposedly the energetic "signature" of that remedy. You insert the card in the slot, crank up the magnet to the desired potency, add a vial of alcohol, and Presto! Out comes your remedy, potentized and ready for use. You may think it's all nonsense, as I did at the time, but I have to tell you, I saw them work lots of times after my own learned prescriptions did nothing. Besides, if you can accept the idea of classical homeopathy, the rest of this stuff isn't so hard to swallow. I'm still interested in such phenomena, which I like to call "experimental" homeopathy, though I have no talent for it myself.

The woman I just spoke of happened to be a gifted psychic, who once found a lost child with her pendulum while I was visiting. A Hispanic lady who lived nearby came in screaming hysterically that she'd lost her kid in the arroyo, which was a genuine emergency in that kind of terrain, where a toddler could get lost for a long time and possibly even die if not found in a hurry. My friend took out a topo map of the area and dowsed with her pendulum until it stopped abruptly over a certain point, and we all went out and found the kid at the exact spot it had indicated.

Ryan: This Rae machine is too far out for me!

Moskowitz: It's interesting how guarded we become in the defense of equally far-out truths that have become vested interests for us. The basic principles of homeopathy, the Law of Similars, the vital force, the single remedy, the infinitesimal dose, and the "Laws" of Cure are every bit as uncanny and strange to most people. One patient recently told me she had dreamed of four numbers in a certain order, which she remembered precisely because she was so unmathematical. A year later she had another dream that she was going to win the lottery, so the next day she played her four numbers and won $5,000. You can say whatever you like, but there has to be a reality out there of which we know very little. Several generations before Hahnemann, Swedenborg, the great polymath of his time, had a vision of Stockholm burning while he was hiking in the north of Sweden, hundreds of miles from the capital, noted the time, and duly recorded it in his journal. When he returned, he discovered that the city was indeed in flames at the very hour he had documented, a feat of telepathy for which he became famous all over Europe.

Though we know very little about paranormal phenomena, homeopaths have always been interested in them and even pioneered in their study. Hahnemann himself was fascinated with mesmerism, and in the 1920's Guy Beckley Stearns, a well-known classical homeopath, discovered the phenomenon and invented the diagnostic procedure we now know as kinesiology or muscle testing. At this point I have no difficulty imagining such a thing, but at no time when I've worked with a pendulum myself have I shown the slightest hint of any talent along that line. Maybe it's sour grapes, but I prefer my books and my computer.

I guess what I'm driving at is that the homeopathic point of view can also lead to fruitful deviations beyond the strict rules and limits of the classical method, like the Bach flower remedies. Although he began as a good homeopath, Bach eventually dropped out and became a saint, picking flowers and intuiting their healing properties directly, without any provings; and for some reason I have a certain trust both for what he found and the process by which he found it. But in doing so he also opened up a big can of worms. What do we do with the dozens of new remedies "discovered" by Guru Das and others? Whom can we trust, and on what basis? I can't give a formulaic answer about that for myself or anyone else. On the other hand, I've often asked myself why we have to go through the enormous hassle of choosing the perfect remedy when we could just as well use Bach flowers, which are much easier to find, simpler in their preparation, and more spiritual in their focus.

The answer for myself is that I love to study. I enjoy comparing and trying out different remedies them in a careful and painstaking manner. This method has sustained me in a fruitful practice for more than 25 years. Its principles are still valid today, in some ways maybe even more so than when Hahnemann first articulated them. But there's a lot of interesting stuff out there, like electro-diagnostic machines.

Ryan: I know nothing about this stuff, I'm like a virgin. [Laughter.]

Moskowitz: That's OK, too. I'm just fascinated by it, that's all. I would welcome a good electro-diagnostic practitioner in my office. I have lots of patients with a paucity of symptoms insufficient to arrive at a remedy, some of whom are grievously ill. As primitive as it may be, this stuff is or could be the laboratory of homeopathy. There's a lot of promise out there. The problem with all these techniques is that they require a good deal of skill on the part of the operator, that the operator is an important part of the circuit. But so does finding the *simillimum.* Go to any homeopathic meeting, and you're likely hear four or five remedies proposed that sound equally plausible for a patient. For myself, that's a big part of what makes what we do artful and exciting. When we get to the point of superior knowledge, where the choice of the remedy becomes cut and dried, with no more room for divergent interpretations, I fear I'll lose interest in it, again purely on aesthetic grounds, and probably take up some other line of work. I also revere homeopathy purely as an intellectual construction, but for me to go on practicing it requires a certain amount of uncertainty.

Ryan: How come this reverence of uncertainty?

Moskowitz: It boils down to how I keep nagging myself when I'm bumbling around with my patients, when I'm certain the right remedy could help them but I can't find it. Such is the luxurious folly I've just been talking about, which my patients also have to live with. It's exactly the same aesthetic criterion that first came up in medical school. Like all other healers, even the allopathic physicians we almost became, homeopaths perforce deal with patients, with particular individuals. Strictly speaking, there ain't no science of these either; that's my last bastion, and my last straw. To the extent that that ceases to be true, I guess I'll retire and write a novel or two before I pack it in.

Ryan: As if homeopathy were so cut and dried. . . .

Moskowitz: Right! As if we could even agree to practice in the same way! Don't hold your breath! Homeopaths are notoriously self-righteous because we feel we're in the possession of absolute, quasi-religious truth. Remember that homeopathy is also a philosophy, not just in the ordinary, loose sense of a general set of propositions about health and disease, but also in a more narrow, technical sense. We start with a few axioms that can't themselves be proven, but from which all else follows. If you accept these premises, homeopathy is indeed as absolute as mathematics. If we accept the vital force, the Law of Similars, and the totality of symptoms, then the single remedy, the *materia medica,* the minimum dose, and the Laws of Cure all follow as logically as the propositions of Euclidean geometry.

Right from the beginning, the homeopathic viewpoint has opened up a whole new world of ideas, of theoretical and practical possibilities, that do not necessarily agree with one another. In addition, it inspired a goodly number of deviants, like Rudolph Steiner, who started out as a homeopath but wasn't content until he became a prophet. His followers still think of themselves as homeopaths, but early on he jettisoned the idea of the single remedy. Although he was very influential in the history of the movement, I personally haven't much use for his medical teachings, because the yoga of the single remedy is the basis of the discipline that makes my study of remedies worthwhile.

So, yes, I'm a fundamentalist in respect of the single remedy, but not in the sense that I would kill or die for it, or excoriate others with different points of view. I practice as I do because it suits me, because it makes sense to me, but I'm not ready to ostracize those who think differently about such matters. Debate is healthy and desirable, and there's no reason to be afraid of it. I think it's a big mistake to try to define homeopathy too narrowly at this point, while it's growing and developing so rapidly. Even if we can't come together on the fine points of technique, we can and must do so on the ethics of how we relate to our patients, which we already agree about in large measure, but haven't articulated very well. It's also where we need to take a stand as part of the larger community of health professionals, to affirm the general moral standards that we are prepared to live by, and to punish the practices that discredit us all.

We also need a mechanism for adjudicating the tricky, gray areas, like when someone makes an appointment for a skeptical friend or relative in their absence, in the hope of giving remedies clandestinely. The need for discretion and the potential for abuse is that much greater in the case of radionic devices or electro-diagnostic machines, like the Vega. But from the old, classical method on down, they're all seductive to the extent that we feel we have the absolute truth, so that we all need to be especially careful about laying them on people without asking just because we think it will do them some good. I still remember a criminal prosecution against a lay homeopath for using a Vega machine on a reluctant patient with disastrous results.

As is often the case, what disgraced the profession had nothing to do with homeopathy *per se,* but only with a fanatical belief in the virtues of the therapy, which in her eyes took precedence over any need for a consensual relationship with her client. It's like those Cuban exiles and their right-wing Congressional allies, for whom the sacrament of American citizenship for a six-year-old boy trumped even the parental rights of his own father.

Ryan: Really, I'm pretty ignorant about these other practices, I've only studied with Paul Herscu and Vassilis Ghegas.

Moskowitz: I'll never forget the 1987 LIGA meeting in Washington, when the current President of the International League of Homeopathic Physicians had a tantrum worthy of a 3-year-old and walked out over some point of methodology, taking the entire French delegation with him, because he felt personally insulted by the disagreement. As a group, French homeopaths tend to use polypharmacy and take a keen interest in modern scientific research, which is fine. But their infantile posturing was something else again.

Another example was the recent putdown of Sankaran by Vithoulkas in much the same vein as Vithoulkas was himself was put down by Eizayaga and the French in days gone by. In America today we're still innocent about all this stuff. I've learned a lot from Vithoulkas, Sankaran, Eizayaga, and the lot of them: we're still babes in the wood, and we need and want to learn from everybody. You're too young to know this, but when I first got into homeopathy in 1974, it seemed almost moribund, and could easily have died out in a short time. Very few of my teachers were actually making their living by practicing it. They were either retired or saints who also accepted a few donations on the side, talking about something they no longer did very much, while the intermediate generation of active practitioners who should have been carrying the main teaching load were simply not there. There were no pharmacies or retail stores to send patients to, no teaching clinics, and no schools. It looked as if the whole business was going down the tubes, and fast.

In recent years there's been something of a revival, but to me, and perhaps to Bill Gray, Bob Schore, Dave Wember, and other veterans of that era, this more recent history still has an air of unreality about it much of the time, like some stock market bubble that is bound to come crashing down again. In a certain funny way I'm a bit ambivalent about the passing of that time, when homeopathy was so out to lunch, so far beyond the pale, that it required a special, quirky sort of mentality to be drawn to it. Now it's become so damned reasonable and sensible that I doubt you guys coming up today can appreciate what it meant to us.

Yet the mainstreaming of homeopathy has also changed it for the better in some ways. I was especially aware of this when I went to Cuba recently. Cuba was the first place I've been where the homeopaths are what I would call "real" or "straight" doctors, the kind who wear white lab coats, wholeheartedly believe in the goals and methods of medical science, and are pursuing their studies with the blessing and support of the government. In all these respects, they're already miles ahead of us. They're studying homeopathy not out of any alienation from the medical viewpoint, as is generally the case in North America, but simply because there are no cash reserves or other resources to buy the drugs and medical supplies they need. I feel fortunate to have been given the chance to teach them something, in spite of my own very different history; and I can tell you that they eagerly ate up every last morsel that we could offer them and digested them with relish. The fact that we could find common ground even under these circumstances also speaks well for the cogency and relevance of the basic homeopathic message for almost any modern audience, an experience that was at least as inspiring for us as for them.

*EPILOGUE: On Homeopathic Research**

I want to discuss the special problem of clinical and basic research, a major obstacle to the public acceptance of homeopathy in the past, which presents timely and useful lessons for the medical system of the future. In what follows, I will not concern myself with the "quackbusters," who never venture beyond their article of faith that homeopathy *can't possibly* work; the audience I aspire to is the literate public at large, who even if fair and open-minded may be inclined to judge it by the standards of valid knowledge about human health now prevailing, based on strict physico-chemical causality.

For those who regard homeopathy as out-and-out fraud, it is enough to show that our infinitesimal doses are capable of doing *something* not reproducible by suggestion alone, and a good deal of research of this type has already been done and repeatedly verified. In bioassays and physical experiments carried out on high dilutions over the past fifty years, French, German, British, and American scientists have shown, among other things, that

1) rats poisoned with arsenic or lead and treated with dilutions of *Arsenicum* or *Plumbum* excrete these toxins more rapidly than their untreated controls;[1,2]

2) various bacterial species exposed to increasingly dilute attenuations of *Cuprum sulph.* show repeating, sinusoidal patterns of enhanced growth, normal growth, and inhibited growth at regular intervals across a range of dilutions from 3C to 30C, with distinct periodicities for each organism;[3] and

3) when exposed to Raman lasers, ultradilute solutions of homeopathic remedies exhibit distinct spectroscopic patterns that are recognizably different from those of the solvent alone.[4]

* Epilogue, "On Homeopathic Research," ***Resonance: the Homeopathic Point of View,*** 2001, pp. 339-343.

For the general public, however, more clinical research is needed to document the effect of dilute remedies on human illness, while the favored double-blind model selects for a kind of forcible causation that can override the individual sensitivity of the patient and is thus wholly exceptional in normal human physiology, as well as often injurious to the gentler, more facultative influences that homeopathy seeks to provide.[5]

After truly heroic efforts to overcome these methodological obstacles and win support from the research community, several investigators have shown positive and statistically significant results from the use of classical homeopathy in controlled clinical trials, such as the following:

4) Jacobs and co-workers showed that Nicaraguan children with epidemic diarrhea and gastroenteritis recovered more rapidly on rehydration and homeopathic remedies classically chosen than on rehydration alone;[6]

5) Fisher, Taylor-Reilly, and colleagues in the UK found that adult patients with fibrositis, hay fever, and allergic asthma experienced greater and more sustained relief from homeopathy than from aspirin or placebo;[7,8,9] and

6) Dorfman and her French team proved that homeopathic medicines given late in pregnancy shortened labor and prevented dysfunctional patterns and both intrapartum and postpartum complications better and more consistently than placebo alone.[10]

Unfortunately, even when such studies are convincing, they require large study populations that are difficult to manage, and are unlikely to do justice to the clinical reality for several reasons:

7) because even the controls are interviewed homeopathically, and are therefore likely to show enhanced responses on the placebo side, while in allopathic studies the controls lack this advantage;

8) because the goal of successful homeopathic treatment is to promote self-healing, which is logically indistinguishable from the "placebo effect," and thus to enhance the unique, individualizing features of the patient in lieu of imposing a solution by force, as the double-blind model calls for;

9) because homeopathic criteria for improvement and worsening are based on the total symptom-picture, including subjective feelings, mood, and well-being,

and more global objective assessments like school attendance and job performance, not just narrowly technical standards like normal lab tests or the absence of particular symptoms, which is as far as double-blind tests need to or indeed can reliably go; and

10) because enforcing a rigid separation between the technical effect of the medicine and the healing power of the interview, the attitude of the patient, and other aspects of the treatment experience as a whole is so artificial and unnatural as to detract from the quality and value of that experience.

For all of these reasons, measuring the positive effects of homeopathic treatment by allopathic standards will tend to understate them to a significant extent, and achieving a greater accuracy will require the development of a more global standard, based on the totality of symptoms, which has been systematically excluded from the start.[11] Whereas double-blind trials are designed mainly to identify treatments powerful enough to compel a desired response of which the organism was not naturally capable, homeopathy and other holistic modalities are based on self-healing, on various attempts to stimulate, assist, and enhance whatever natural responses are already under way.[12]

Finally, I submit that the medical system is itself in dire need of broader, more permissive standards based on the totality of symptoms, because even positive double-blind studies must limit their findings to the specific technical variables the investigator seeks to control, leaving ambiguous and indeed unanswerable the decisive question of their overall effect on the energy, mood, vitality, and optimal functioning of the patient as a whole.[13] Therefore I offer the following very different research model, based on friendly rivalry or competition between pharmaceutical drugs or surgery, on the one hand, and treatment with classical homeopathy on the other, refereed by qualified and impartial judges mutually agreed upon beforehand, and conducted according to the following rules:

1) *nobody is blinded,* doubly or singly: all subjects know what form of treatment they will receive, having chosen it for themselves precisely because of their belief, interest in, or personal experience with it, and thus *maximizing* the placebo effect, rather than seeking to defeat or overpower it;

2) everybody in both groups receives the treatment they asked for, such that *nobody gets placebo,* and the treating physicians are similarly chosen and encouraged to use suggestion, shamanic incantation, or whatever else they feel will most effectively enhance it. In other words, *each group will serve as the control group of the other;*

3) *using the totality of symptoms over time,* including *lab tests, subjective and objective reports of patients, their families, friends, colleagues, teachers, employers, etc., as to how well or badly they are measuring up in their own lives, and according to the standards that they set for themselves or at least agree to be measured by, both groups of patients will be followed and evaluated for months or years,* to include not only the acute phase, but also the aftermath, including any sequelæ, and the chronic dimension in general; and

4) *the judges then determine which of the two groups comes out ahead in which respects,* and publish the results in a friendly, fair, and unbiased journal of good repute, to be agreed upon in advance.

The outcome of such experiments will thus simply be that the best of both methods will be made freely available to all those who want them, which is all that I have ever argued or hoped for. Classical homeopathy requires too much time, skill, and knowledge, and the number of skilled practitioners is at present far too small, to replace the prevailing method of controlling and managing chronic illness on a large scale in the foreseeable future. At present, and under these circumstances, its most enduring contributions to the medical profession may well be its coherent model of health and illness, its distinctive conception of medicinal substances, its excellent track record in treating the acute diseases of everyday practice, and its humanistic style of doctoring, all of which fit our ordinary experience of illness much more closely than the prevailing model of separate disease entities, each requiring separate diagnosis and treatment. In the spirit of mutual co-operation, and for the sake of a health care system that is accessible to everyone, I offer this vision of the homeopathic point of view, which merits an honored place in an integrated healing profession of the future.

NOTES.

1. Cazin, J., et al., "A Study of the Effect of Dilutions of Arsenic on the Retention and Mobilization of Arsenic in the Rat," *Human Toxicology* 6:315, 1987.
2. Fisher, P., "The Influence of the Homeopathic Remedy *Plumbum met.* on the Excretion Kinetics of Lead in the Rat," *Human Toxicology* 6:321, 1987.
3. Noiret, P., "Activity of Several Dilutions of Copper Sulfate in Different Microbial Species," *Proceedings,* 31st Congress of the International Homeopathic Medical league, 1976, pp. 137-147.
4. Boiron, J., Studies of the Physical Structure of Homeopathic Dilutions Utilizing the Raman Laser Effect," ibid., pp. 459-474.
5. Cf. Moskowitz, R., "Some Thoughts on the Malpractice Crisis," *British Homeopathic Journal* 77:17, 1988.
6. Jacobs, J., et al., "Treatment of Childhood Diarrhea with Homeopathic Medicine: a Randomized Clinical Trial in Nicaragua," *Pediatrics* 93:719, 1994.
7. Fisher, P., et al., "Effect of Homeopathic Treatment on Fibrositis," *British Medical Journal* 299:365, 1989.
8. Taylor-Reilly, D., et al., "Is Homeopathy a Placebo Response? Controlled Trial of a Homeopathic Potency, with Hay Fever Pollen as Model," *Lancet* 328:881, 1986.
9. Taylor-Reilly, et al., "Is the Evidence of Homeopathy Reproducible?" *Lancet* 344:1601, 1994.
10. Dorfman, P., et al., "Preparation for Childbirth by Homeopathy," *Cahiers de Biothérapie* 94:77, 1987.
11. Cf. Moskowitz, op. cit., 1988.
12. Cf. Moskowitz, "Who Needs the American Institute of Homeopathy?" *Journal of the AIH* 87:193, 1994.
13. Ibid.

*APPENDIX: Historical Development**

Hahnemann's Achievement and Legacy.

In spite of his distinguished reputation as physician, chemist, and authority on the preparation of medicinal substances, Hahnemann's unorthodox claims and discoveries were greeted with silence by most of his colleagues, and aroused particularly active opposition amongst the local apothecaries, whose livelihood seemed directly threatened by his insistence on physicians using single remedies and preparing them themselves.[1] Even after his success in treating epidemic diseases won him a lectureship and made him famous throughout Europe, he continued to be ridiculed and persecuted for his heresies, although in 1822 a wealthy patron finally gave him shelter and a comfortable stipend to publish his writings.[2] In addition to the *Organon of Medicine,* his original text, which ran to six editions, and the *Materia Medica Pura* and *Chronic Diseases,* his other major works, he wrote a host of technical articles and monographs, maintained a voluminous correspondence, and continued to teach, practice, and conduct experimental research until the end of his life.

Late in life, many years after the death of his first wife, he married a young Frenchwoman and moved with her to Paris, where he enjoyed wealth and celebrity in his final years and died secure in the knowledge that his students and followers were practicing quality homeopathy in most countries of Europe and in the New World. Over fifty years after his death, his body was exhumed, brought back to Paris, and laid to rest in the Père Lachaise, crowned by his own epitaph, *Non inutilis vixi,* "I have not lived in vain." Gifted by intellect and driven by ambition, he left behind a philosophy, methodology, and body of work that have stood the test of time, such that today, two hundred and fifty years after his birth, even his

* Appendix, "Historical Development," ***Resonance: the Homeopathic Point of View,*** 2001, pp. 345-358.

most illustrious successors are still content merely to add to our knowledge of the subject whose outlines he so clearly and thoroughly delineated.

At the same time, his autocratic style and imperious temper alienated many promising students, and engendered a plethora of opposing factions and interpretations, each claiming inspiration and legitimate descent from his own all-encompassing viewpoint. Modern polemics against "mongrels" clinging to allopathic philosophy, "pluralists" using several remedies simultaneously, and "pathological prescribers" advocating the lower dilutions to treat the disease rather than the patient all originated with diatribes emanating from the pen of the master himself.[3]

Defending homeopathy as sacred, revealed truth, Hahnemann and his chief disciples were, as many still remain, harshly intolerant of all who even appeared to deviate from his vision, creating a sectarian mentality that has always invited persecution, and a tradition of ideological warfare that continues to divide the movement through both success and decline.

Homeopathy in the United States.

Several factors contributed to the rapid growth and development of American homeopathy in the middle and late nineteenth century, when the United States became the epicenter of the movement and produced some of its greatest masters, whose works are still used throughout the world today.

The first was simply the youth of the country, the absence of laws or bureaucracy licensing and regulating the practice of medicine, and a more tolerant, "live-and-let-live" attitude born of the general yearning to break free from the oppressive economic, social, and political constraints of the Old World. In the 1830's, when the first school of homeopathy opened in Pennsylvania, American physicians were organized on a voluntary basis, and most state legislatures were reluctant to favor or discriminate against any faction or ideology, or to prevent uneducated or lay healers from helping anyone who requested their services.[4]

The second was the great westward migration of those seeking land, so that untrained lay people were obliged to take care of themselves and their families, friends, and animals in times of need. Under frontier conditions, the special affinity of homeopathy for the ordinary language and experience of the patient was ideally suited to educate the public in basic self-care, and popular manuals of first aid for homeopathic treatment of injuries and common domestic ailments appeared almost immediately.[5]

The third was the distinctive concept of the *materia medica,* which gave both physicians and laypeople a critical methodology for learning about their own folk traditions, as well as the indigenous remedies they were hearing about or found ready-to-hand. Introducing dozens of Native American herbs into the pharmacopœia, American homeopaths both learned from and added to the botanical lore of midwives and medicine men, eclectics, Thomsonians, and native herbalists, most of whom were self-taught, and many of whose recipes are still in use today.[6]

In these primitive circumstances, homeopathy grew and prospered in the United States as never before, creating its own medical schools, hospitals, and insane asylums, enjoying broad popularity, and recording notable victories against major diseases attracting public attention.[7] In epidemics of cholera, typhus, scarlet fever, and the like, pure homeopathic treatment repeatedly proved its superiority over the more drastic methods then in vogue,[8] and physicians adhering to the classical principles often rose to social prominence, treating many of the rich and famous of the time, including writers, intellectuals, industrialists, and even Presidents and Cabinet ministers.[9]

Yet the so-called "Golden Age" of American homeopathy in the late Nineteenth Century was also to a great extent a fiction, created by the large majority of practitioners who practiced in its name but knew little of its fundamentals, as well as the eclectic and often unprincipled schools that trained them.[10] By the turn of the century, although between 10 and 15% of all physicians used homeopathic remedies to some extent in their practices, the great majority of them were ignorant or even contemptuous of the totality of symptoms, the single remedy, the minimum dose, and in some cases the Law of Similars itself, having been trained to use specific remedies for particular diseases in the allopathic mode.[11]

Meanwhile, the tremendous expansion of American industry during and after the Civil War generated new pressures and influences that utterly transformed the nature of medical practice within a few decades. As successive waves of mass immigration inundated city and country alike, the long, detailed interviews and immaterial doses of hand-made remedies began to seem like old-fashioned luxuries that few could still afford, and could not keep up with the more streamlined, high-volume approach of the "regulars," utilizing mass-produced chemicals and the assembly-line efficiency of the Machine Age.[12]

At the same time, modern experimental science based on strict physicochemical causality was producing impressive technical achievements like antisepsis, anesthesia, and modern surgery, which in turn engendered the new sciences of microbiology, vaccines, antibiotics, and the detailed anatomy, physiology, and biochemistry of the human body, and inexorably led in our own day to bio-technology and the deciphering of the genetic code.

In contrast, using nothing but infinitesimal doses at rare intervals, with only their fundamentalist principles and laborious methodology to sustain them, the relatively small number of American homeopaths adhering to classical principles never succeeded in generating a large or profitable industrial base capable of financing educational, research, or training institutions on a national scale, while the vast majority of their less scrupulous colleagues found it increasingly difficult to resist the lure of success or the excitement of power when the AMA opened its doors to them after 1900.[13]

Although the AMA was formed in 1847 specifically to combat the spread of homeopathy and other kindred heresies, and the various state medical societies had excluded homeopaths for many decades and forbidden its members to consult or fraternize with them,[14] such persecutions had little effect until the end of the century, when state legislatures undertook to license physicians and accredit medical schools, and the "regulars," backed by the money and power of the pharmaceutical industry, won control of the process.[15] By inviting homeopaths, eclectics, and botanical physicians to become members and obtain licensure, the AMA attempted to create a unified medical profession as in effect a guild monopoly against competition from lay healers, midwives, and herbalists.

In 1914, with the publication of the Flexner Report, it duly proposed a uniform standard of medical education for all licensed physicians, based on the latest research and laboratory facilities and a permanent clinical faculty, using its power of accreditation to phase out the homeopathic colleges that failed to meet these standards and adhered to the older apprenticeship model.[16]

On both fronts, the AMA strategy was completely successful. By the 1920's, all of the homeopathic schools had either closed down or converted to the new guidelines, such that homeopathy was demoted to a postgraduate specialty for the increasingly few physicians who were prepared to swim against the tide of four years of allopathic indoctrination. Apart from the small cadre of devoted physicians who continued to practice quality homeopathy, the movement as a whole declined rapidly over the next forty years, until by the early 1970's it seemed quite moribund, with its best teachers either dead or semi-retired, few new physicians being trained, and the one or two generations in between simply missing.[17]

Against all odds, American homeopathy has begun to flourish yet again in the past twenty years or so, thanks largely to the crisis of our misnamed "health-care system," the rebirth of the self-care movement, and what Ivan Illich called the increasing "medicalization" of life that has inspired them.[18] By successfully persecuting and eliminating lay healers of every stripe, and by aspiring to control every identifiable aspect of the life process using purely technical means,[19] American medicine has itself become an industrial colossus of Gargantuan proportions, thriving on high-cost, high-tech, high-risk solutions, generating more iatrogenic illness,[20] and consuming a far greater share of GNP than anywhere else in the world.[21] Facing interrelated crises in health insurance, malpractice litigation, and the doctor-patient relationship,[22] the public and even the medical profession itself have increasingly been drawn to acupuncture, homeopathy, chiropractic, and other more holistic alternatives.[23]

With world-class homeopaths like Vithoulkas, Sankaran, Scholten, and Mangialavori now teaching or having taught in the United States, their students have reintroduced homeopathy into family medicine as a workable, patient-centered model for primary care. Notably inexpensive, safe, and effective enough to sustain busy practices even without third-party reimbursement, classical homeopathy has become increasingly popular with the new crop of family physicians, whose instant waiting lists attest to the huge and still growing demand for their services.

Finally, the method has also proven a godsend to nurses, nurse-practitioners, and physician-assistants as a vehicle for their own increasingly independent and free-standing practices, and also to midwives, naturopaths, osteopaths, acupuncturists, chiropractors, psychologists, and social workers, as an added service that they can provide. Yet not far beneath these optimistic signs looms the serious and mounting crisis in the maldistribution of health care, and especially in the health-insurance industry, whose poor or at best uneven record of reimbursement for homeopathic care augurs trouble and conflict for the future.

Much as in frontier days, the resurgence of American homeopathy today could not have happened without the efforts of dedicated lay people, first in using remedies for their own self-care, then in organizing study groups in their communities and teaching their friends and neighbors. While the infrastructure they helped build now supports the practices of physicians, nurses, and other licensed health professionals, as above, more than a few of these talented and dedicated amateurs have become professional educators, counselors, and practitioners in their own right, at all levels of proficiency, and with no laws either to protect or regulate them.

At the retail level, both the expanding self-care market and the publication of new texts for the lay public[24] have helped to make single remedies profitable for the first time and more widely available in health-food stores, food co-ops, herb and natural cosmetic shops, and even in regular pharmacies all over the country.

Unfortunately, the same economic forces have emboldened some manufacturers to produce and market ostensibly homeopathic combinations with exaggerated or outlandish claims, even for serious chronic diseases, and often containing substances not included in the Pharmacopœia, or not prepared in conformity with its standards, with no effective policing or enforcement mechanism within the industry itself.[25] In short, the exponential growth of American homeopathy in recent years has exposed the need and created the opportunity to resolve many of the same problems and difficulties that weakened it in the past.

Homeopathy Abroad.

At present, homeopathy is practiced by physicians and licensed health professionals all over the world, especially in Europe, the Americas, the British Commonwealth, and the Indian subcontinent. In the UK, where it has been sponsored by the Royal Family for a hundred and fifty years, it is practiced by family physicians using an admixture of conventional drugs within the National Health Service, and also by registered lay homeopaths completing a four-year course, according to the time-honored British custom of self-healing without government or medical interference. Similar medical and non-medical options are available in Canada, Australia, New Zealand, South Africa, and other present or former countries of the British Commonwealth with strong traditions of self-care.

On the European continent, homeopathy is practiced mainly by licensed physicians and naturopaths, as in parts of the U. S., and also certified lay or folk healers in some places, notably Germany. In most countries of the European Union, homeopathic remedies are available for sale in many pharmacies, and homeopathy is frequently taught as an elective course in medical schools, where it enjoys a certain scientific standing and has prompted advanced research in biophysics, chemistry, and various biomedical sciences.[26] With practically universal health coverage and popular, efficient systems for delivering it, most Western Europeans enjoy unrestricted access to homeopathic medicine, albeit commonly sanitized to varying degrees with low dilutions, polypharmacy, and liberal helpings of antibiotics, hormones, and other pharmaceutical drugs, as in Britain.

In Greece, homeopathy dates mainly from the 1970's, with the opening of the top-rated Vithoulkas graduate school for licensed physicians exclusively. Under the protection of the Greek government, classical homeopathy is now practiced everywhere in the country, including hospitals and medical schools. In the former Soviet bloc, where state and party bureaucracies had done nothing to support and in some cases actively discouraged it, the use of homeopathic remedies has made significant gains since the fall of Communism, most notably in Russia, the Ukraine, Poland, Hungary, Rumania, and the Czech Republic, more or less on the continental model, and often with the help of established Western teachers.

In Latin America, homeopathy has been widely taught and practiced since the late 1800's, emanating from the main teaching centers in Mexico, Argentina, and Brazil. In Mexico, as in the United States a century ago, it grew up with and has also contributed to the study of indigenous plants and folk healers and remedies. Popular with Mexicans of all classes, homeopathy is practiced mainly by licensed physicians and enjoys a relatively high social standing, with varying admixtures of allopathic drugs and procedures, much as in Europe. The same is true in Argentina and Brazil, where distinctive national styles have been developing for generations, and qualified practitioners enjoy more or less cordial relationships with non-homeopathic colleagues. In general, despite widespread economic hardship and political unrest, the future of homeopathy throughout Central and South America seems quite stable, promising, and secure.

In the last half-century or so, India has become the world capital of homeopathy, both in regard to the large number of physicians practicing it, an in its collective influence on the culture. Widely practiced in hospitals and taught in medical schools, it has also engendered a vast network of dispensaries and infirmaries staffed by trained homeopaths under medical supervision, which bring affordable health care to millions of people in dire need. In Muslim Pakistan and Bangladesh, and even in war-torn Sri Lanka, the homeopathic tradition is equally popular and serves analogous functions.

Now both recognized and supported by the Indian government, homeopathy also admirably complements the ancient Ayurvedic system, with its own indigenous pharmacopoeia of over a thousand traditional remedies, many still awaiting provings to ascertain their full therapeutic range.

With their unparalleled experience in treating the gravely and critically ill, Indian homeopaths have successfully weaned patients from renal dialysis and intractable congestive heart failure, as well as palliating or curing others with metastatic cancer, life-threatening blood dyscrasias, multiple sclerosis, and other degenerative diseases widely regarded as incurable.[27] Its intermediate position between modern Western medicine, likewise highly esteemed in India, and its ancient traditions of religious and folk healing has facilitated communication and cross-fertilization between these often divergent and seemingly incompatible points of view.

Non-Classical Methods.

Progressive and forward-looking in its philosophy, homeopathy offers not only a strict methodology, but also a radically new way of looking at health and illness, which has in turn inspired a large number and wide variety of experimental and clinical techniques, by no means all of them obedient to the totality of symptoms, the single remedy, the minimum dose, and other Hahnemannian principles.

As we saw, some of the most important deviations first appeared in the master's own lifetime and drew scathing criticism from him, especially the practice of using more than one remedy at a time, usually in the lowest dilutions, and routinely for specific diseases and complaints, all of which still flourish today in the mixed practices of many part-time homeopaths and the combination remedies available for self-care in every health food store.

Later in the Nineteenth Century, loyal Hahnemannians stoutly opposed the pathological prescribing of Dr. Richard Hughes and his followers in England, who emphasized the physiological properties of the lower dilutions and tended to discount the importance of mental and emotional symptoms altogether.[28] Hughes' more medically-oriented style nevertheless exercised considerable influence over many good classical prescribers in England and America, such as the great Compton-Burnett, who not infrequently prescribed organ-specific remedies concurrently with remedies based on the totality of symptoms.[29]

Still very popular in Europe and Latin America today, especially in cases involving serious organic pathology, the organopathic approach is ably represented by the elaborate method of Dr. Francisco Eizayaga, for example, who gives only one remedy at a time, but first in a low dilution, from a limited totality based on the pathological diagnosis, before proceeding to higher dilutions based on more classical or "constitutional" criteria.[30] In the same low-potency or physiological tradition, Schuessler used twelve of the mineral remedies, called "tissue salts," to treat *all* illnesses,[31] thus dispensing entirely with the rest of the *materia medica,* whose size and diversity do indeed bedevil any who would master it, but also provide its incomparable richness and glory.

At the end of the Nineteenth Century, the Austrian philosopher and polymath Dr. Rudolph Steiner (1861-1925), the creator of Waldorf education, biodynamic agriculture, and eurhythmics, developed an elaborate method of prescribing homeopathically-prepared combination remedies on partly esoteric and spiritual indications, revealed to him by direct intuition in most cases.[32] Proclaiming his elegant, almost poetic system as a kind of perfected homeopathy, Steiner and the "anthroposophical" physicians who still use it have always professed to be homeopaths in spite of choosing not to follow Hahnemannian principles, thus raising anew the vexatious question of how to define the method, over which much ink and bile continue to be spilled.

On the other hand, the deeply humanistic and spiritual emphasis of anthroposophy have strongly influenced modern classical homeopaths as well, from Wheeler and Twentyman in England to Elizabeth Wright-Hubbard, Edward Whitmont, Henry Williams, and their lineage in America. As a further dimension for understanding the relationships between groups of remedies in the natural world, it has also helped lay the foundations for the important work of Scholten, Sankaran, and Mangialavori on the general characteristics of mineral, plant, and animal remedies, which have already been discussed in the text.

An even more radical yet less contentious departure from the classical method, the Bach flower remedies have become popular and widely available for self-care throughout the world. Trained as a pathologist, Edward Bach, M.D. (1886-1936), began his tragically short career as a homeopath, doing pioneering work on the intestinal flora, as "nosodes," or pathological remedies in their own right.[33] Not long afterward, he closed his practice and became a saintly pilgrim, wandering the English countryside, literally smelling the flowers to which he was mystically drawn, intuiting their healing properties, and using them to help the sick he encountered along the way.[34]

Focusing mainly on the psychospiritual properties of these "flower remedies," he also developed a simple and elegant method of preparing them, by simply floating the petals in water and setting them out in the sun to "potentize" them, thus avoiding the laborious process of homeopathic dynamization, just as his beautifully poetic descriptions distilled the totality of symptoms into a purely spiritual whole.[35] Because his flower essences appeared to work primarily in the ethereal realm, without obvious intereference to or from other medicines, whether homeopathic or otherwise, he felt justified in disregarding not only the physical symptoms but also the principle of the single remedy, and began giving the indicated remedy or remedies as often as desired, even indefinitely.[36]

With documented and at times truly remarkable success, even in severe or allegedly incurable diseases, these remedies and the simplified method for preparing and selecting them should challenge all good homeopaths to ask themselves why they adhere to the elaborate rigamarole of dilution and succussion, choosing one remedy according to the totality of symptoms, and giving it as infrequently as possible. Speaking for myself, I enjoy learning about remedies through study, not only to train and correct my intuition, but also for its own sake, for the sheer pleasure of doing so. Even more important, I am reluctant to stipulate in advance that only the emotional or psycho-spiritual aspects of the case need to be considered, important though they so often are. Laborious as it is, I still prefer the classical discipline of recording all the symptoms, physical, mental, and emotional, just as I find them, i. e., typically mixed up together. But it is always a fair and relevant question, which others might answer differently.

Now that Bach's flower-essence concept and methodology are being applied wholesale to many other plants by various newcomers claiming his mantle,[37] neither the purity of Bach's life nor the simplicity of his experiments is sufficient to bless or validate the efforts of his imitators, which will need to be evaluated objectively and scientifically like all other such claims, including those of homeopathy itself.

In like manner, the partly esoteric realm presupposed, envisioned, and exemplified by homeopathy has given rise to a long history of technical and quasi-scientific innovations, from Hahnemann's early experiments with dilution and succussion to a variety of mechanical "potentizing" devices that were patented and used by his successors in the Nineteenth Century, and including several generations of as yet poorly authenticated, futuristic technology in our own time.

Ever since the early 1900's, a small number of investigators have sought to develop experimental methods for detecting, measuring, and harnessing the "vital force" or life energy that underlies not only homeopathy, but all other varieties of holistic healing as well. Designed to measure bioelectric potentials on the body surface, both the original Abrams machine and the later Boyd Emanometer were early versions of the electrodiagnostic machines used by clinicians of today to identify and assesss deep pathological conditions for which elaborate symptomatology is lacking, such as advanced cancer and various degenerative diseases.[38] Such forerunners of what I like to call "experimental homeopathy" have also helped to explore and open up the vast, uncharted territory that is now being touted and appropriated as the brand-new field of "energy medicine."[39]

Building on the work of Reinhard Voll in the 1940's, sophisticated mapping devices give electronic readings at various acupuncture points that their proponents claim can provide accurate diagnoses of deeper levels of etheric or "subtle-body" energies by utilizing the enormous database of traditional Chinese and Japanese medicine.[40] Although admirable for the ingenuity of their design and the vast range of phenomena they encompass, and at times capable of uncanny accuracy on a par with that of the greatest Oriental masters, these electrodiagnostic machines still require a degree of intuitive skill and sensitivity on the part of the operator that limits their usefulness and undercuts their claim to measuring something objective that exists independently of the process.

An important area of bioenergetic research dating from Hahnemann himself is the phenomenon of magnetism, associated in his time with the charismatic spiritualism of Pierre Mesmer and the long tradition of religious healing, including the "laying on of hands." In the final paragraphs of the *Organon,* Hahnemann proposed a careful investigation of mesmerism and other forms of "animal magnetism" as a scientific phenomenon,[41] and he and his followers later developed a whole new group of remedies he called the *imponderabilia,* by exposing vials of alcohol to physical forces and non-material energies such as sunlight, moonlight, electricity, and the north and south poles of a magnet, and then diluting and succussing them in the usual way.[42] Ever since the discovery of X-Rays in the 1890's, homeopaths have valued and used this form of radiation as a remedy, based on extensive provings.[43]

In the 1920's, Guy Beckley Stearns, a top-notch classical homeopath with a strong interest in physics, devised a subtle test of the correctness of the seemingly-indicated remedy by its measurable effect on the pulse and various reflexes when simply held in the hand, one of the earliest known instances of kinesiology.[44] In related attempts to make use of the electromagnetic field emanating from all living organisms, a hand-held pendulum has been used by many psychically-gifted homeopaths to dowse for the correct remedy, like a divining rod for locating the ground water before digging a well.

Still further down this slippery slope, more complex radionic devices claim to prepare homeopathic remedies wholly "etherically," based on their distinctive magnetic interference patterns, without using the parent chemical substances at all.[45] Although lacking the talent or inclination to use such techniques myself, I have learned from personal experience not to dismiss or ridicule them either, since I have actually witnessed remedies so chosen and prepared on the spot work effectively in labor, for example, when my own learned prescriptions had utterly failed to do so. Since classical homeopathy already lives on both sides of the frontier separating immaterial doses from the "real world" of chemistry, atoms, and molecules, the more ethereal realms of clairvoyance, telepathy, radionics, faith healing, and the like should pose no insuperable obstacles to anyone who has stayed with me this far!

The neatest and most repeatable demonstration of the vital force to date is the technique of Kirlian "photography," devised many years ago by a Russian scientist with a homeopathic background, which provides eerily beautiful images of the "aura" or bioenergetic field emanating from and surrounding all living tissue,[46] and could well become a useful instrument of diagnosis and treatment alike, even in the modern, quantitative sense.

Partly because of these explorations, the definition of homeopathy has never been agreed upon by all those who study and practice under the vast umbrella that its name has come to provide. Ever since the time of Hahnemann, a bewildering array of adaptations and modifications have arisen to claim descent from some aspect of his work, with many of them still at odds to the point of keeping the family divided, unwilling and unable to accept, give allegiance to, or even try to articulate the common ground of what we all believe. As a bioenergetic science still in its infancy, it is still growing and evolving so rapidly that it may even be an enormous mistake to try to define it too rigidly or exclusively at this point, much less to be willing to kill or die for such a purely doctrinal cause.[47]

I have presented homeopathy from the classical or Hahnemannian point of view for the same reason that I have chosen to practice in accordance with it, because it is elegant and beautiful as it stands, and even the formidable challenge of learning to use it with skill only adds depth to its vision. But I have never claimed for it any monopoly on the truth or the healing process, or any exemption from the basic human need to grow and learn from one another.

NOTES.

1. Bradford, T. L., *Life and Letters of Hahnemann,* Boericke & Tafel, 1895, pp. 113-116.
2. Ibid., pp. 120-134.
3. Ibid., pp. 300-302.
4. Starr, P., *The Transformation of American Medicine,* Basic, 1982, pp. 30-59.
5. Hering, C., *The Domestic Physician,* 1844, still the classic of the genre.
6. Hale, E. M., *Materia Medica of the New Remedies,* 1867.
7. Coulter, H., *Divided Legacy,* vol. 3, 1974, pp. 285-316.
8. Bradford, *The Logic of Figures,* 1900, pp. 141-145, *passim.*
9. Coulter, op. cit., 1974, pp. 140-238.
10. Cook, D., and Naudé, A., "The Ascendance and Decline of Homeopathy in America, *Journal of the AIH* 89:125, 1996.
11. Ibid.
12. Winston, J., *The Faces of Homeopathy,* Great Auk, NZ, 1999, pp. 214-215.
13. Starr, op. cit., 1982, pp. 99-123.
14. Coulter, op. cit., 1974, pp. 140-238.
15. Starr, op. cit., 1982, pp. 99-123.
16. Ibid.
17. Kaufman, M., *Homeopathy in America,* Johns Hopkins, 1971.
18. Illich, I., *Medical Nemesis,* Pantheon, 1976, p. 39ff.
19. Moskowitz, R., "Some Thoughts on the Malpractice Crisis," *British Homeopathic Journal* 77:17, 1988.
20. Steel, K., et al., "Iatrogenic Illness on a General Medical Service at a University Hospital," *New England Journal of Medicine* 304:638, 1981.
21. Starr, *The Logic of Health Care Reform,* Grand Rounds, 1992, pp. 16-19.
22. Moskowitz, 1988, op. cit.
23. Eisenberg, D., et al., "Unconventional Medicine in the United States, *New England Journal of Medicine* 328:246, 1993.
24. Lockie and Geddes, *Complete Guide to Homeopathy,* DK, 1995, and Jonas and Jacobs, *Healing with Homeopathy*, Warner, 1996.
25. Moskowitz, "Ethics in Homeopathic Practice," *Journal of the AIH* 86:238, 1993.
26. Resch, G., "Physical Chemistry of Highly-Attenuated Remedies," *Proceedings,* 42nd Congress, International Homeopathic Medical League, Washington, 1987, pp. 300-304; Davenas, E., et al., "Human Basophil Degranulation Triggered by Very Dilute Antiserum against IgE," *Nature* 333:816, 1988; Resch and Gutmann, *Scientific Foundations of Homeopathy,* Barthel & Barthel, Germany, 1987; and Bellavite, P., and Signorini, A., *Homeopathy: a Frontier in Medical Science,* North Atlantic, Berkeley, 1995.
27. Chand, D. H., "Clinical Cases," and Ramakrishnan, A. U., 'Experience with Hemorrhagic Disorders in Homeopathy," *Proceedings,* 1987, 42nd LIGA Congress, 1987, op. cit., pp. 191-206.

28. Hughes, R., *Principles and Practice of Homeopathy,* Leath & Ross, 1902.
29. Compton-Burnett, J., *Curability of Tumours by Medicines,* Boericke & Tafel, 1901.
30. Eizayaga, F. X., *Treatise on Homeopathic Medicine,* Marecel, 1991, pp. 211-220.
31. Boericke and Dewey, *The Twelve Tissue Remedies*, Boericke & Tafel, 1920.
32. Steiner, R., *Four Lectures to Doctors,* Anthroposophical Press, 1928; Bott, V., *Anthroposophical Medicine,* Thorsons, 1984; and Glas, N., *Conception, Birth, and Early Childhood,* Anthroposophical Press, 1972.
33. Bach, E., and Wheeler, C., *Chronic Disease,* 1926.
34. Weeks, N., *The Medical Discoveries of Edward Bach,* Daniel, 1950.
35. Bach, *Heal Thyself* and *The Twelve Little Healers,* Daniel, 1931, 1933.
36. Ibid.
37. Gurudas, *Flower Essences and Vibrational Healing,* Brotherhood of Life, 1983.
38. Bellavite and Signorini, *Homeopathy: a Frontier in Medical Science,* North Atlantic, 1995.
39. Gerber, R., *Vibrational Healing,* Bear Press, 1988.
40. Voll, R., "Twenty Years of Electroacupuncture," *American Journal of Acupuncture,* March and December, 1975.
41. Hahnemann, *Organon,* Aphorisms 286-290.
42. Allen, H. C., *Materia Medica of the Nosodes,* Boericke & Tafel, 1910, "Electricity," pp. 41-48, and "The Magnet," pp. 206-256.
43. Ibid., "Provings of the X-Ray," pp. 552-583.
44. Stearns, G. B., "Body Reflexes as a Means of Selecting a Remedy," *Homeopathic Recorder* 47:781, 1932.
45. Tansley, D., *Radionics: Science or Magic?* Daniel, 1982.
46. Moskowitz, op. cit., 1993.

Bibliography

Books.

1. ***Homeopathic Medicines for Pregnancy and Childbirth,*** 288 pp., Index, North Atlantic, Berkeley, 1992; German version, ***Homöopathie für Schwangerschaft und Geburtshilfe,*** Haug, Heidelberg, 1998.
2. ***Resonance: The Homeopathic Point of View,*** 372 pp., with Epilogue & Appendix, Xlibris, Philadelphia, 2001; German version, ***Das Resonanzgesetz der Heilung,*** Kai Kröger Verlag, Groß Wittensee, 2012.
3. ***Plain Doctoring: Selected Writings, 1983-2013,*** 397 pp., with Bibliography, CreateSpace, Charleston, SC, 2013.
4. ***More Doctoring: Selected Writings,*** Volume 2, 1977-2014, CreateSpace, 2014.

Articles.

1. "Drug Reactions and Biological Individuality," ***Homeotherapy*** 3:1, August 1977.
2. "When *Not* to Give a Remedy," ***Journal of the AIH*** 73:11, March 1980.
3. "Homeopathic Remedies vs. the Placebo Effect," ***Homeotherapy*** 6:99, July-August 1980.
4. "Homeopathic Reasoning," Lecture to Symposium, "Homeopathy: the Renaissance of Cure, San Francisco, April 1980; published in ***Homeotherapy*** 6:135, September 1980.
5. "Two Obstetrical Remedies," ***Homeopathy Today,*** July 1981.
6. "Homeopathic Remedies in Pregnancy and Childbirth," ***Homeopathy Today,*** January 1983.
7. "*Magnesia Phosphorica,*" ***Homeopathy Today,*** February 1983.
8. "The Case Against Immunizations," ***Journal of the AIH*** 76:7, March 1983; reprinted as NCH and UK Society of Homœpaths pamphlets; included in Robert Mendelsohn, ed., ***Dissent in Medicine,*** Contemporary Books, Chicago, 1985.

9. Vague, Long-Term Diagnosis: the *Nocebo* Effect," ***Journal of the AIH*** 76:26, March 1983.
10. "Peculiar and Characteristic Symptoms," ***Homeopathy Today,*** April 1983.
11. "Postscript on Immunizations," ***Journal of the AIH*** 76:101, September 1983.
12. "Unvaccinated Kids: What's Next for Them (and Us)?" ***Mothering*** Magazine, January 1987.
13. "AIDS: Chronic Immune Failure," ***Resonance*** (Journal of the International Foundation for Homeopathy), January 1988.
14. "Some Thoughts on the Malpractice Crisis," ***British Homœopathic Journal*** 77:17, January 1988; reprinted in ***Journal of the AIH*** 81:22, March 1988, and ***The Homœopath*** (Journal of the UK Society of Homeopaths), September 1992.
15. "What Is Homeopathy?" in Robin Larsen, ed., ***Emanuel Swedenborg: a Continuing Vision,*** Swedenborg Foundation, New York, 1988, p. 475.
16. "Is There More than One Correct Remedy?" ***Resonance***, January 1989.
17. "More on *Similia Similibus Curentur,*" ***Journal of the AIH*** 82:22, March 1989.
18. "Hospital Ethics Committees: the Healing Function," ***HEC Forum*** 1:309, January 1990; reprinted in Stuart Spicker, ed., ***The Hospital Ethics Committee Experience,*** Kluwer, 1998.
19. "Options in Homeopathic Self-Care," ***EastWest Journal,*** January 1990.
20. "Two Childbirth Remedies," ***Journal of the AIH*** 83:72, September 1990; reprinted in ***British Homœopathic Journal*** 79:206, October 1990; German version, ***Zeitschrift für Klassische Homöopathie,*** 1991.
21. "Whose Life Is It, Anyway? Some Thoughts about the Doctor-Patient Relationship," ***Chrysalis*** (Journal of the Swedenborg Foundation) 6:103, Summer 1991.
22. "Vaccination: a Sacrament of Modern Medicine," lecture to the Society of Homeopaths Annual Conference, 1991; published in ***Journal of the AIH*** 84:96, December 1991; reprinted in ***The Homœopath*** 12:137, March 1992.

23. "Ethics in Homeopathic Practice," lecture to the AIH Conference, 1993; published in *Journal of the AIH* 86:238, December 1993.
24. "Vaccinations," in Barbara Katz Rothman, ed., ***Encyclopedia of Childbearing,*** Oryx Press, Phoenix, AZ, 1993.
25. "Childhood Ear Infections," lecture to the AIH Conference, 1994; published in *Journal of the AIH* 87:137, Autumn 1994; reprinted in *The Homœopath*, 1994.
26. "Homeopathy," with Jennifer Jacobs, M. D., in ***Fundamentals of Complementary and Alternative Medicine,*** Marc Micozzi, ed., Churchill Livingstone, London, 1995.
27. "Plain Doctoring," ***Resonance*** 19:30, March-April 1997.
28. "Hahnemann's Achievement and Legacy," Lecture at the Dedication of the Hahnemann Monument, Washington, D. C., spring 2000; published in *American Homeopath* 6:65, Summer 2000.
29. "To Have and Have Not: Homeopathy in Cuba," *Journal of the AIH* 93:59, Summer 2000; reprinted in ***Homeopathy Today,*** July-August 2000, and ***New England Journal of Homeopathy*** 9:115, Spring-Summer 2000.
30. "Illness as Metaphor (with Apologies to Susan Sontag)," *Journal of the AIH* 94:176, Autumn 2001.
31. "Innovation and Fundamentalism in Homeopathy," ***American Journal of Homeopathic Medicine*** (formerly *Journal of the AIH*) 95:91, Summer 2002; reprinted in ***Simillimum*** (Journal of Homeopathic Academy of Naturopathic Physicians) 15:17, Fall 2002.
32. "Epiphany: the Quantum Mechanics of the Spiritual Life," published as "Housecalls," ***Chrysalis Reader,*** Swedenborg Foundation, New York, December 2002.
33. "The Fundamentalist Controversy: an Issue That Won't Go Away," lecture to Society of Homeopaths Annual Conference, Keele, UK, May 2003; published in ***American Journal of Homeopathic Medicine*** 97:28, Spring 2004, reprinted in ***The Homeopath,*** Winter 2004.
34. "Hidden in Plain Sight: the Rôle of Vaccines in Chronic Disease," lecture to the 60th LIGA Congress, Berlin, 2005; published in ***American Journal of Homeopathic Medicine*** 98:15, Spring 2005.
35. "Advisory on Bird Flu," ***American Journal of Homeopathic Medicine*** 99:16, Spring 2006.

36. "Diagnosis," ***American Journal of Homeopathic Medicine*** 102:7, Spring 2009, and 102:56, Summer 2009; reprinted in ***Medical Studies*** (Netherlands) 2:121, 2010.
37. "Vaccines, Drugs, and Other Causes: a Homeopath Looks at the Medical System," lecture to 65th LIGA Congress, Los Angeles, May 2010; published in ***American Journal of Homeopathic Medicine*** 103:214, Winter 2010, and 104:13, Spring 2011.
38. "Hidden in Plain Sight: Vaccines as a Major Risk Factor for Chronic Disease," abridged version of op. cit., ***AJHM,*** 2005, ***American Journal of Homeopathic Medicine*** 106:107, Fall 2013.
39. "Some Thoughts on the Beginnings of Life," ***Spectrum of Homeopathy*** (Germany) Spring 2013; reprinted in ***American Journal of Homeopathic Medicine*** 106:147, Winter 2013.

Case Reports.

1. "Plague and Pregnancy: a Case Report," with Jonathan Mann, M. D., ***Journal of the American Medical Association*** 237:1854, 25 April 1977.
2. "A Sampling of Animal Cases," ***Homœopathic Links*** 16:15, Spring 2003.
3. "A Wound Heals - after 25 Years," ***Homeopathy Today,*** February 2007.
4. "A 42 Year Old Man with Bronchiectasis, Among Other Things," ***American Journal of Homeopathic Medicine*** 102:78, Summer 2009.
5. "An Autistic Boy," ***American Journal of Homeopathic Medicine*** 102:117, Autumn 2009.
6. "A Woman with Lupus, and a Whole Lot More," ***American Journal of Homeopathic Medicine*** 103:22, Spring 2010.

Reviews.

1. Book Review: Dana Ullman and Stephen Cummings, *Everybody's Guide to Homeopathic Medicines,* ***Homeopathy Today,*** March 1985.
2. Book Review: Adelaide Suits, *Brass Tacks: an Oral Biography,* ***Homeopathy Today,*** December 1985.

3. Book Review: Alain Horvilleur, *The Family Guide to Homeopathy,* ***Homeopathy Today,*** May 1987.
4. Conference Review: "The Scientific Sessions," 42nd LIGA Congress, Washington, May 1987, ***Homeopathy Today,*** July-August 1987.
5. Book Review: Larry Dossey, *Beyond Illness,* ***Chrysalis*** 4:117, Spring 1989.
6. Book Review: Catherine Coulter, *Portraits of Homeopathic Medicines,* Volume 2, ***Homeopathy Today,*** April 1989.
7. Book Review: George Vithoulkas, *A New Model of Health and Disease,* ***Homeopathy Today,*** January 1993.
8. Book Review: George Vithoulkas, *Materia Medica Viva,* Volume 1, ***Journal of the AIH*** 86:257, December 1993.
9. Book Review: Harris Coulter, *The Controlled Clinical Trial,* ***Journal of the AIH*** 86:254, December 1993.
10. Book Review: Roger Morrison, *Desktop Guide to Keynotes and Confirmatory Symptoms,* ***Homeopathy Today,*** January 1994.
11. Video Review: Julian Winston, *The Faces of Homeopathy,* ***Journal of the AIH*** 88:158, Spring 1995.
12. Book Review: Nancy Herrick, *Animal Mind, Human Voices: Provings of Eight New Animal Remedies,* ***Homeopathy Today,*** January 1999.
13. Book Review: Roger Morrison, *Desktop Guide to Physical Pathology,* ***Homeopathy Today,*** April 1999.
14. Book Review: Julian Winston, *The Faces of Homeopathy,* ***Homeopathy Today,*** October 1999.
15. Book Review: Judyth Reichenberg-Ullman and Robert Ullman, *Rage-Free Kids,* ***Homeopathy Today,*** July-August 2000.
16. Book Review: A. U. Ramakrishnan and Catherine Coulter, *A Homeopathic Approach to Cancer,* ***Homeopathy Today,*** November 2001; reprinted in ***Homœopathic Links*** 15:60, Spring 2002.
17. Book Review: Julian Winston, *The Heritage of Homeopathic Literature,* ***Homeopathy Today,*** April-May 2002.
18. Book Review: Isaac Golden, *Vaccination & Homeoprophylaxis,* ***American Journal of Homeopathic Medicine*** 99:149, Summer 2006.
19. Seminar Review: Russell Malcolm, "Introduction to Homeopathy" and "The Bowel Nosodes," ***American Journal of Homeopathic Medicine*** 102:27, Spring 2009.

20. Book Review: Dana Ullman, *The Homeopathic Revolution,* ***Journal of Alternative and Complementary Therapies*** 16:517, April 2010.
21. Book Review: Massimo Mangialavori, *Praxis,* ***Spectrum of Homeopathy***, 2010, p. 134; reprinted in ***American Journal of Homeopathic Medicine*** 104: 218, Winter 2011.
22. Book Review: Catherine Coulter, "The Power of Vision: a Life of Samuel Hahnemann," ***Spectrum***, Spring 2012; reprinted in ***Homeopathy Today,*** Spring 2012.
23. Book Review: Rajan Sankaran, *The Synergy in Homeopathy,* ***American Journal of Homeopathic Medicine*** 105:138, Autumn 2012.
24. Seminar Review: Karl Robinson, et al., "Prafull Vijayakar's Predictive Homeopathy," ***American Journal of Homeopathic Medicine*** 106:56, Summer 2013.
25. Seminar Review: Prafull and Ambrish Vijayakar, "Predictive Honeopathy," ***American Journal of Homeopathic Medicine*** 107:77, Summer 2014.
26. Book Review: Karl Robinson, *Small Doses, Big Results,* ***American Journal of Homeopathic Medicine*** 107:145, Autumn 2014.

Obituaries

1. "Henry Waters, 1899-1986," ***Homeopathy Today,*** July-August 1986.
2. "Elinore Peebles, 1897-1992," ***Homeopathy Today,*** October 1992.
3. "Maesimund Panos, M. D., 1912-1999: Stateswoman, Friend, Mother of Us All," ***Homeopathy Today,*** October 1999.
4. "Julian Winston, 1941-2005, In Loving Memory," ***Homeopathy Today,*** July August 2005.
5. "Christine Luthra, M. D. (1951-2006): Dedicated Homeopath, Dear Friend, and Inspiration to Many," ***Homeopathy Today,*** November December 2006.
6. "Harris Coulter, Ph. D. (1932-2009): Devoted Scholar, Keen Intellect, Soldier for the Cause," ***American Journal of Homeopathic Medicine*** 103:7, Spring 2010.
7. "David Warkentin (1951-2010): An Appreciation," ***American Journal of Homeopathic Medicine*** 103: 179, Winter 2010.
8. "Catherine Coulter (1934-2014): A Remembrance," ***Homeopathy Today***, Summer 2014.

Political Statements.

1. "On Lay Prescribing," ***Homeopathy Today,*** April 1982.
2. President's Message, ***Homeopathy Today,*** June 1985.
3. President's Message, "Lay Practice," ***Homeopathy Today,*** October 1985.
4. President's Message, ***Homeopathy Today,*** January 1986.
5. "Homeopathy on the Line," ***Homeopathy Today,*** April 1986.
6. President's Report, ***Homeopathy Today,*** September 1986.
7. Open Letter to President Clinton, ***Homeopathy Today,*** February 1993.

Letters and Rebuttals.

1. "The Great Malpractice Scandal," ***Santa Fe Reporter,*** 16 April 1981.
2. Open Letter to Prof. Harold Morowitz, in reply to his article, "Much Ado about Nothing," in *Hospital Practice,* July 1982, ***Homeopathy Today,*** October 1982.
3. Reply to letter from John Coker, ***Homeopathy Today,*** September 1984.
4. Letter to the Editor, "Sample Living Will Addendum," ***Journal of the AIH*** 85:10, March 1992.
5. Open Letter to Gerald Weissman, M. D., in reply to his article, "Dancing with Fairies, Sucking with Vampires," in *MD Magazine,* November 1992, ***Homeopathy Today,*** March 1993.
6. "Animal Testing in Homeopathy," Open Letter to Jennifer Jacobs, M. D., and the Homeopathic Research Network, ***Journal of the AIH*** 88:8, Spring 1995.
7. "More on Vaccinations," Letter to the Editor, ***Mothering*** Magazine, Spring 1997.
8. Reply to letter from Domenick Masiello, D. O., ***Homeopathy Today,*** December 2000.
9. "For Homeopathy: a Practicing Physician's Perspective," in rebuttal to Kevin Smith's article, "Against Homeopathy: a Utilitarian Perspective," in *Bioethics* (UK), February 2011, ***American Journal of Homeopathic Medicine*** 104:125, Autumn 2011; German version, ***Homöopathie Zeitschrift,*** 2012, p. 99.

Lectures.

1. "Homeopathic Reasoning," lecture to Symposium, "Homeopathy: the Renaissance of Cure, San Francisco, April 1980; published in ***Homeotherapy*** 6:135, September 1980.
2. "Whose Birth Is It, Anyway?" lecture to Cæsarean Prevention Movement Conference, Newark, 1984; CPM videotape.
3. "What Homeopathy Can Teach, and What It Has to Learn," lecture to NCH Annual Conference, 1986, summarized in ***Homeopathy Today,*** September 1986.
4. "Poverty in the Midst of Plenty: American Homeopathy in 1987," Lecture to NCH Annual Conference, 1987, summarized in ***Homeopathy Today,*** October 1987; NCH audiotape.
5. "How Can It All Be Done?" lecture to NCH Annual Conference, 1987, summarized in ***Homeopathy Today,*** September 1987; NCH audiotape.
6. "Beyond Curing," Julia Green Memorial Lecture, NCH Summer School, July 1988, NCH audiotape.
7. "Vaccination: a Sacrament of Modern Medicine," lecture to Society of Homeopaths Annual Conference (UK), 1991; published in ***Journal of the AIH*** 84:96, December 1991; reprinted in ***The Homœopath*** (UK)12:137, March 1992.
8. Homeopathic Philosophy Lecture Series, NCH Summer School, 1991,1992; NCH audio- tapes.
9. "Childhood Ear Infections," lecture to AIH Conference, 1994; published in ***Journal of the AIH*** 87:137, Autumn 1994; reprinted in ***The Homœopath*** (UK), 1994.
10. "Illness as Conflict, Health as Resolution," lecture to Boston Graduate School of Psychoanalysis Annual Conference, Santa Fe, 1997, unpublished.
11. "Samuel Hahnemann: the Man and His Impact," lecture at Centenary of the Hahnemann Monument, Washington, May 2000, AIH audiotape.
12. "Hidden in Plain Sight: the Rôle of Vaccines in Chronic Disease," lecture to 60th LIGA Congress, Berlin, 2005; published in ***American Journal of Homeopathic Medicine*** 98:15, Spring 2005.

13. "Vaccines, Drugs, and Other Causes: a Homeopath Looks at the Medical System," lecture to 65th LIGA Congress, Los Angeles, May 2010; published in ***American Journal of Homeopathic Medicine*** 103:214, Winter 2010, and 104:13, Spring 2011.

Panels and Symposia.

1. "Malpractice," ***Firing Line,*** William F. Buckley, moderator, WNET, New York, October 1982, WNET videotape.
2. Symposium, "Vaccination: The Issue of Our Time," ***Mothering*** Magazine, Spring 1996.
3. "The Vaccination Debate," with Andrew Weil, M. D., ***Natural Health*** Magazine, November- December 1997.
4. "Report on Bioterrorism," AIH Bioterrorism Committee, Richard Moskowitz, M. D., Ed., ***American Journal of Homeopathic Medicine*** 96:94, Summer 2003.

Miscellaneous.

1. Memoir, "Why I Became a Homeopath," ***Homeopathy Today,*** December 1982.
2. Interview with Peggy O'Mara, ***Mothering*** Magazine, April 1988.
3. Memoir, "Why I Became a Homeopath," ***Journal of the AIH*** 89:74, Winter 1996; reprinted in ***The Homœopath*** (UK),1997, p. 712.
4. "What Is Homeopathy?" unpublished patient handout, 1996.
5. Interview with Jane Ryan, C. N. M., ***New England Journal of Homeopathy*** 9:83, Spring- Summer 2000.
6. "Advisory on Anthrax," unpublished patient handout, 2002.
7 "Advisory on Smallpox," unpublished patient handout, 2002.
8. Foreword, Nancy Herrick, ***Sacred Plants, Human Voices: Provings of Seven New Plant Remedies,*** Hahnemann Clinic Publishing, San Francisco, 2003.
9. "Hidden in Plain Sight," expanded version of op. cit., ***American Journal of Homeopathic Medicine,*** 2005, unpublished.
10. "Advisory on Swine Flu," unpublished patient handout, 2009.

About the Author:

Richard Moskowitz earned his B. A. from Harvard in 1959, where he was elected to Phi Beta Kappa, and his M. D. from New York University in 1963. Receiving a U.S. Steel Foundation Fellowship, he then completed two years of graduate study in Philosophy at the University of Colorado in Boulder and qualified for the Ph. D. in 1965. After serving an internship at St. Anthony's Hospital in Denver, he obtained his medical license in 1967, and has practiced general and family medicine ever since.

Attending over 600 home births in the 1970's, mostly in Colorado and New Mexico, he studied Japanese acupuncture with Sensei Masahilo Nakazono in Santa Fe, and classical homeopathy with many teachers, mainly Prof. George Vithoulkas in Greece and Dr. Rajan Sankaran and his school in India. He has practiced homeopathic medicine since 1974.

Author of three previous books and numerous articles on homeopathy, midwifery, and the philosophy of medicine, Dr. Moskowitz has also taught and lectured widely, and served on the Board of the National Center for Homeopathy from 1980-87, as its President in 1985-86, and more recently on the Board of the American Institute of Homeopathy since 2006, and as its Secretary since 2007. He lives and practices in the Boston area.

www.ingramcontent.com/pod-product-compliance
Lightning Source LLC
Chambersburg PA
CBHW071354170526
45165CB00001B/43
9781502426680